Springer
Berlin
Heidelberg
New York
Barcelona
Hong Kong
London
Milan
Paris
Singapore
Tokyo

The Skin and Gene Therapy

Ulrich R. Hengge · Beatrix Volc-Platzer

Editors

The Skin and Gene Therapy

With 41 Figures, Some in Color, and 16 Tables

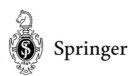 Springer

Associate Professor
Dr. med. ULRICH R. HENGGE
Department of Dermatology,
Venerology and Allergology
University of Essen
Hufelandstr. 55
45122 Essen
Germany

Associate Professor
Dr. med. BEATRIX VOLC-PLATZER
Division of Immunology,
Allergy and Infectious Diseases
Department of Dermatology
University of Vienna Medical School
Währinger Gürtel 18–20
1090 Vienna
Austria

ISBN 3-540-66760-1 Springer-Verlag Berlin Heidelberg New York

Library of Congress Cataloging-in-Publication Data

The skin and gene therapy/Ulrich Hengge, Beatrix Volc-Platzer (eds.).   p.; cm.
  Includes bibliographical references and index.
  ISBN 3-540-66760-1
  1. Skin Dieseases – Gene therapy. 2. Skin Diseases – Immunotherapy. I. Hengge,
Ulrich, 1963. II. Volc-Platzer, Beatrix, 1954. [DNLM: 1. Skin Diseases – immunology. 2. Gene Therapy – methods. 3. Gene Transfer. 4. Skin Diseases – therapy. WR
140 S6272 2001]   RL120.G45 S58 2000   616.5′042–dc21   00-038802

Springer-Verlag is a company in the BertelsmannSpringer publishing group.
© Springer-Verlag Berlin · Heidelberg 2001
Printed in Germany

Cover-Design: Erich Kirchner, Heidelberg; Markus Ibs, Essen
Typesetting: K+V Fotosatz GmbH, Beerfelden
Printing: Saladruck, Berlin
Binding: Stürtz AG, Würzburg

Printed on acid-free paper   SPIN 10732879   24/3130/PF   5 4 3 2 1 0

Preface

Gene therapy is a novel concept of treating diseases at the molecular level by rescuing genetic defects through the introduction of corrective genes. The knowledge of genetic defects underlying various diseases is being rapidly accumulated, and new genotypic findings are being reported with striking frequency. The elucidation of the genetic background of many diseases, including hereditary blistering and hyperkeratotic skin disorders, has provided the necessary knowledge to correct inborn genetic aberrations in animal models and patient-derived tissue. However, skin is not only a target organ for gene therapy of cutaneous disorders. Due to its biological properties, easy accessibility, and convenient, established culture conditions and grafting techniques, skin has rapidly become an important target for correcting other diseases as well.

Both skin fibroblasts and epidermal keratinocytes have been successfully transfected ex vivo and in vivo using viral and nonviral gene transfer methods. Notably, in the first corrective gene therapy approach in 1987, fibroblasts from adenosine-deaminase (ADA)-deficient humans with severe combined immunodeficiency (SCID) syndrome were transduced using retroviral vectors. Moreover, skin cells are capable of synthesizing various proteins that are therapeutic, either locally or systemically. Human epidermal grafts expressing human growth hormone after retroviral gene transfer and grafting onto athymic mice released human growth hormone into the bloodstream of the transplanted mice, for a limited time. These studies demonstrated the formation of a differentiated epidermis from genetically modified keratinocytes and the continuous production of therapeutic proteins accessing the bloodstream. In addition to producing missing or correct functional proteins, the skin may also provide the necessary enzymes to detoxify metabolic products ("metabolic sink"). Other constituents of the skin, such as the epidermal Langerhans cells (members of the dendritic cell family) with their powerful antigen-presenting capacity, are potentially effective for "genetic immunization," i.e., DNA vaccination or "gene vaccines" against cancer and infectious diseases. In concert with the advancement of innate immunology, DNA vaccination is about to revolutionize traditional vaccinology.

Despite recent molecular biological and technical achievements, several problems with regard to gene therapy remain. Current in vivo gene transfer generally leads to transient expression of the transferred gene, and thus it is not suitable for long-term correction and improvement of inborn genetic errors despite the considerable progress which has been made in targeting of gene expression to various organs or cells using tissue-specific promotors. Among the viral gene delivery systems, retroviral gene transfer has been shown to persist long-term, but the transgene was gradually inactivated. Nonviral delivery systems using lipoplexes, polyplexes, or receptor-mediated gene transfer have been explored in parallel. The ultimate goal for this therapeutic approach is to overcome the epidermal barrier for the purpose of gene delivery to interfollicular keratinocytes. Furthermore, a strategy that may improve durable protein expression is to repopulate the epidermis with epidermal stem cells transduced with lentiviral vectors (ex vivo transduction).

Since the first therapeutic attempts in 1970, more than 350 clinical gene therapy trials were approved, and more than 4000 patients have been treated worldwide. As usual, new approaches in medicine are controversial until unequivocal evidence of clinical success has been demonstrated. Malignant melanoma was one of the first tumors targeted by transfer of genes encoding accessory molecules and cytokines. The initial clinical phase I/II studies in stage III/IV tumor patients showed good tolerability of these cancer vaccines, without overt toxicity. However, in order to provide realistic therapeutic options and not to impair outcome by harmful side effects, more extensive studies are needed. Particular emphasis has to be placed on the safety aspects of nonviral and particularly viral vectors. By substantially supporting biosafety investigations through major research authorities, and by making scientific information available to the public, wider acceptance of this novel biomedical field will hopefully be achieved.

Every rapidly evolving field in biomedical and particularly genetic science warrants ethical vigilance to guarantee proper implementation and clinical application of newly developed techniques. Therefore, the new and important biomedical approach of gene therapy requires a team effort on the part of experts in basic biology, biochemistry, immunology, microbiology (including virology), clinical medicine, and ethics.

With this book we hope to add to the interdisciplinary understanding between basic researchers and physicians caring for patients and to provide basic information for further developments in the field of gene therapy.

August 2000   ULRICH R. HENGGE
                                                      BEATRIX VOLC-PLATZER

Contents

Systemic Effects of Skin Gene Therapy

Genetic Vaccination Using the Skin

List of Contributors

ARIN, MERAL J.
e-mail: marin@bcm.tmc.edu
Tel.: +1-713-798-6350, Fax: +1-713-798-3800
Department of Molecular and Cellular Biology,
Baylor College of Medicine, One Baylor Plaza,
Houston, TX 77030, USA

BERTON, THOMAS R.
e-mail: tberton@sprd1.mdacc.tmc.edu
Tel.: +1-512-237-9473, Fax: +1-512-237–9566
Anderson Cancer Center, Department of Carcinogenesis,
Science Park – Research Division, P.O. Box 389,
Smithville, TX 78957, USA

BICKENBACH, JACKIE R.
e-mail: Jackie-bickenbach@uiowa.edu
Tel.: +1-319-335-6719, Fax: +1-319-335-7198
Department of Anatomy and Cell Biology,
and Department of Dermatology, University of Iowa,
Iowa City, IA 52242, USA

CAO, TONGYU
e-mail: tcao@bcm.tmc.edu
Tel.: +1-713-798-6350, Fax: +1-713-798-3800
Department of Molecular and Cellular Biology,
Baylor College of Medicine, One Baylor Plaza,
Houston, TX 77030, USA

CORR, MARIPAT
e-mail: mcorr@ucsd.edu
Tel.: +1-858-534-7817, Fax: +1-858-534-5399
Department of Medicine, University of California,
and The Sam and Rose Stein Institute for Research on Aging,
9500 Gilman Drive,
La Jolla/San Diego, CA 92093-0663, USA

CSAKY, KARL G.
e-mail: kcsaky@helix.nih.gov
Tel.: +1-301-402-0896, Fax: +1-301-402-0485
Laboratory of Immunology, National Eye Institute,
National Institutes of Health,
Bethesda, MD 20892-1908, USA

DAVIDSON, JEFFREY M.
e-mail: jeff.davidson@vanderbilt.edu
Tel.: +1-615-322-0126, Fax: +1-615-322-0122
Department of Pathology, Vanderbilt University,
Nashville, TN 37212-2561, USA

DEXLING, BJÖRN
e-mail: dexling@uni-essen.de
Tel.: +49-201-723-2847, Fax: +49-201-723-2847
Department of Dermatology, Venerology and Allergology,
University of Essen,
Hufelandstr. 55,
45122 Essen, Germany

ELIAS, PETER M.
e-mail: eliaspm@itsa.ucsf.edu
Tel.: +1-415-750-2091, Fax: +1-415-751-3927
Department of Dermatology,
University of San Francisco School of Medicine,
San Francisco, CA 94121, USA

EMING, SABINE A.
e-mail: sabine.eming@uni-essen.de
Tel.: +49-221-478-4518, Fax: +49-221-478-4538
Department of Dermatology and Venerology,
University of Cologne,
Joseph-Stelzmann-Str. 9,
50931 Cologne, Germany

GOOS, MANFRED
e-mail: manfred.goos@uni-essen.de
Tel.: +49-201-723-2430, Fax: +49-201-723-5935
Department of Dermatology, Venerology and Allergology,
University of Essen,
Hufelandstr. 55,
45122 Essen, Germany

HENGGE, ULRICH R.
e-mail: ulrich.hengge@uni-essen.de
Tel.: +49-201-723-3634, Fax: +49-201-723-2847
Department of Dermatology, Venerology and Allergology,
University of Essen,
Hufelandstr. 55,
45122 Essen, Germany

JENSEN, THOMAS G.
e-mail: thomas@humgen.au.dk
Tel.: +45-8942-1686, Fax: +45-8612-3173
Institute of Human Genetics, The Bartholin Building,
University of Aarhus,
8000 Aarhus C, Denmark

KALLMAN, JAMES E.
e-mail: j_kallman@yahoo.com
Tel.: +1-215-505-1914, Fax: +1-215-485-2862
Department of Otorhinolaryngology, Head and Neck Surgery,
Hospital of the University of Pennsylvania,
505 Stellar-Chance Building, 422 Curie Boulevard,
Philadelphia, PA 19104-6100, USA

KIM, JONG J.
Tel.: +1-215-662-2352, Fax: +1-215-573-9436
Department of Pathology and Laboratory Medicine,
Hospital of the University of Pennsylvania,
505 Stellar-Chance Building, 422 Curie Boulevard,
Philadelphia, PA 19104-6100, USA

KRIEG, ARTHUR M.
e-mail: arthur-krieg@uiowa.edu
Tel.: +1-319-335-6841, Fax: +1-319-335-6887
Department of Internal Medicine,
University of Iowa College of Medicine,
540 EMRB,
Iowa City, IA 52242, USA

KRIEG, THOMAS
e-mail: thomas.krieg@uni-koeln.de
Tel.: +49-221-478-4500, Fax: +49-221-478-4538
Department of Dermatology and Venerology,
University of Cologne,
Joseph-Stelzmann-Str. 9,
50931 Cologne, Germany

LEE, DELPHINE J.
e-mail: djlee@ucsd.edu
Tel.: +1-858-534-5377, Fax: +1-858-534-5399
Department of Medicine, University of California,
and The Sam and Rose Stein Institute for Research on Aging,
9500 Gilman Drive,
La Jolla/San Diego, CA 92093-0663, USA

MAGUIRE JR., HENRY C.
e-mail: hmaguire@mail.upenn.edu
Tel.: +1-215-955-8874, Fax: +1-215-955-2340
Department of Otolaryngology, Head and Neck Surgery,
Jefferson Medical College,
Hospital of the University of Pennsylvania,
111 South 11th Street,
Philadelphia, PA 19107, USA

MENEGUZZI, GUERRINO
e-mail: meneguzz@unice.fr
Tel.: +33-493-3777-77, Fax: +33-493-8114-04
U385 INSERM, Faculté de Médecine, Hôpital de l'Archet 2,
Avenue de Valombroise,
06107 Nice Cedex 2, France

MENON, GOPI K.
e-mail: gopi.menon@avon.com
Tel.: +1-845-369-2904, Fax: +1-845-369-2402
Avon Products Inc., Avon Place,
Suffern, NY 10901-5605, USA

MEYER, HELMUT E.
e-mail: helmut.e.meyer@ruhr-uni-bochum.de
Tel.: +49-234-700-2427, Fax: +49-234-700-2427
Institute of Physiological Chemistry, Medical Faculty MA2/143,
Ruhr-University Bochum,
Universitätsstr. 150,
44780 Bochum, Germany

MIRMOHAMMDSADEGH, ALIREZA
e-mail: mirmohammadsadegh@uni-essen.de
Tel.: +49-201-723-3894, Fax: +49-201-723-2847
Department of Dermatology, Venerology and Allergology,
University of Essen,
Hufelandstr. 55,
45122 Essen, Germany

PASCHEN, ANNETTE
e-mail: a.paschen@dkfz-heidelberg.de
Tel.: +49-621-383-2177, Fax: +49-621-383-2163
Clinical Cooperation Unit of Dermato-Oncology (DKFZ),
Department of Dermatology, University of Mannheim,
Medical Faculty of the University of Heidelberg,
Theodor-Kutzer-Ufer 1,
68135 Mannheim, Germany

RAZ, EYAL
e-mail: eraz@ucsd.edu
Tel.: +1-858-822-3358, Fax: +1-858-534-5399
Department of Medicine, University of California,
and The Sam and Rose Stein Institute for Research on Aging,
9500 Gilman Drive,
La Jolla/San Diego, CA 92093-0663, USA

ROOP, DENNIS R.
e-mail: roopd@bcm.tmc.edu
Tel.: +1-713 798-4966, Fax: +1-713 798-3800
Department of Cell Biology, Room 123D,
Baylor College of Medicine, One Baylor Plaza,
Houston, TX 77030, USA

SAWAMURA, DAISUKE
e-mail: smartdai@cc.hirosaki-u.ac.jp
Tel.: +81-138-23-8651, Fax: +81-172-37-6060
Department of Dermatology,
Hirosaki University School of Medicine,
Hirosaki 036, Japan

SCHADENDORF, DIRK
e-mail: d.schadendorf@dkfz-heidelberg.de
Tel.: +49-621-383-2126, Fax: +49-621-383-2163
Clinical Cooperation Unit of Dermato-Oncology (DKFZ),
Department of Dermatology, University of Mannheim,
Medical Faculty of the University of Heidelberg,
Theodor-Kutzer-Ufer 1,
68135 Mannheim, Germany

SCHNEEBERGER, ACHIM
e-mail: achim.schneeberger@akh-wien.ac.at
Tel.: +43-1-40400-7726, Fax: +43-1-403-1900
Division of Immunology, Allergy and Infectious Diseases,
Department of Dermatology,
University of Vienna Medical School,
Währinger Gürtel 18–20,
1090 Vienna, Austria

STINGL, GEORG
e-mail: georg.stingl@akh-wien.ac.at
Tel.: +43-1-40400-7704, Fax: +43-1-403-1900
Division of Immunology, Allergy and Infectious Diseases,
Department of Dermatology,
University of Vienna Medical School,
Währinger Gürtel 18–20,
1090 Vienna, Austria

SUN, YUANSHENG
e-mail: y.sun@dkfz-heidelberg.de
Tel.: +49-621-383-2177, Fax: +49-621-383-2163
Clinical Cooperation Unit of Dermato-Oncology (DKFZ),
Department of Dermatology, University of Mannheim,
Medical Faculty of the University of Heidelberg,
Theodor-Kutzer-Ufer 1,
68135 Mannheim, Germany

TAKABAYASHI, KENJI
e-mail: ktakabayashi@ucsd.edu
Tel.: +1-858-822-3090, Fax: +1-858-534-5399
Department of Medicine, University of California,
and The Sam and Rose Stein Institute for Research on Aging,
9500 Gilman Drive,
La Jolla/San Diego, CA 92093-0663, USA

TSCHAKARJAN, ETIENA
e-mail: etiena@gmx.de
Tel.: +49-201-723-2847, Fax: +49-201-723-2847
Department of Dermatology, Venerology and Allergology,
University of Essen,
Hufelandstr. 55,
45122 Essen, Germany

UDVARDI, ASTRID
e-mail: astrid.udvardi@akh-wien.ac.at
Tel.: +43-1-40400-7794, Fax: +43-1-403-1900
Division of Immunology, Allergy and Infectious Diseases,
Department of Dermatology,
University of Vienna Medical School,
Währinger Gürtel 18–20,
1090 Vienna, Austria

VAILLY, JOËLLE
e-mail: vailly@unice.fr
Tel.: +33-493-37-7648, Fax: +33-493-8114-04
U385 INSERM, Faculté de Médecine, Hôpital de l'Archet 2,
Avenue de Valombrose,
06107 Nice Cedex 2, France

VOLC-PLATZER, BEATRIX
e-mail: Beatrix.Volc-Platzer@univie.ac.at
Tel.: +43-1-40400-7725, Fax: +43-1-403-0224
Division of Immunology, Allergy and Infectious Diseases,
Department of Dermatology,
University of Vienna Medical School,
Währinger Gürtel 18–20,
1090 Vienna, Austria

WAGNER, STEPHAN N.
e-mail: stephan.wagner@uni-essen.de
Tel.: +49-201-723-2532, Fax: +49-201-723-5935
Department of Dermatology, Venerology and Allergology,
University of Essen,
Hufelandstr. 55,
45122 Essen, Germany

WANG, XIAO-JING
e-mail: xwang@bcm.tmc.edu
Tel.: +1-713-798-6350, Fax: +1-713-798-3800
Department of Molecular and Cellular Biology,
Baylor College of Medicine, One Baylor Plaza,
Houston, TX 77030, USA

WEINER, DAVID B.
e-mail: dbweiner@mail.med.upenn.edu
Tel.: +1-215-662-2352, Fax: +1-215-573-9436
Department of Pathology and Laboratory Medicine,
Hospital of the University of Pennsylvania,
505 Stellar-Chance Building, 422 Curie Boulevard,
Philadelphia, PA 19104-6100, USA

YANG, JOOS S.
Tel.: +1-215-662-2352, Fax: +1-215-573-9436
Department of Pathology and Laboratory Medicine,
Hospital of the University of Pennsylvania,
505 Stellar-Chance Building, 422 Curie Boulevard,
Philadelphia, PA 19104-6100, USA

ZHOU, ZHIJIAN
e-mail: zzhou@bcm.tmc.edu
Tel.: +1-713-798-4967, Fax: +1-713-798-3800
Department of Molecular and Cellular Biology,
Baylor College of Medicine, One Baylor Plaza,
Houston, TX 77030, USA

Abbreviations

$\alpha 1$AT	$\alpha 1$-Antitrypsin
AAV	Adenovirus-associated virus
Ad5	Adenovirus type 5
ADA	Adenosine deaminase
ADCC	Antibody-dependent cellular cytotoxicity
APC	Antigen-presenting cell
ApoE	Apolipoprotein E
AVET	Adenovirus-enhanced transferrinfection
β-gal	β-Galactosidase
BCG	*Bacillus Calmette Guerin*
BPAG1	Bullous pemphigoid antigen 1
$CaPO_4$	Calcium phosphate
CBER	Center for Biologics, Evaluation and Research
CCR	Chemokine receptor
CDK	Cyclin-dependent kinase
CE	Cornified envelope
CEA	Carcinoembryonal antigen
CHS	Contact hypersensitivity
CIE	Congenital ichthyosiform erythroderma
CMV	Cytomegalovirus
CpG	Cytosine-p-Guanine
Cre	Cre recombinase of bacteriophage P1
CTL	Cytotoxic T-lymphocyte
DC	Dendritic cell
DEB	Dystrophic epidermolysis bullosa
DNCB	Dinitrochlorobenzene
DTH	Delayed-type hypersensitivity
EB	Epidermolysis bullosa
EBS	Epidermolysis bullosa simplex
EBS-DM	Epidermolysis bullosa simplex Dowling-Meara
EGF	Epithelial growth factor
EHK	Epidermolytic hyperkeratosis
Epo	Erythropoietin
ES	Embryonic stem cells
FDA	Food and Drug Administration

FGF	Fibroblast growth factor
GA	Gyrate atrophy
GFP	Green fluorescent protein
GM-CSF	Granulocyte-macrophage colony stimulating factor
GPI	Glycosylphosphatidylinositol
hCG	Human chorionic gonadotropin
hGH	Human growth hormone
HIV	Human immunodeficiency virus
HK1	Human keratin 1
HLA	Histocompatibility leukocyte antigen
HMG	High mobility group
HMG CoA	3-Hydroxy-3-methyl-glutaryl coenzyme A
HSVtk	Herpes simplex virus thymidine kinase
HVJ-liposome	Hemagglutinating virus of Japan liposome
i.d.	Intradermal
IE	Immediate early
IF	Intermediate filament
IFN	Interferon
IGF-1	Insulin-like growth factor-1
IL	Interleukin
IL-1ra	Interleukin-1 receptor antagonist
i.m.	Intramuscular
iNOS	Inducible nitric oxide synthase
ISS	Immunostimulatory sequences
JEB	Junctional epidermolysis bullosa
K5	Keratin 5
K10	Keratin 10
K14	Keratin 14
KLH	Keyhole limpet haemocyanin
LAK	Lymphokine-activated killer cells
LB	Lamellar bodies
LI	Lamellar ichthyosis
loxP	Locus of crossover of bacteriophage P1
LRCs	Label-retaining cells
LTR	Long terminal repeat
MAPKs	Mitogen-activated protein kinases
MDR	Multi-drug resistance
MHC	Major histocompatibility complex
MR	Minor response
NFκB	Nuclear factor κB
NK	Natural killer cell
NMF	Natural moisturizing factors
NO	Nitric oxide
NP	Nucleoprotein
OAT	Ornithine aminotransferase
ODN	Oligodeoxynucleotide

OsO$_4$	Osmium tetroxide
P5C	Pyrroline-5-carboxylate
PAF	Platelet-activating-factor
PCNA	Proliferating cell nuclear antigen
PDGF	Platelet-derived growth factor
PEM	Polymorphic epithelial mucin
PF-4	Platelet factor 4
poly-I	Polyinosine
PPK	Palmoplantar keratoderma
PR	Partial response
PRRs	Pattern recognition receptors
PSA	Prostate-specific antigen
Rb	Retinoblastoma
RDEB	Recessive dystrophic epidermolysis bullosa
RES	Reticulo-endothelial system
ROS	Reactive oxygen species
RPE	Retina pigment epithelium
RS	Rous sarcoma
RuO$_4$	Ruthenium tetroxide
SALT	Skin-associated lymphoid tissue
SB	Stratum basale
SC	Stratum corneum
SCID	Severe combined immunodeficiency
SD	Stable disease
SG	Stratum granulosum
SLS	Sodium lauryl sulfate
SPT	Serine palmitoyl transferase
SS	Stratum spinosum
TCR	T-cell receptor
TEWL	Transepidermal water loss
TGase 1	Transglutaminase 1
TGF	Transforming growth factor
Th$_1$	T helper 1
Th$_2$	T helper 2
TIL	Tumor-infiltrating lymphocytes
TNF	Tumor necrosis factor
UV	Ultraviolet
VEGF	Vascular endothelial growth factor

Basic Aspects

1   The Epidermal Barrier and Strategies for Surmounting It: An Overview

G. K. Menon, P. M. Elias

Introduction

As the largest organ comprising more than 10% of the body mass in humans, the skin serves as the physical barrier for the body. The bulk of it is made up of dermis, but it is the epidermis that is vested with the function of producing, maintaining and renewing the superficial and crucial compartment, the stratum corneum (SC). This layer of terminally differentiated keratinocytes provides the physical basis for several types of barrier functions including: barrier to water permeability, penetration of xenobiotics, and microbial and parasitic invasion. Additionally the SC barrier helps to maintain the integrity of other components by providing 1) defense against UV radiation and free radical injury, 2) the immune barrier and 3) crucial skin functions such as thermoregulation, waste elimination and sensory transduction (heat, cold, pain, etc.).

The wear and tear associated with protection is solved by continuous renewal of the outermost exposed layer, the SC. In the majority of mammals the SC is covered by integumentary appendages such as a coat of pelage. However, the species that are of interest to clinical and basic dermatological researchers (humans, hairless mice, etc.) have essentially glabrous skin and their SC is exposed directly to the external milieu. Being the interface of the organism and the environment, the SC has evolved into a versatile tissue: a marvelous biopolymer with unique functionalities, an autopoietic system and a composite material of unprecedented biological and physical attributes. As discussed in the following chapter, the epidermal stem cells and the transiently amplifying cells generate the keratinocytes whose terminal differentiation results in the production and constant renewal of the SC. In turn, the SC protects these underlying cells and restrains keratinocyte proliferation to maintain levels required by unperturbed skin. This "Yin" and "Yang" effectively maintains the homeostasis of the epidermal barrier.

Formation of the Stratum Corneum: The Basis of the Barrier

It has been firmly established that the structural basis of the cutaneous permeability barrier of mammals (and other tetrapod vertebrates) is the SC. Its architecture resembles a "brick and mortar" organization, wherein the corneocytes form the "bricks" partly attached together by desmosomes and partly by a "mortar" of lipids sequestered in the extracellular domains. The formation, maintenance and renewal of the SC is the most important function of the epidermal keratinocytes that proliferate and synthesize structural proteins (keratins that form the bulk of the bricks) and lipids (secreted and sequestered in the extracellular domains to form the mortar). We will first review the sequence of events that leads to the formation of SC, before discussing its unique organization and properties.

Excellent and comprehensive reviews on permeability barrier (Downing 1992, Schaefer and Redelmeier 1996), ultrastructural features of the permeability barrier (Landmann 1988, Elias and Menon 1991, Holbrook 1994) and epidermal keratinization (Eckert 1989) have appeared relatively recently and the reader is referred to these for detailed information. Currently, we focus on the essential features of the dual process of keratinization and lipogenesis that give rise to the "bricks" and "mortar" of the SC.

The epidermis rests on the basement membrane and is divisible into the basal layer (stratum basale, SB); the spinous layer (stratum spinosum, SS), the granular layer (stratum granulosum, SG), and the stratum corneum (SC). Cells of the basal layer show keratin filaments in their cytosol, oriented in a plane perpendicular to the skin surface. As the keratinocytes proliferate and leave the basal layer, they form the SS, so designated due to the histological appearance of being joined by spines. Ultrastructurally, the spines resolve to be desmosomes with keratin filaments (tonofilaments) radiating into the cytosol. The large dense bundles of keratin filaments within the spinous cells are the result of newly synthesized, differentiation-specific polypeptides that are added to the pre-existing keratin filaments. The keratins of the SS are arranged in a concentric pattern around the nucleus, with small bundles extending into the cell periphery to insert into the desmosomal plaques. Due to shrinkage of the cells during tissue processing for histology, the intercellular spaces between individual desmosomal junctions appear widened, thus exaggerating the appearance of the spines.

Specific lipid markers of keratinocyte differentiation, the epidermal lamellar bodies (LB), derived from the Golgi apparatus first appear in the SS. Morphologically, these are 0.2 to 0.5 micrometers in diameter and contain parallel stacks of lipid enriched disks enclosed by a trilaminar membrane. In near perfect cross-sections, each lamella shows a major electron dense band that is shared by electron lucent material divided centrally by a minor electron dense band (Fig. 1.1 b, inset). In the upper layers of the SS, cells begin to elongate. Above the SS layer is the SG, so named due to the distinct histological appearance of homogeneous dark staining keratohyalin granules in the cytoplasm. The thickness of the SG layer varies depending upon the area examined with the thickest skin (e.g. palms and soles) having significantly more SG cells. Electron micro-

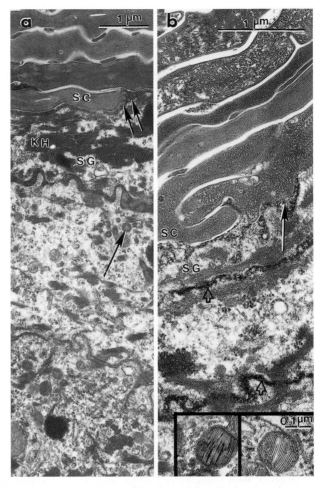

Fig. 1.1. a Low magnification electron micrograph of murine epidermis showing the stratum granulosum (SG) and part of stratum corneum (SC). Lamellar bodies (LB) in cytosol (arrow) and secreted LB contents at SG-SC interface (double arrows) are marked. Lipid structures are not visualized within the SC domains (OsO_4 post-fixation) that appear electron lucent and empty. **b** Colloidal lanthanum, a water-soluble tracer, permeates outward (open arrows) from the dermis following subcutaneous injection. The egress of tracer stops where secreted contents of LBs occlude the intercellular space (arrows). Note the absence of tracer within the SC domains. Insets: Lamellar bodies, post-fixation with RuO_4 (left) and OsO_4 (right). Reproduced with permission of Wiley-Liss from Menon and Ghadially (1997)

scopy reveals the keratohyalin as electron dense and irregular to stellate shaped granules that are composed of profilaggrin, an intermediate filament-associated protein, deposited at the points of intersection of keratin filament bundles. The granules become progressively larger in the upper SG due to a quantitative increase in keratin synthesis. The filaggrin subunits of profilaggrin play the role of a matrix molecule to aggregate and align the keratin filaments. Keratin filaments in upper granular cells are highly phosphorylated and have extensive disulfide bonds, compared to the cell layers below. The increase in protein synthesis is accompanied by an upregulation in lipogenesis, reflected in the boost in number of LB reaching their highest density in the uppermost granular cells. In this layer they occupy about 20% of the cell cytosol, and, as seen in electron micrographs of oblique sections, they are highly polarized in the apical cytosol of the upper SG. Biochemical characterization of LBs by preparing an enriched fraction as well as by cytochemical studies (reviewed in Elias and Menon 1991) show that they are enriched in glucosyl ceramides, phospholipids and cholesterol, and hydrolytic enzymes such as lipases, β-glucosylcerebrosidase, sphingomyelinase and phosphodiesterases. At the SG-SC interface, responding to appropriate signals, LBs fuse with the apical membrane of SG cells and release their disk contents into the extracellular domains. This secretion lays the foundation for establishment of the epidermal permeability barrier as illustrated by electron microscopy (Fig. 1.1 a, b), showing the egress of water soluble tracers such as lanthanum blocked at this level. Following secretion, the LB derived disks align themselves in an orderly pattern and fuse end-to-end with adjacent disks. Desmosomes, as well as the covalently bound lipid enveloping the cornified membrane of the corneocyte, may aid this alignment of the disks (Fartasch et al. 1993). Fusion of adjacent disks may involve enzymes such as phospholipases (co-secreted with the lipids) as well as ionic calcium. Static images in electron micrographs provide a glimpse, albeit a frozen moment, of the dynamic post-secretory modulations in the pro-barrier lipids (Fig. 1.2 inset, Fig. 1.3 lower inset). Whereas the proximal parts of SG-SC interface contain separate disks or those in the process of fusing with each other, close to the membrane of the first corneocyte layer, the fused LB disks have already formed continuous lipid bilayers (Fig. 1.3, lower inset). The basic unit pattern of the bilayers consists of a series of six electron lucent lamellae alternating with five electron dense lamellae (Fig. 1.3, upper inset). Double and triple basic units occur frequently. The basic units' structures persist all the way to the outermost layers of SC, although contamination with sebum (and other topical contaminants) results in loss of the tight arrays of bilayers. Additionally, the structural relation of the bilayers to the corneodesmosomes shows gradual changes associated with the progressive degeneration of desmosomal structures. Ultrastructurally, the process of desmosomal breakdown involves: 1) formation of electron lucent areas in their core and 2) eventual expansion or ballooning of the cores to form 3) the 'lacunar domains', which are gradually engulfed by the extracellular bilayers. These different stages are shown in Fig. 1.4 (upper inset).

It was previously thought that the terminal differentiation of the granular cell involved proteolytic degradation of its cytosol and large scale secretion of lamellar bodies that is coordinated with the formation of the cornified envelope (CE), but it is now clear that the granular cell is a secretory cell, continuously synthesizing and maintaining a basal rate of secretion of the LB, while waiting for appropriate signals to cornify. The deep invaginations functioning as portals of LB secretion are an adaptation allowing continuous secretion even while the thickened envelope is being formed. The CE is formed from precursors such as involucrin and loricrin

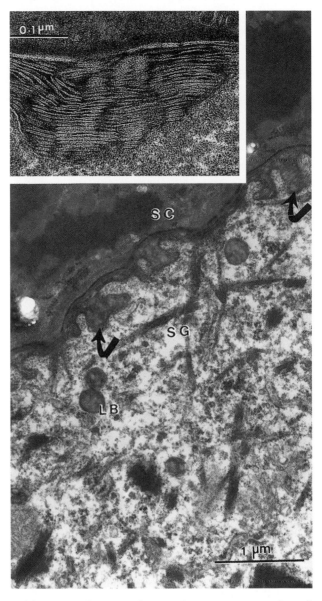

Fig. 1.2. The SG-SC junction of human epidermis is showing the outermost granular cell and a cornifying cell. Note portals of LB secretion as deep invaginations in the plasma membrane of the granular cell (arrow) as well as nascent LBs within the apical cytosol (OsO_4 post fixation). Inset: High magnification view of the appearance of secreted LB contents filling the SG-SC domains (Murine epidermis-RuO_4 post-fixation)

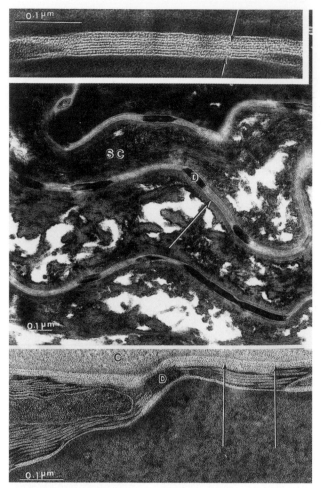

Fig. 1.3. Electron micrograph of the human SC revealing it as a composite structure. Note the tortuous extracellular (intercellular) domains filled with mortar lipid bilayers (arrows) and desmosomes (D) that rivet the corneocytes (C). The large 'holes' within some corneocytes are artifacts (due to keratin digestion by the highly reactive RuO_4 used in post-fixation). Lower inset: High magnification view of post-secretory unfurling and end-to-end fusion of LB contents in the lowermost SC domains. Note distinct and separate bilayers below, and the formation of broad, compact bilayers at distal portions of the intercellular domain. The relation of desmosomes to lipid disks that anchor onto them is also evident (murine epidermis, RuO_4 post-fixation). Reproduced with permission of Wiley-Liss from Menon and Ghadially 1997. Upper inset: A high magnification view of intercellular bilayer structures with repeat pattern of lucent and dense bands (arrows) in normal human SC

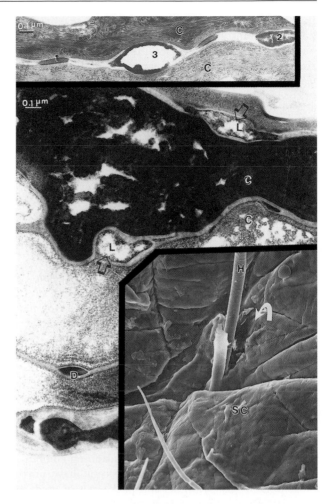

Fig. 1.4. Transmission and scanning electron micrographs of SC illustrate 'pores' at the micro- and macro-levels of organization. Transmission EM of murine SC following a brief (10 s) microwave assisted fixation and RuO_4 post-fixation reveal lacunae that are expanded by the microwave energy (open arrows, L). Undegraded desmosomal structures (D) are not altered by the fixation procedure. Scanning EM of a surface replica of human skin shows a hair follicle, a pore (white arrow) at the macro-level of organization, and a potential route for targeting delivery of genes/vaccines. (See text for details)

that undergo extensive cross-linking mediated by the enzyme transglutaminase, which is activated by calcium. Coincident with cornification, the plasma membrane of the outermost SG cell is replaced by a solvent-resistant envelope. This structure is enriched in ω-hydroxyceramides, which are covalently bound to the outer CE (primarily glutamine/glutamic acid residues in involucrin). The origin of this structure is uncertain, i.e., lamellar contents, limiting the envelope of sphingomyelin residues in the plasma membrane. The last two options would allow transglutaminase 1, the calcium dependant enzyme required for CE peptide cross-linking, to transesterify ω-hydroxyceramides in situ. The function of the covalently bound lipid envelope, whether it is required for barrier function, corneocyte cohesion, and/or regulation of access/egress of molecules from the corneocyte cytosol, is unknown. The nature of signals for terminal differentiation of the granular cells to corneocytes is still being elucidated. One such signal that triggers the process is a massive influx of ionic calcium. The rapid transformation of granular cells into a corneocyte, involving the activation of several proteases has been termed 'diffpoptosis' (Whitfield 1997) to distinguish it from the classic apoptotic pathway.

The ontogeny of the epidermal barrier has been studied primarily using late gestation fetal rats (reviewed by Williams et al. 1998). These studies have delineated the roles of various hormones, nuclear receptors and ionic signals in the development of the barrier around birth. Additionally, the patterned acquisition of the barrier reflects the developmental sequence of pattern formation that characterize integument and its derivatives in general (Hardman et al. 1998).

Barrier Homeostasis and Barrier Repair

Local perturbation in the epidermal barrier sets in motion a series of events that signal secretion of nascent LB, upregulation of lipid synthesis and assembly of new LB. The nature of ionic and cytokine signals involved in barrier restoration/homeostasis have been well studied (see reviews by Feingold 1997, Elias and Feingold 1998). Yet, the origin and mechanisms of apical trafficking/targeting and the mechanics of organelle secretion from a highly keratinized cytosolic matrix are only incompletely understood.

Very recently, the subcellular distribution and organization of the epidermal LB have been examined in vitro and in vivo by a variety of investigative techniques (Elias et al. 1998, Madison et al. 1998). These studies, utilizing fluorescently labeled ceramides, fluorescent dyes, scanning confocal microscopy, ultrastructural cytochemistry and electron microscopy, have provided new insights into the biogenesis of LBs, synthesis and packaging of lipids within LBs, and the spatial organization of a LB secretory system within individual cells of the SG. The picture that emerges now is that of LB budding off from a modified trans-Golgi like network within individual secretory granular cells (immediately subjacent to the SC) that are poised to respond to barrier requirements via an appropriate degree of LB secretion. The portals of such secretion appear as deep invaginations from the apical cell membrane, so that the formation of the CE does not impede the ability of cells to continue secretion while in transit (i.e. waiting for signals for terminal differentiation). It is extremely difficult, if not impossible, to quantify the secretory response using the currently available investigative techniques. However, several studies on barrier repair have contributed pieces of evidence towards solving the puzzle of barrier repair response.

Stratum Corneum: Its Unique Organization and Properties

The stratum corneum is a unique biological structure with remarkable physical and biological properties unsurpassed by other organ-systems. This paper-thin wrap, crucial for life, is a composite material made of proteins (85% dry weight) and lipids. Proteins are sequestered inside individual corneocytes embedded within a lipid matrix, analogous to a "brick-and-mortar" arrangement. The human SC typically has about 18 to 21 cell layers. Individual corneocytes are 20 to 40 micrometers in diameter, compared to 6 to 8 micrometers for the basal cell, due to the extreme flattening during cornification. Corneocytes differ in their thickness, packing of keratin filaments, number of desmosomes (corneodesmosomes) etc. depending on the body site, and to a lesser extend, their location within the SC (lower vs. upper layers). These features also influence the degree of hydration of the cell, normally about 10–30% bound water. Corneocytes have ridges and undulations that aid the overlapping cells to interdigitate and enhance the stability of the layers. Corneodesmosomes, important for the cohesion of the SC, are intact in stratum compactum (lower layers of SC). Cornified cells are attached to a plasma membrane that is reinforced by a layer of highly cross-linked and resistant protein, the cornified cell envelope. The interior of the cell is packed with keratin filaments (85%) surrounded by a matrix composed mainly of filaggrin. Lipid bilayers derived from the probarrier lipids of the LBs surround the individual corneocytes. As shown in Fig. 1.3, the lamellar body contents fuse end-to-end upon secretion, forming elongated bilayer structures that go through chemical and structural modulations mediated by a battery of lipolytic enzymes. These enzymes include acid and neutral lipases, esterases, sphingomyelinase, phospholipases and β-glucocerebrosidase (Elias and Menon 1991). At the SG-SC interface, a string of fused LB disks can still be identified, but closer to the membrane of the first layer of corneocytes the individual disk outlines have disappeared, and long continuous bilayer structures have already been formed. The desmosomes are surrounded by the lipid lamellae, but in the SG-SC interface desmosomes appear to provide anchorage to the disk contents of LBs. LB-derived proteases are involved in degradation of desmosomes leading to the orderly desquamation of the outermost corneocytes (Menon et al. 1992 a, Sondell et al. 1995), but the lipid bilayers initially protect the desmosomes of the stratum compactum from proteolytic degradation ensuring the integrity of this stratum crucial for barrier function. The exceptionally low permeability of the SC is the consequence of a highly convoluted and tortuous extracellular pathway (Potts and Francoeur 1991), packed with the mortar lipids. The bilayered arrangement of the lipids and the segregation of various lipid molecules into domains displaying different physical and chemical characteristics (the "domain mosaic model" (Forslind 1994)) add further degrees of complexity to the tortuous pathway. Clearly, the scaffolding of corneocytes is crucial for the barrier organization (anchoring the lipids and creating the tortuosity of the hydrophobic path), but much of the barrier research has been focussed on lipids, the universal waterproofing molecules in nature.

The near total segregation of lipids to intercellular domains of SC was confirmed by isolating SC membrane 'sandwiches' that contained trapped intercellular lipids (Grayson and Elias 1982). These preparations comprised about 50% lipid by weight accounting for over 80% of SC lipids, and had the same lipid profile of whole SC (Grayson et al. 1985). Additionally, it had the same freeze fracture pattern (broad lamellae) and X-ray diffraction pattern of whole SC (Elias and Feingold 1988). These lipids are composed mainly of ceramides, cholesterol and fatty acids (Wertz and Downing 1991) present in a roughly equimolar ratio (Man et al. 1993), in addition to small amounts of triglycerides, glycosphingolipids and cholesterol sulfate that are detected in the SC (Schurer and Elias 1991). Ceramides amount to approximately 50% of the total lipid mass and 40% of the total number of lipids, and are crucial to the lipid organization of the SC barrier (Bouwstra et al. 1996). Of the 6 major ceramide classes, ceramide 1 is believed to be uniquely significant in the formation of the covalently bound lipid envelope of corneocytes (Wertz and Downing 1983). Ceramide 1 consists of sphingosine and long chain, saturated, mono- and di-unsaturated ω-hydroxy acids in the amide linkage. Cholesterol is the second most abundant lipid in SC accounting for approximately 25 weight % or 30 mol % of SC (Norlan et al. 1999). It is crucial for promoting the intermixing of different lipid species and its 'phase' behavior is complex. Cholesterol decreases the chain mobility and reduces the mean molecular polar head group area of lipids in the liquid crystalline state. By so doing it increases the chain mobility of lipids in the gel state. Free fatty acids account for about 10% of SC lipids or 15 mol % and consist predominantly of long chain saturated fatty acids having more than 20 carbon atoms. Oleic (6%) and linoleic (2%) are the only unsaturated fatty acids detected in the SC (Wertz and Downing 1991).

A decrease in the concentrations of any of these critical lipid species affects the barrier integrity (see review by Menon and Ghadially 1997). Several excellent papers and reviews on the biophysical aspects of barrier lipids have been published (Kitson et al. 1994, Bouwstra et al. 1995 and 1996, Wertz and van den Bergh 1998, Norlan et al. 1999) and have contributed to our present day understanding of the mechanics of barrier function. Two of the recent models of barrier lipid organization are the "domain mosaic model" (Forslind 1994) and the "plastic mosaic model" (Norlan 1999).

The "domain mosaic model" of Forslind (1994) considers the SC lipid matrix as a lamellar two phase system with a discontinuous lamellar crystalline structure embedded in a continuous liquid crystalline structure. If the crystalline areas are considered impermeable while the liquid crystalline areas are permeable (to diffusing substances), and the water is primarily located in the liquid crystalline areas, the diffusion of compounds (both hydrophilic and hydrophobic) would be restricted to the liquid crystalline structures. As a result, the molecules would perform a 'random walk' in the 'channels' of liquid crystalline structures separating the two crystalline domains. The only way of moving up to the next layer (of the SC stacks) is when two 'channels' cross. Thus the diffusing molecule has to follow a highly tortuous pathway, due to the long diffusion pathlength in the lateral direction and/or small area available for diffusion in the vertical direction. The latest model proposed for mammalian barrier is the "plastic model" of Norlan (1999). This is based on his findings that only long alkyl chain, saturated lipids together with cholesterol are present in the SC extracellular domain – a finding that questions the existence of a separate liquid crystalline structure. As the skin barrier should be as tight as possible (with the exception of a minor 'leakage' adequate to maintain the hydration of corneocytes), and optimized for a wide range of ambient conditions, sudden phase transitions and phase separations would not be biologically advantageous. Consequently, the barrier lipids should be as homogeneous as possible. This state is achieved by impurities in the lipid composition that broaden the transition zones and stabilize the ideal lipid morphology (i.e., a plastic crystalline state) to ensure that the lamellar structures are intact and that no pores or non-lamellar structures are induced. The model proposes that barrier lipids are in a lamellar arrangement that are in a "plastic" crystalline state with or without water being present between the lamellae. As the upper SC lipids are mixed in with the sebaceous lipids, and as its lower water content promotes phase transitions and phase separations, the true (ideal) barrier is located in the lower SC.

The "domain mosaic model" advocates a meandering route of polar pathway for water through the grain boundaries of the lipid mosaic, thus adding another level of complexity to the tortuous lipid pathway of the simple "brick and mortar" model. The morphological basis of the aqueous pore pathway, much debated based on theoretical calculations of the molecular weight of compounds that traverse the SC and their activation energies (Flynn 1989), remained uncertain. Menon and Elias (1997), based on transmission EM studies of tracer permeation under various permeabilization strategies, identified the lacunar domains embedded within the lipid bilayers as the morphological basis of the pore pathway. The lacunae mostly – but not entirely – correspond to the sites of desmosome degradation (Haftek et al. 1998), and hence remain as scattered and discontinuous aqueous domains within the mortar lipids (Fig. 1.5), but transiently become interconnected, forming a continuous "pore pathway" (Fig. 1.6) under appropriate conditions of permeabilization (sonophoresis, iontophoresis, prolonged hydration). The pore pathway reverts back to its original discontinuous state once the permeabilizing stimuli are turned off (as in the case of sonophoresis) or no longer exist (as in hydration). Such a lacunar system does not correspond to the grain boundaries of the "domain mosaic model", but instead forms an "extended macrodomain mosaic" within the SC (Menon et al. 1998).

In the context of gene delivery techniques, the morphological organization of the SC, its biophysical properties as a composite material, and its responses to chemical and physical manipulations are of interest. What emerges from cytochemical studies of experimental and comparative aspects of SC is the picture of a complex tissue that is 1) not a uniform layer, 2) not a static or dead tissue, but rather one that is in a dynamic state with ongoing structural modifications and 3) a tissue that senses and responds to the physical environment and brings about modifications in its own physical/chemical properties.

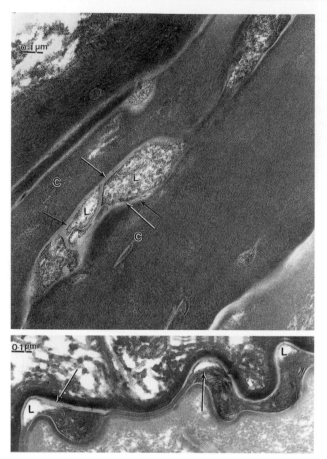

Fig. 1.5. Highly expanded lacunae (L) in murine SC (corneocyte = C) following acetone treatment. Inset: Changes in lipid organization of lower SG of murine epidermis following sonophoresis

SC As a Non-uniform Layer

The outermost layers of the SC, the stratum disjunctum, are easily removed by tape stripping but not so the lower layers – the stratum compactum with more functional desmosomes, and where the lipid bilayers are more compact and uniform. Natural moisturizing factors (NMF), the peptide breakdown products of filaggrin, which become more abundant in the outer corneocytes depending on variations in external humidity, may account for the non-uniformity of corneocytes that is evident in conventional electron micrographs. In particular, some corneocytes have dense packing of keratin, while others have a much looser and sparser packing of filaments. Whether these differences are related to the hydration state or other functional differences among corneocytes has not been determined.

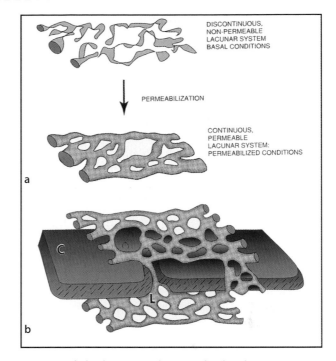

DISCONTINUOUS, NON-PERMEABLE LACUNAR SYSTEM BASAL CONDITIONS

PERMEABILIZATION

CONTINUOUS, PERMEABLE LACUNAR SYSTEM: PERMEABILIZED CONDITIONS

a

b

Fig. 1.6. a Schematic representation of the lacunar pathway under basal versus permeabilized conditions. Reprinted from Menon and Elias 1997, with permission from S. Karger, AG Basel. **b** Schematic representation of a continuous lacunar pathway (L) in relation to corneocytes (C) (not drawn to scale). Lipid bilayers are not represented

SC As a Dynamic Tissue

There has been much debate as to whether the SC is a dead tissue or not. Semantics apart, there is clear evidence of ongoing enzymatic processes within the bricks as well as the mortar. As noted above, degradation of filaggrin to give rise to NMF, crucial for water holding properties of corneocytes, is triggered by differences in hydration level that is somehow sensed by the SC. The extracellular processing of pro-barrier lipids, largely originating from LB secretion involves a battery of enzymes (acid and neutral lipases, esterases, β-glucocerebrosidase, sphingomyelinase, phospholipase, steroid sulfatase) which, when inhibited, lead to alterations in the lipid morphological appearance and barrier functions of the SC. Specific proteases, localized in the LBs, (Lundstrom and Egelrud 1991, Sondell et al. 1995) play a role in desmosomal degradation and orderly desquamation of the outer SC, and, perhaps, in other as yet unrecognized functions. The versatility of SC responses to environmental stress is illustrated by the rapid improvement of barrier functions in aves when xerically challenged (Menon et al. 1996).

SC As a Composite Material

A composite material is defined as being made of two or more dissimilar materials combined to optimize the properties of the composite. The combination of different properties yields a third property to the composite. Stress concentration is achieved by combining stiff and compliant phases in parallel. Many man-made composites (stainless steel, plywood) and structural engineering designs are built on this principle. Such materials are abundant in nature e.g., the protective exoskeleton of molluscan shells, where the brick and mortar arrangement of calcified plates glued with a highly deformable protein provides impact resistance. SC is a more flexible and versatile example of such a protective composite material, and, from a biomaterial perspective, is a self-cleaning and self-renewing biopolymer (Hoath et al. 1993). Individual corneocytes can absorb water and swell, and then release the water and revert back to their original dimensions without breaking apart. The mortar lipids coupled with the cornified envelope maintain the biopolymer during hydration-dehydration cycles. The shape memory of this biopolymer as well as its ability to sense and respond to the environment in an adaptive manner qualifies the SC to be considered a "smart material". "Passively smart" and "actively smart" materials are recognized based on their responses (Newnham and Ruschau 1996). Passive smartness involves the ability to respond to environmental conditions in a useful manner (the proteolytic production of NMF by corneocytes is an example). Active smartness is defined with reference to sensing and actuating functions. SC and SG layers together form an actively smart system, responding to barrier requirements, and indeed barrier disruption, by enhanced LB secretion triggered by cytokine signals from SC or ionic milieu of SG (Feingold 1997). Like many smart systems, SC is also known to exhibit certain piezoelectric and pyroelectric properties (Athenstaedt et al. 1982). An appreciation of SC as a composite biopolymer with "intelligence" will no doubt contribute greatly to improved bioengineering approaches for effective transcutaneous delivery of drugs, vaccines and genes.

Strategies to Overcome the Barrier

Several approaches and strategies to overcome the barrier have been devised for transdermal delivery with varying degrees of success. Briefly, these have been classified as either physical, chemical, mechanical or metabolic approaches. Combinations of these strategies can also be employed for increasing the efficacy (Johnson et al. 1996, Tsai et al. 1996, Choi et al. 1999) or for extending the time available for transdermal delivery. The techniques vary from very straightforward approaches (e.g. occlusion, tape stripping) to the highly sophisticated instrumentation and miniaturization (e.g. iontophoresis, electroporation).

Physical Techniques

Tape Stripping

The simplest way of decreasing barrier efficacy of the SC is by removing a large part of it by stripping off the corneocytes with either an adhesive tape or cyanoacrylate glue. Sequential stripping increases the transepidermal water loss (TEWL), an indicator of a barrier defect, which coincides with increased permeability (Spruit and Malten 1966). Tape stripping removes both corneocytes and extracellular lipid, reducing the tortuous path length that substances have to traverse. Moreover, stripping induces varying degrees of mechanical disruption (of the lipid lamellae and the packing of the secreted lamellar discs at the SG-SC interface) focally, even in the lower retained SC layers. Together, these alterations provide pathways for delivering drugs, vaccines or genes (naked DNA) into the viable cells below. Such barrier disruption with tape stripping is easily done in animal models where TEWL values increase to >50 times of normal depending on the number of strippings. However, human skin needs many more strippings to obtain comparable results. As a result, mast cell degranulation and inflammation can occur leading to discomfort and pain. Tape stripping in humans is complicated by the fact that its efficacy is dependent on pigmentation, as darker/pigmented skin not only takes more strippings to disrupt (Reed et al. 1995) but also exhibits a greater propensity for post-inflammatory pigmentary changes. Finally, tape stripping causes a loss of the calcium ion gradient, which signals a localized barrier repair response in vivo (Menon et al. 1992b). Still, a window of opportunity for transdermal delivery across the treated area for up to 6 hours may be available. This window can be extended for several more hours (up to 24 h) by simple occlusion with a vapor impermeable film or chamber that inhibits (at best) or slows down (at worse) the barrier repair mechanisms (Proksch et al. 1991). The decreased thickness of SC following tape stripping (or laser ablation) could also enable the use of the gene gun at lower pressures than are usually employed.

Occlusion

Prolonged (24 h) occlusion of normal mammalian skin alters the barrier properties of SC (van den Merwe and Ackermann 1987, Mikulowska 1992) and this effect is used in the patch testing of potential irritants. Occlusion with a vapor-impermeable membrane/chamber leads to increased local hydration and alters SC organization. Electron microscopy studies have shown that the corneocytes swell, intercellular spaces become distended and that the lacunae become dilated following 24–48 hours of occlusion and resultant hydration. It is the distention of lacunae leading to continuities within an otherwise non-continuous system, which creates "pores" through which polar and non-polar substances can penetrate the SC. Such patches or chambers (Finn chambers, Hilltop chambers) offer relatively simple approaches for the potential topical delivery of vaccines or genes. Although lacking the technological appeal of a gene gun, occlusion or pretreatment with occlusion can be expected to improve the uptake of either topically applied naked DNA or anti-sense oligonucleotides.

Chemical Techniques

A variety of solvents (ethanol, methanol, chloroform, acetone) and detergents can extract SC barrier lipids and permeabilize the SC to varying degrees (Fig. 1.5). Morphological changes in human SC following in vitro exposure to a variety of solvents and chemical agents have been described by Menon et al. (1998). These include phase separation of lipids, derangement of SC lamellar bilayers and LB derived disks at the SC-SG interface as well as creation of "holes" within corneocytes (following exposure to phenolic compounds). Moreover, surfactants such as sodium lauryl sulfate (SLS) and vehicles like propylene glycol create extensive expansion of the existing lacunar domains. Several other penetration enhancers such as azone, sulfoxides, urea, essential oils, fatty acid, etc. alter the SC lipid organization and aid in transdermal delivery (Santus and Baker 1993).

Liposomes/Transfersomes

The use of liposomes to deliver specific genes via or to hair follicles has been reported (Yarosh et al. 1994, Domashenko and Cotsarelis 1999). However, the efficacy of liposomes in transdermal delivery has been questioned as well (Lasch et al. 1991). Many studies have shown that liposomes do not penetrate the SC as intact structures and that they fuse with SC lipids releasing their contents in the upper SC (Korting et al. 1995). Transfersomes, a patented technology, are claimed to be able to penetrate the SC intact (perhaps via the lacunae?) due to the deformable nature of these liposomes (Cevec et al. 1998). However, the successful use of transfersomes by others remains undocumented. Very recently, elastic liquid-state vesicles have been developed that were shown to modify the SC lipid organization when applied non-occlusively (van den Bergh 1999). These may prove promising either as carriers for drugs or as penetration enhancers for topical delivery across the SC.

Metabolic Approaches

This approach entails creating a focal intrinsic barrier defect by blocking the synthesis of any or all of the crucial barrier lipid species such as cholesterol, ceramides or fatty acids (Tsai et al. 1996) or their precursors. Repeated topical application of selective inhibitors of enzymes such as 3-hydroxy-3-methyl-glutaryl-(HMG) CoA-reductase, serine palmitoyl transferase (SPT) or fatty acyl CoA carboxylase, inhibits synthesis of cholesterol, ceramides and free fatty acids, respectively (Man et al. 1993, Holleran et al. 1991). This is accompanied by morphological and physiological changes in SC lamellar bilayers, leading to increased transepidermal water loss and permeation of tracers through the SC (Tsai et al. 1996). The underlying defects in the LB system and SC lipid organization have been well-characterized in murine models. The deficient LB contents show a moth-eaten appearance, incomplete processing of the precursor bilayers and/or lipid phase separations within the SC as well as enlargement of the lacunar pathway. Induction of such abnormalities in normal skin takes about a week of twice daily applications of the inhibitors, but the process can be accelerated if inhibitors are applied following barrier abrogation with a lipid solvent. This will inhibit the barrier repair response and sustain the defective window in the barrier for a longer duration, besides accelerating delivery of the inhibitors to the SG where they target sites of lipid synthesis. Combinations of inhibitors can theoretically also be effectively used as metabolic approaches for areas of skin predetermined for topical gene delivery.

Yet, another metabolic strategy is to use lipolytic enzymes (Patil et al. 1996) or inhibitors of enzymes that are crucial for the lipid modulations or processing of the LB derived disks such as bromoconduritol epoxide that inhibit β-glucocerebrosidase (Holleran et al. 1993). The metabolic strategy, although validated in animal models, is yet to be evaluated for safety concerns before human application. Some of the inhibitors are approved drugs (e.g. statin, and phospholipase A2 inhibitors), while others are not. There may also be additional regulatory issues of simultaneous use of two different drugs.

Iontophoresis and Electroporation

These techniques are based on electrically assisted delivery of drugs/macromolecules into or across the skin (Banga et al. 1999). Iontophoresis uses a small amount of electric current (<100 V) to drive the drugs through the skin, and has been known for several decades. Electroporation (electropermeabilization) is relatively new and employs ultrashort but large transmembrane voltages (~100 V or more) to induce structural rearrangement and conductance changes in membranes leading to the formation of 'pores' (Banga et al. 1999).

Iontophoresis uses an electrode with the same polarity as the charge of the drug, to drive charged drugs across the SC. The predominant pathway of iontophoretic transport is trans-appendegeal (hair follicles, sweat glands) although SC extracellular routes have been demonstrated using tracer studies (Monteiro-Riviere et al. 1994). Iontophoretic delivery is considered to occur via water filled pores, and thus the pore pathway in skin can be considered to occur at the macro- (appendegeal) and the micro- (lacunae) levels of organization. As drug delivery is proportionate to the current, iontophoresis offers an opportunity for programmable drug delivery (Green 1996), especially with the development of miniaturized microprocessor systems and disposable hydrogel pads.

Electroporation is essentially the physical cell transfection method of opening pores in cell membranes with a brief electrical pulse to insert DNA or other macromolecules into the cytoplasm. Although most effective for unilamellar cell membranes, recent studies show the feasibility of this method for permeabilizing the SC (Prausnitz et al. 1993). Weaver and Chizmadzev (1996) conclude that the SC with about 100 multilamellar bilayers needs about 100 V pulses (or 1 V per bilayer). Electroporation is thought to be non-thermal and pore formation is considered to be the mechanism, although the pores have not yet been visualized by any microscopic technique.

A related technique, claimed to be effective is termed electro-incorporation (Zhang et al. 1997). Drugs encapsulated in vesicles/particles are applied to the skin and pulsed with electrodes placed on top of the particles. The resulting electric field is claimed to cause a 'breakdown' of SC by an as yet unknown mechanism (Hofmann et al. 1995). Particles varying from 0.2 to 4.5 micrometers in size were shown to be embedded in hairless mouse skin when pulsed with 3 exponential decay pulses of 120 V and 1–2 ms pulse length. However, with the reported ineffectiveness of the technique (Chen et al. 1999) and in the absence of what defines "SC breakdown", this technique lacks clear validation.

Phonophoresis (Sonophoresis)

Ultrasound, extensively used in medical diagnostics and physical therapy, is considered safe with no short- or long-term side effects. Ultrasound (especially high frequency ultrasound) undergoes a loss of energy upon encountering a different medium (such as SC) causing an increased energy concentration there and generating defects in SC structure (Wu et al. 1998) leading to permeabilization of the SC. Numerous studies have examined the effects of ultrasound at various frequencies on penetration of substances across the SC with inconsistent results. Most of these studies used ultrasound in frequency ranges of 1–3 MHz mainly due to technical limitations in the available equipment. Bommannan et al. (1992a) investigated the use of 10 and 16 MHz frequencies on hairless guinea pigs and obtained significantly enhanced drug delivery. The low intensities used prevented local heating of the skin. In follow-up studies, the pathway of permeation of tracers such as lanthanum and FITC-conjugated dextrans during sonophoresis was investigated in the skin of hairless guinea pigs as well as mice (Bommannan et al. 1992b, Menon et al. 1994a). The tracers penetrated into the epidermis and dermis within 5 minutes of sonophoresis with no apparent damage to the keratinocytes. Longer exposure (20 min) was damaging the cells. Ruthenium tetroxide (RuO_4) staining confirmed that ultrasound caused dilation of the lacunae located within the SC extracellular bilayers creating a transiently continuous channel or pore pathway (Fig. 1.6a). This has been postulated as the mechanism for overcoming the barrier, albeit temporarily, with the use of ultrasound. In the lowermost layers of SC, the LB derived disks showed physical separation in their otherwise tightly packed pattern. These defects persisted even after 24 hours post treatment, although the transepidermal water loss (TEWL) values were back to base line. The return of TEWL to base values is postulated as due to 1) the collapse of the pore pathway as well as 2) an accelerated LB secretion by the SG responding to ultrasound-induced changes in its calcium milieu (Menon et al 1994b). The combined effect of this "actively smart" response of the SG-SC unit is the rapid return of the functional barrier.

Mitragotri et al. (1995a and b) and Johnson et al. (1996) examined the effects of low frequency and therapeutic ultrasound as well as synergistic effects of chemical enhancers and ultrasound on human cadaver skin. They concluded that ultrasound induces cavitation within the SC, disordering the lipid bilayers, and thus enhances penetration of lipophilic drugs. However, in these ex vivo studies, the SC was subjected to extensive freeze-thaw cycles (–80 °C storage), thawing followed by heat separation of SC (at 60 °C), followed by several days of storage at 4–5 °C before continuous ultrasound exposure (up to 24 hours) in a fully hydrated state occurred. These treatments and conditions can be expected to abolish even the passively smart responses of the SC. In the light of the "actively smart" cutaneous response in vivo mentioned above it is clear that the influence of experimental design and conditions of sonophoresis on epidermal morphology and response cannot be overemphasized. Another significant issue is the finding from Tachibana's lab that following short ultrasound exposure in a water bath, profound changes occur in the hair follicle structure, including large-scale loss of the SC that exposes the SS (Yamashita et al. 1997). These changes may be due to the extensive surface area that is exposed to ultrasound in combination with the high degree of hydration.

Photomechanical Waves

This is a recently developed technique utilizing laser beams (Lee et al. 1998 and 1999). The photomechanical (stress) waves, generated by high power pulse lasers, are broad band compressive waves that interact directly with the tissue in ways that are different from that of ultrasound. The waves are generated by ablation of a target material (polystyrene) covering the solution to be delivered across the skin. The target absorbs the laser radiation, and the solution serves as a coupling medium for the stress waves to be propagated into the SC. In murine models, 40 kD dextran molecules and 20 nm latex particles were delivered across the SC by a single photomechanical wave (Lee et al. 1998). These laser stress waves were generated using a 23 ns Q-switched Ruby laser. A single (110 ns) photomechanical compression wave reportedly modulates the permeability of human SC transiently, and the barrier function recovers within minutes following the exposure. Very recently, this method has been used to deliver small molecules such as 5-aminolevulenic acid in human skin without causing pain or discomfort and without adverse effects with regard to the skin structure or viability (Lee et al. 1999). The pathway of permeation is thought to be intercellular, as is known for phonophoresis.

Particle-Mediated Gene Delivery (Gene Gun)

The mode of barrier disruption in particle-mediated gene delivery "biolistic" via a gene gun differs from the above-described methods. With the use of the gene gun, the particles (gold) physically penetrate the SC (Williams et al. 1991) traversing the corneocytes as well as the mortar lipids (Fig. 1.7) leaving many

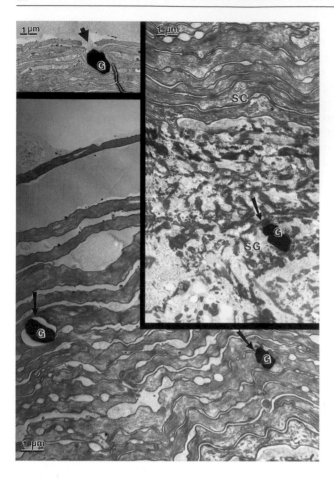

Fig. 1.7. Transmission electron microscopic image of human SC following gene gun application at 500 psi. Gold particles (G) are embedded in the SC. Inset shows gold particles within the SG as well as in SC. Upper left inset: A gold particle lodged in the uppermost layers of SC, as well as the physical gap in the corneocyte created by the biolistic process

"microwounds" or physical channels open. Very few, if any, studies have characterized the SC morphology following gene gun treatment. Menon et al. (1997) showed that the human SC presents a formidable barrier to the penetration of gold particles at 350 to 500 psi. Using scanning and transmission EM, the majority of gold particles were detected in the surface layers, though a few particles penetrated to the basal layers and even the dermis. This observation underscores the significance of the bricks in the physical barrier (including impact resistance) in addition to the well-recognized function of providing the scaffolding for the organization of barrier lipids that are crucial for the permeability barrier. The application of the gene gun could be effectively followed by topical application of naked DNA at the treated sites to maximize gene delivery through the physical channels created by particle bombardment. Indeed, pores at the macrolevel of organization, i.e. hair follicles aid effective topical gene transfer as demonstrated recently (Fan et al. 1999).

Acknowledgements. We acknowledge Drs. B. Bommannan (Palo Alto, CA), A. Doukas (Harvard, Boston) and L. Norlan (Geneva) for freely sharing information and checking parts of the manuscript for accuracy. P.M. Elias acknowledges support from NIH Grant AR 19098. Dr. J. Menon (William Paterson University, NJ) provided partial support with electron microscopy, and Dr. P. Attar (Avon Products, NY) provided comments and editorial help.

References

Athenstaedt H, Claussen H, Schaper D (1982) Epidermis of human skin: Pyroelectric and piezoelectric sensor layer. Science 216:1018–1020

Banga AK, Bose S, Ghosh TK (1999) Iontophoresis and electroporation: comparisons and contrasts. Int Natl J Pharmaceut 179:1–19

Bommannan D, Okuyama H, Stauffer P, Guy RH (1992a) Sonophoresis. I. The use of high-frequency ultrasound to enhance transdermal drug delivery. Pharmacol Res 9:559–564

Bommannan D, Menon GK, Okuyama H, Elias PM, Guy RH (1992b) Sonophoresis. II. Examination of the mechanism(s) of ultrasound-enhanced transdermal drug delivery. Pharmacol Res 9:1043–1047

Bouwstra JA, Gooris GS, Bras W, Downing DT (1995) Lipid organization in pig stratum corneum. J Lipid Res 36:685–695

Bouwstra JA, Gooris GS, Cheng K, Weerheim A, Bras W, Ponec M (1996) Phase behaviour of isolated skin lipids. J Lipid Res 37:999–1011

Cevec G, Gebauer D, Stieber J, Schatzlein A, Blume G (1998) Ultraflexible vesicles, transfersomes, have extremely low pore penetration resistance and transport therapeutic amounts of insulin across the intact mammalian skin. Biochim Biophys Acta 1368:201–215

Chen T, Langer R, Weaver JC (1999) Charged microbeads are not transported across the human stratum corneum in vitro by short high-voltage pulses. Bioelectrochem Bioenerg 48:181–192

Choi EH, Lee SH, Ahn SK, Hwang SM (1999) The pretreatment effect of chemical skin penetration enhancers in transdermal drug delivery using iontophoresis. Skin Pharmacol Appl Skin Physiol 12:326–335

Domashenko A, Cotsarelis G (1999) Transfection of human hair follicles using topical liposomes is optimal at the onset of anagen. J Invest Dermatol 112:552

Downing DL (1992) Lipid and protein structures in the permeability barrier of mammalian epidermis. J Lipid Res 33:301–313

Eckert RL (1989) Structure, function and differentiation of the keratinocyte. Physiol Rev 69:1316–1345

Elias PM, Feingold KR (1988) Lipid-related barriers and gradients in the epidermis. Ann N Y Acad Sci 548:4–13

Elias PM, Feingold KR (1998) A dynamic view of the stratum corneum: applications to skin care. In: Tagami II, Parrish JA, Ozawa T (eds) Skin: Interface of a living system. Elsevier Science B.V. pp. 141–150

Elias PM, Menon GK (1991) Structural and biochemical correlates of the epidermal permeability barrier. In: Elias PM (ed) Advances in lipid research. Academic Press, San Diego, pp. 1–26

Elias PM, Cullander C, Mauro T, Rassner U, Komuves L, Brown D, Menon GK (1998) The secretory granular cell: the outermost granular cell as a specialized secretory cell. J Invest Dermatol Symp Proc 3:87–100

Fan H, Morissey GR, Khavari PA (1999) Immunization via hair follicles by topical application of naked DNA to normal skin. Nat Biotechnol 17:870–872

Fartasch M, Bassukas ID, Diepgen TL (1993) Structural relationship between epidermal lipid lamellae, lamellar bodies and desmosomes in human epidermis. Br J Dermatol 128:1–9

Feingold KR (1997) Permeability barrier homeostasis: its biochemical basis and regulation. Cosmetics & Toiletries 112:49–59

Flynn GL (1989) Mechanism of percutaneous absorption from physicochemical evidence. In: Bronaugh RL, Maibach HI (eds) Percutaneous absorption. Dekker, New York. pp. 27–51

Forslind B (1994) A domain mosaic model of the skin barrier. Acta Derm Venereol 74:1–6

Grayson S, Elias PM (1982) Isolation and lipid biochemical characterization of stratum corneum membrane complexes: Implications for the cutaneous permeability barrier. J Invest Dermatol 78:128–135

Grayson S, Johnson-Winegar AG, Wintraub BU, Epstein EH Jr., Elias PM (1985) Lamellar body enriched fractions from neonatal mice: Preparative techniques and partial characterization. J Invest Dermatol 85:289–295

Green PG (1996) Iontophoretic delivery of peptide drugs. J Controlled Release 41:33–48

Haftek M, Teillon MH, Schmitt D (1998) Stratum corneum, corneodesmosomes and ex vivo percutaneous penetration. Microsc Res Tech 43:242–249

Hardman MJ, Sisi P, Banbury DN, Byrne C (1998) Patterned acquisition of skin barrier during development. Development 125:1541–1552

Hoath SB, Tanaka R, Boyce ST (1993) Rate of stratum corneum formation in the perinatal rat. J Invest Dermatol 100:400–406

Hofmann GA, Rustrum WV, Suder KS (1995) Electro-incorporation of microcarriers as a method for the transdermal delivery of large molecules. Bioelectrochem Bioenerg 38:209–222

Holbrook KA (1994) Ultrastructure of the epidermis. In: Leigh IM, Lane EB, Watt FM (eds) The keratinocyte handbook. Cambridge University Press, Cambridge pp. 3–39

Holleran WM, Man M-Q, Gao WN, Menon GK, Cho SS, Elias PM, Feingold KR (1991) Sphingolipids are required for mammalian barrier function: inhibition of sphingolipid synthesis delays barrier recovery after acute perturbation. J Clin Invest 88:1338–1345

Holleran WM, Takagi Y, Feingold KR, Menon GK, Legler G, Elias PM, (1993) Processing of epidermal glucosylceramides is required for optimal mammalian permeability barrier function. J Clin Invest 91:1656–1664

Johnson ME, Mitragotri S, Patel A, Blankschtein D, Langer R (1996) Synergistic effects of chemical enhancers and therapeutic ultrasound on transdermal drug delivery. J Pharm Sci 85:670–679

Kitson N, Thewalt J, Lafleur M, Bloom M (1994) A model membrane approach to the epidermal permeability barrier. Biochemistry 33:6707–6715

Korting HC, Stolz W, Schmidt MH, Maierhofer G (1995) Interaction of liposomes with human epidermis reconstructed in vitro. Br J Dermatol 132:571–579

Landmann L (1988) The epidermal permeability barrier. Anat Embryol 178:1–13

Lasch J, Laub R, Wohlrab W (1991) How deep do intact liposomes penetrate into human skin? J Controlled Release 18:55–58

Lee S, McAuliff DJ, Flotte TJ, Kollias N, Doukas AG (1998) Photomechanical transcutaneous delivery of macromolecules. J Invest Dermatol 111:925–929

Lee S, Kollias N, McAuliffe DJ, Flotte TJ, Doukas AG (1999) Topical drug delivery in humans with a single photomechanical wave. Pharm Res 16:1717–1721

Lundstrom A, Egelrud T (1991) Stratum corneum chymotryptic enzyme: A proteinase which may be generally present in the stratum corneum with a possible involvement in desquamation. Acta Derm Venereol 71:471–474

Madison KC, Sando GN, Howard EJ, True CA, Gilbert D, Swartzendrauber DC, Wertz PN (1998) Lamellar granule biogenesis: a role for ceramide glucosyltransferase, lysosomal enzyme transport, and the Golgi. J Invest Dermatol Symp Proc 3:80–86

Man MQ, Elias PM, Feingold KR (1993) Fatty acids are required for epidermal permeability barrier homeostasis. J Clin Invest 87:1668–1673

Menon GK, Elias PM (1997) Morphological basis for a pore-pathway in mammalian stratum corneum. Skin Pharmacol 10:235–246

Menon GK, Ghadially R (1997) Morphology of lipid alterations in the epidermis: A review. Microsc Res Tech 37:180–192

Menon GK, Williams ML, Ghadially, R, Elias PM (1992a) Lamellar bodies as a delivery system of hydrolytic enzymes. Implications for normal and abnormal desquamation. Br J Dermatol 126:337–345

Menon GK, Elias PM, Lee SH, Feingold KR (1992b). Localization of calcium in murine epidermis following disruption and repair of the permeability barrier. Cell Tissue Res 270:503–502

Menon GK, Bommannan DB, Elias PM (1994a) High-frequency sonophoresis: Permeation pathway and structural basis for enhanced permeability. Skin Pharmacol 7:130–139

Menon GK, Price LF, Bommannan DB, Elias PM, Feingold KR (1994b) Selective obliteration of the epidermal calcium gradient leads to enhanced lamellar body secretion. J Invest Dermatol 102:789–795

Menon GK, Maderson PFA, Drewes RC, Baptista LF, Price LF, Elias PM (1996) Ultrastructural organization of avian stratum corneum lipids as the basis for facultative cutaneous waterproofing. J Morphol 227:1–13

Menon GK, Brandsma J, Schwartz P (1997) Gene gun and the human skin: Ultrastructural study of distribution of gold particles in the epidermis. J Invest Dermatol 110:673

Menon GK, Lee SH, Roberts MS (1998) Ultrastructural effects of some solvents and vehicles on the stratum corneum and other skin components: evidence for an "extended mosaic – partitioning model of the skin barrier". In: Roberts MS, Walters, KA (eds) Dermal Absorption and Toxicity Assessment. Marcel Dekker, Inc. New York-Basel Hong Kong pp. 727–751

Mikulowska A (1992) Reactive changes in human epidermis following simple occlusion with water. Contact Dermatitis 26:224–227

Mitragotri S, Blankschtein D, Langer R (1995a) Ultrasound mediated transdermal protein delivery. Science 269:850–853

Mitragotri S, Edwards DA, Blankschtein D, Langer R (1995b) A mechanistic study of ultrasonically-enhanced transdermal drug delivery. J Pharm Sci 84:697–706

Monteiro-Riviere N, Inman A, Riviere J (1994) Identification of the pathway of iontophoretic drug delivery: light and ultrastructural studies using mercuric chloride in pigs. Pharmaceut Res 11:251–256

Newnham RE, Ruschau GR (1996) Smart Electroceramics. Amer Ceramic Soc Bul 75:51–61

Norlan L (1999) The Skin Barrier, Structure and Physical Function, Thesis. Karolinska Institute, Stockholm, Sweden

Norlan L, Nicander,I, Rozell BL, Ollmar S, Forslind B (1999) Inter- and intra-individual differences in human stratum corneum lipid content related to physical parameters of skin barrier function in vivo. J Invest Dermatol 112:72–77

Patil S, Singh P, Szolar-Platzer C, Maibach H (1996) Epidermal enzymes as penetration enhancers in transdermal delivery? J Pharm Sci 85:249–252

Potts RO, Francoeur, ML (1991) The influence of stratum corneum morphology on water permeability. J Invest Dermatol 96:495–499

Prausnitz MR, Bose VG, Langer R, Weaver JC (1993) Electroporation of mammalian skin: a mechanism to enhance transdermal drug delivery. Proc Natl Acad Sci USA 90:10504–10508

Proksch E, Feingold KR, Man M-Q, Elias PM (1991) Barrier function regulates epidermal DNA synthesis. J Clin Invest 87:1668–1673

Reed JT, Ghadially R, Elias PM (1995) Skin type, but neither race or gender, influence epidermal permeability barrier function. Arch Dermatol 131:1134–1138

Santus GC, Baker RW (1993) Transdermal enhancer patent literature. J Controlled Release 25:1–20

Schaefer H, Redelmeier TE (1996) Skin barrier. Principles of percutaneous absorption. Karger, Basel. p 310

Schurer N, Elias PM (1991) The biochemistry and function of stratum corneum lipids. In: Elias PM (ed) Advances in lipid research. Academic Press. 24, pp 27–56

Sondell B, Thornell LE, Egelrud T (1995) Evidence that stratum corneum chymotryptic enzyme is transported to the stratum corneum extracellular space via lamellar bodies. J Invest Dermatol 104:819–823

Spruit D, Malten KE (1966) The regeneration rate of the water vapour loss of heavily damaged skin. Dermatologica 132:115–123

Tsai JC, Guy RH, Thornfeldt CR, Gao WN, Feingold KR, Elias PM (1996) Metabolic approaches to enhance transdermal drug delivery. 1. Effect of lipid synthesis inhibitors. J Pharm Sci 85:643–648

Van den Bergh B (1999) Elastic liquid state vesicles as a tool for topical drug delivery. Thesis, Leiden University, Leiden

Van Den Merwe E, Ackermann C (1987) Physical changes in hydrated skin. Int Nat J Cosmet Sci 9:237–247

Weaver JC, Chimadzhev Y (1996) Electroporation. In: Polte C, Postow E (eds) Biological effects of electromagnetic fields. CRC Press, Boca Raton, NY, pp 247–274

Weaver JC, Vaughan TE, Chizmadzhev Y (1999) Theory of electrical creation of aqueous pathways across skin transport barriers. Adv Drug Deliv Rev 33:21–39

Wertz PN, Downing DL (1983) Ceramides of pig epidermis: structure determination. J Lipid Res 24:759–765

Wertz PN, Downing DL (1991) Epidermal lipids. In: Goldsmith LA (ed) Physiology, Biochemistry and Molecular Biology of the Skin. Oxford University Press, NY, pp 205–236

Wertz PN, van den Bergh BAI (1998) The physical, chemical and functional properties of lipids in the skin and other biological barriers. Chem Phys Lipids 91:85–96

Whitfield JF (1997) Calcium: cell cycle driver, differentiator and killer. Chapman and Hall, New York

Williams ML, Hanley K, Elias PM, Feingold KR (1998) Ontogeny of the epidermal permeability barrier. J Invest Dermatol Symp Proc 3:80–86

Williams RS, Johnston SA, Riedy M, DeVit MJ, McElligott SG, Sanford JC (1991) Introduction of foreign genes into tissues of living mice by DNA-coated microprojectiles. Proc Natl Acad Sci USA 88:2726–2730

Wu J, Chappelow J, Yang J, Weimann L (1998) Defects generated in human stratum corneum specimens by ultrasound. Ultrasound Med Biol 24:705–710

Yamashita N, Tachibana K, Ogawa K, Tsujita N, Tomita A (1997) Scanning electron microscopic evaluation of the skin surface after ultrasound exposure. Anat Rec 247:455–461

Yarosh D, Bucana C, Cox P, Alas L, Kibitel J, Kripke M (1994) Localization of liposomes containing a DNA repair enzyme in murine skin. J Invest Dermatol 103:461–468

Zhang L, Li LN, An ZL, Hofmann GA (1997). In vivo transdermal delivery of large molecules by pressure-mediated electroincorporation and electroporation: a novel method for drug and gene delivery. Bioelectrochem Bioeng 42:283–292

2   Stem Cells, Differentiation and Renewal Kinetics of Keratinocytes: Implications for Cutaneous Gene Therapy

J. R. Bickenbach

Basal Cell Kinetics Are Related to Tissue Structure in Stratified Squamous Epithelia

Stratified squamous epithelia such as the epidermis of the skin are continuously renewing tissues with structures that are maintained by division of cells in the proliferative basal layer to replace cells in the outer stratum corneum layer that are sloughed into the environment. This mechanism of balancing the rate of cell division with the rate of cell loss is essential for epithelial homeostasis and must be maintained for life (Potten 1981). However, the mechanisms for controlling the relationship between cell division and cell differentiation are not clear. Early work on cell proliferation in the basal layer of rat esophageal epithelia concluded that in normal homeostasis only the basal cells could divide, that all of the basal cells divided, and that they appeared to do so randomly (Leblond et al. 1964). Furthermore, migration from the basal layer into the differentiation compartment was a random event, probably related to squeezing out of cells as a result of population pressure from adjacent dividing cells. Subsequent work by Iverson (Iverson et al. 1968) studying mouse epidermis indicated that migration from the basal layer was restricted to the oldest cell in the G1 phase of the cell cycle that was in the vicinity of a cell undergoing mitosis. This finding suggested that the population of basal cells might contain post-mitotic differentiating cells which are committed to migration but which might require a period of preparation before that event occurs.

In the late sixties and early seventies, it was also shown that the suprabasal strata of the epidermis had a highly-ordered pattern of structure (Mackenzie 1969, Christophers 1971). The flattened cells of the spinous, granular and cornified layers were shown to be stacked and aligned to form a series of hexagonal units of structure, measuring 30–40 µm across. The normal formation of these cell columns appeared to be related to a low rate of cell proliferation. Typically, cell columns were not formed in epithelia with a naturally high, or experimentally or pathologically raised mitotic rate (Christophers 1971, Mackenzie 1975). About ten small basal cells lay beneath each columnar unit of structure and it was shown that basal cells in mitosis were located principally beneath the periphery of such units (Mackenzie 1975). A similar non-random position of S-phase cells was also suggested (Potten 1974). Initially, it was thought that mitotic activity in the ring of cells beneath the column periphery produced cells that moved centrally to migrate from the basal layer in alignment with the overlying cell stacks. However, Christophers (Christophers 1971) using fluorescein isothiocyanate as a differential stain for maturing cells showed that basal cell migration into the suprabasal strata occurred from the peripheral region. This finding led to the assumption that the central non-mitotically active basal cells were the epidermal stem cells (Potten and Hendry 1973), and it was proposed that the number of stem cells directly corresponded to the number of epidermal cell columns (Potten 1974). Today, it is accepted as fact that stratified squamous epithelia consist of a hierarchy of dividing basal cells maintained by a small subpopulation of stem cells (for reviews see Cairnie et al. 1976, Potten 1997, Potten and Lord 1983). However, the exact number and distribution of these stem cells is still debated.

Stem Cells in Stratified Squamous Epithelia

Basically, a stem cell is considered to be a cell that is self-maintaining and is also ultimately the source of all differentiating cells in the tissue. With this definition, all continuously replicating tissues clearly can be said to have stem cells, and it was in this sense that Leblond et al. (Leblond et al. 1964) considered all basal epithelial cells to be potential stem cells. Whether they in fact remained as stem cells depended on whether they were forced from the basal region by external pressure due to dividing cells. There is now strong evidence that a stem cell pattern of regeneration exists for several types of epithelia, and only a small fraction of the proliferative cells are stem cells (for review see Cairnie et al. 1976, Potten 1997, Potten and Lord 1983). Stem cells are thought to be undifferentiated cells that divide to produce two types of daughter cells: one that maintains the stem cell phenotype and one called a transient amplifying cell that undergoes a finite number of cell divisions before differentiating and leaving the proliferative compartment. Only the stem cells persist throughout the lifetime of the organism (Cairns 1975). In 1979 proposed a two-compartment proliferative model in which stem cells made up a very small percentage of the proliferative compartment and transient amplifying cells comprised the larger population with fast proliferative rates (Lajtha 1979). Thus, sustained fast proliferative rates would be avoided in stem cells, the cells responsible for self and tissue maintenance, and thereby the stem cells would be less likely to accumulate DNA mutations (Cairns 1975). Although stem cells are considered to progress through the cell cycle at a slower rate than transient amplifying basal cells, they have a higher proliferative potential, and it is thought that they proliferate at times of tissue regeneration, such as during fetal development and wound healing (for reviews see Cairnie et al. 1976, Potten 1997). In the first direct demonstration of heterogeneity in the epithelial basal cell compartment, a small population of label-retaining cells (LRCs) was identified in various mouse epithelia (Bickenbach 1981; Fig. 2.1). These epithelial LRCs retained a tritiated thymidine label for up to 240 days, indicating that the cells were very slowly cycling. LRCs were shown to have the stem characteristics of immaturity in that they were smaller and contained few organelles, that they were clonogenic, and that they were slowly cycling

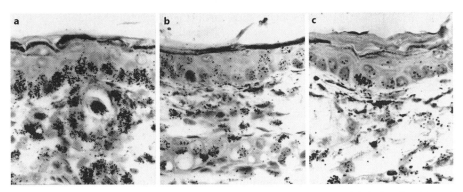

Fig. 2.1 a–c. Label-retaining cells in mouse ear epidermis. Mice were labeled with trititated thymidine on the tenth and eleventh days after birth. **a** One hour after labeling, 90% of basal keratinocytes in ear skin showed a heavy trititated thymidine label. **b** By 10 days the label was significantly diluted through cell division. **c** By 30 days most of the keratinocytes had only slight residual labeling. However, about 2% were still heavily labeled

(Bickenbach 1981). Using this tritiated thymidine label-retention method, many researchers have now identified and localized stem cells in a variety of epithelia from several species (Bickenbach 1981, Lavker and Sun 1982, Bickenbach and Mackenzie 1984, Bickenbach et al. 1987, Cotsarelis et al. 1989 and 1990, Morris et al. 1990). Although this method marks the putative stem cell population, it involves a long procedure and cannot be used to easily mark human epidermal stem cells. Antibodies against cell surface markers in conjunction with fluorescence activated cell sorting (FACS) have been used extensively to isolate functionally-distinct subpopulations of the immune and hematopoietic cell populations (Civin and Loken 1987, Spangrude et al. 1988, Bernstein et al. 1994, Orlic et al. 1994), but no specific cell surface antibodies for epidermal stem cells or for transient amplifying cells have been identified. Previously, it was proposed that epidermal stem cells expressed a higher level of $\beta 1$ integrin on their cell surface than did the transient amplifying cells (Jones and Sharpe 1994, Jones et al. 1995). The authors showed that the $\beta 1$-bright population represented approximately 40% of the total basal cells. However, as the authors point out, it had been predicted that less than ten percent of basal cells could be true stem cells (Potten and Morris 1988), thus this integrin-bright population was too large to contain only stem cells. Other reported stem cell markers, such as c-myc, either affected cells other than just stem cells (Gandarillas and Watt 1997) or were shown to be upregulated in the proliferatively active transient amplifying population and thus not a stem cell marker, such as telomerase (Bickenbach et al. 1998). Two groups have reported that by using a combination of markers they could enrich the epidermal stem cell population. The first study was based on a cell surface monoclonal antibody that differentially stained proliferative basal cells so that they could be sorted by FACS according to how brightly they were stained (Mackenzie et al. 1989). The second study used high expression of $\alpha 6$ integrin and low expression of a proliferation-associated cell surface marker and resulted in an epidermal population highly enriched for proliferative cells (Li et

Table 2.1. Mouse ear epidermis contains three distinct populations of basal cells

Cell type[a]	% of total basal cells[b]	% LRCs[b,c]
Stem	3.4±0.2	95.3±2.1
Transient amplifying	89.2±1.1	0.1±0.1
Other basal	7.4±0.9	0

[a] Mouse ear epidermal basal cells were dissociated, stained with Hoechst 33342 and propidium iodide, and sorted into three populations with an EPICS 753 flow cytometer
[b] Mean ± standard deviation for 6 experiments
[c] LRCs is % of each group that was BrdU label-retaining cells

al. 1998). Unfortunately, neither method yielded a pure population of stem cells. Rapid adhesion to collagen type IV also yielded a population of epidermal cells that showed very high proliferative capacity (Jones and Sharpe 1994, Jones et al. 1995, Bickenbach and Chism 1998). These methods resulted in an enriched population of epidermal stem cells, but again not a pure population. To overcome the lack of a stem cell marker, we modified a previously published method that resulted in a pure population of hematopoietic stem cells (Goodell et al. 1996). This modified sorting method resulted in a virtually pure population of label-retaining cells, the putative epidermal stem cell population (Dunnwald et al. 2000, in press). Based upon dye characteristics, adult mouse epidermal basal cells could be easily sorted into stem and transient amplifying cell populations (Table 2.1). Both types of cells expressed K14, a keratin marker of basal cells (Fuchs 1990) and did not express K1, a keratin upregulated when basal cells leave the proliferative pool and commit to differentiation (Chung et al. 1994). The stem cell fraction represented about 4% of the basal cell population and about 90% of the stem cells were in the G1 phase of the cell cycle, suggesting that stem cells are slowly-cycling, rather than non-cycling.

Stem Cells and the Consequences for Gene Therapy

One of the main problems with designing a gene therapy approach for a continuously renewing tissue, such as the epidermis, is that most of the cells transfected with target genes are eventually sloughed into the environment (Morgan et al. 1987, Vogt et al. 1994, Huber and Hohl 1995, Choate et al. 1996, Fenjives et al. 1996, Freiberg et al. 1997, Dellambra et al. 1998, Seitz et al. 1999). Since it is generally accepted that of all keratinocytes only the stem cells remain for the lifetime of the epidermis (Cairns 1975), it becomes important to target stem cells, especially when considering how to treat several of the genetically inherited skin diseases (for reviews see Korge and Krieg 1996, Blau and Khavari 1997). In a renewing tissue, such as the epidermis, cells are continuously sloughed into the environment and in human epidermis most of the cells are replaced every twenty days (Halprin 1972, Gelfant 1982). Any persistent genetic defect must be present in the stem cells with expression passed onto daughter cells at each cell division. Thus, any permanent genetic treatment must be directed toward the stem cell genome.

Fig. 2.2. Epidermal stem cells show long term expression of transduced retroviral LacZ. Epidermal stem cells preselected by rapid adhesion to collagen type IV were transduced with MFG-LacZ in submerged culture, grown on the dermal substrate AlloDerm™ in organotypic culture for 12 weeks, then stained with X-gal, which stains LacZ expressing cells blue

Although several studies have reported introduction of recombinant genes into continuously renewing epithelial tissues (Sanes 1989, Garlick et al. 1991) in most cases long term gene expression was not achieved (Morgan et al. 1987, Sanes 1989, Garlick et al. 1991, Vogt et al. 1994, Fenjives et al. 1996). It did not matter whether the gene transfer technique involved shooting the DNA directly into the tissue via a gene gun or transducing cultured epithelial cells and grafting the transduced cells to host animals. Loss of expression in these studies might be due to selective methylation of viral promoters, especially retroviral promoters (Fenjives et al. 1996). On the other hand, the real problem might be loss of the transfected cells due to differentiation (Kolodka et al. 1998), since in most of these studies stem cells were not transfected. To introduce genes into stem cells one must either achieve 100% transfection efficiency in a population of total basal cells (Choate et al. 1996, Dellambra et al. 1998) or separate the stem cells from the transient amplifying cells before transfection. The first method is most commonly used, but it appears to transfect very few stem cells. This may be because the most common transfection method uses retroviruses and integration of the DNA into a host genome occurs only if there is active cell division at the time of infection (Miller et al. 1990). In this case the slowly-cycling stem cells would be less likely to be transfected than the more rapidly cycling transient amplifying basal cells, the cells destined to differentiate. This argues for preselecting stem cells before attempting gene therapy. Previous work, exploiting various enrichment procedures, demonstrated that substantial enrichment of stem cells before transfection is possible (Bickenbach 1998). When human keratinocytes, enriched for stem cells by rapid adherence to collagen type IV, were transfected with a retroviral vector carrying the LacZ reporter gene, they showed persistent expression of the LacZ reporter gene throughout twelve weeks of growth in organotypic culture (Bickenbach and Roop 1999; Fig. 2.2). Furthermore, the enriched human stem cells recombined with AlloDerm®, an acellular dermal substrate, reformed a long lasting skin. More recently, a new sorting technique yielded pure populations of mouse epidermal stem and transient amplifying cells, which were transfected with a retroviral LacZ recombinant gene (Dunnwald et al. 2000). Both cell types were transfected with an efficiency of 15%, and both showed expression of the recombinant LacZ gene in culture. However, only the epidermis engineered from the stem cells showed long term expression in organotypic culture. The tissue engineered from the transient amplifying cells completely differentiated by two months. Thus, it seems likely that total loss of recombinant gene expression in a continuously renewing tissue, such as the epidermis, is due to the failure to transfect stem cells, indicating that any method that increases the percentage of stem cells in the population should increase the possibility of transfecting stem cells, thereby improving gene therapy approaches.

Acknowledgements. I would like to thank Ann Tomanek-Chalkley and Dana Alexandrunas of my laboratory for their excellent assistance, and Dr. Martine Dunnwald for her invaluable discussions; also the members of The University of Iowa Flow Cytometry Facility for their assistance in establishing the appropriate gates for sorting mouse epidermal stem cells and The University of Iowa Vector Core (NIH-NIDDK-P60-DK54759 and Carver Foundation) for supplying the retroviral LacZ for transduction. This work was supported by NIH-NIAMS-RO1-AR45259, NIH-NIDR-RO1-DE-13001, NIH-NIAMS-NO1-AR-62228 Subcontract, and by The University of Iowa Center for Gene Therapy NIH-NIDDK-P60-DK54759.

References

Bernstein ID, Andrews RG, Rowley S (1994) Isolation of human hematopoietic stem cells. Blood Cells 20:15–23

Bickenbach JR (1981) Identification of label-retaining cells in oral mucosa and skin. J Dent Res 122 C:1611–1620

Bickenbach JR (1998) Selection and growth of epidermal stem cells. In: Savage LM (ed) Bioengineering of Skin Substitutes, IBC Library Series, Southborough, MA, pp. 75–92

Bickenbach JR, Chism E (1998) Selection and extended growth of murine epidermal stem cells in culture. Exp Cell Res 244:184–915

Bickenbach JR, Holbrook KA (1987) Label-retaining cells (LRCs) in human embryonic and fetal epidermis. J Invest Dermatol 88:42–46

Bickenbach JR, Mackenzie IC (1984) Identification and localization of label-retaining cells in hamster epithelia. J Invest Dermatol 82:618–622

Bickenbach JR, Roop DR (1999) Transduction of a preselected population of human epidermal stem cells: consequences for gene therapy. Proc Assoc Amer Physicians 111:184–189

Bickenbach JR, Vormwald-Dogan V, Bachor C, Bleuel K, Schnapp G, Boukamp P (1998) Telomerase is not an epidermal stem cell marker and is downregulated by calcium. J Invest Dermatol 111:1045–1052

Blau H, Khavari P (1997) Gene therapy: progress, problems, prospects. Nat Med 3:612–613

Cairnie AB, Lala PK, Osmond DUG (1976) Stem Cells of Renewing Cell Populations. Academic Press, New York

Cairns J (1975) Mutation selection and the natural history of cancer. Nature 255:197–200

Choate KA, Khavari PA (1997) Sustainability of keratinocyte gene transfer and cell survival in vivo. Human Gene Therapy 8:895–901

Choate KA, Medalie DA, Morgan JR, Khavari PA (1996) Corrective gene transfer in the human skin disorder lamellar ichthyosis. Nat Med 2:1263–1267

Christophers E (1971) Cellular architecture of the stratum corneum. J Invest Dermatol 56:165–170

Chung SY, Cheng CK, Rothnagel JA, Yu SH, Nakazawa H, Mehrel T, Hohl D, Rosenthal DS, Steinert PM, Yuspa SH, Roop DR (1994) Expression of the human keratin gene (K1) in transgenic mice is tissue- and developmental-specific but altered with respect to differentiation state. Mol Cell Diff 2:61–81

Civin CI, Loken MR (1987) Cell surface antigens on human marrow cells: dissection of hematopoietic development using monoclonal antibodies and multiparameter flow cytometry. Internat J Cell Cloning 5:267–288

Cotsarelis G, Cheng S-Z, Dong G, Sun T-T, Lavker RM (1989) Existence of slowly-cycling limbal epithelial basal cells that can be preferentially stimulated to proliferate: implications on epithelial stem cells. Cell 57:201–209

Cotsarelis G, Sun T-T, Lavker RM (1990) Label-retaining cells reside in the bulge area of pilosebaceous unit: implications for follicular stem cells, hair cycle, and skin carcinogenesis. Cell 61:1329–1337

Dellambra E, Vailly J, Pellegrini G, Bondanza S, Golisano O, Macchis C, Zambruno G, Meneguzzi G, De Luca M (1998) Corrective transduction of human epidermal stem cells in laminin-5-dependent junctional epidermolysis bullosa. Hum Gene Ther 9:1359–1370

Dunnwald M, Tomanek-Chalkey A, Alexandrunas D, Fishbaugh J, Bickenbach JR (2000) Isolating a pure population of stem cells for use in tissue engineering. Exp Dermatol, in press

Fenjives ES, Yao S-N, Kurachi K, Taichman LB (1996) Loss of expression of a retrovirus-transduced gene in human keratinocytes. J Invest Dermatol 106:576–578

Freiberg RA, Choate KA, Deng H, Alperin ES, Shapiro LJ, Khavari PA (1997) A model of corrective gene transfer in X-linked ichthyosis. Hum Mol Genet 6:927–933

Fuchs E (1990) Epidermal differentiation: the bare essentials. J Cell Biol 111:2807–2814

Gandarillas A, Watt FM (1997) c-Myc promotes differentiation of human epidermal stem cells. Genes Dev 11:2869–2882

Garlick JA, Katz AB, Fenjives ES, Taichman LB (1991) Retrovirus-mediated transduction of cultured epidermal keratinocytes. J Invest Dermatol 97:824–829

Gelfant S (1982) "Of mice and men" the cell cycle in human epidermis in vivo. J Invest Dermatol 78:296–299

Goodell MA, Brose K, Paradis G, Conner AS, Mulligan RC (1996) Isolation and functional properties of murine hematopoietic stem cells that are replicating in vivo. J Exp Med 183:1797–1806

Halprin KM (1972) Epidermal turnover time – a re-examination. Brit J Dermatol 86:14–19

Huber M, Hohl D (1995) Mutations of keratinocyte transglutaminase in lamellar ichthyosis. Science 267:525–528

Iverson OH, Bjerknes R, Devik F (1968) Kinetics of cell renewal, cell migration, and cell loss in the hairless mouse dorsal epidermis. Cell Tiss Kinet 1:351–367

Jones KT, Sharpe GR (1994) Thapsigargin raises intracellular free calcium levels in human keratinocytes and inhibits the coordinated expression of differentiation markers. Exp Cell Res 210:71–76

Jones PH, Harper S, Watt FM (1995) Stem cell patterning and fate in human epidermis. Cell 80:83–93

Kolodka TM, Garlick JA, Taichman LB (1998) Evidence for keratinocyte stem cells in vitro: Long term engraftment and persistence of transgene expression from retrovirus-transduced keratinocytes. Proc Natl Acad Sci USA 95:4356–4361

Korge BP, Krieg T (1996) The molecular basis for inherited bullous diseases. J Mol Med 74:59–70

Lajtha G (1979) Stem cell concepts. Differentiation 14:23–34

Lavker RM, Sun TT (1982) Heterogeneity in epidermal basal keratinocytes: morphological and functional correlations. Science 215:1239–1241

Leblond CP, Greulich RC, Marques-Pereira JP (1964) Relationship of cell formation and cell migration in the renewal of stratified squamous epithelia. Adv Biol Skin 5:39–67

Li A, Simmons PJ, Kaur P (1998) Identification and isolation of candidate human keratinocyte stem cells based on cell surface phenotype. Proc Natl Acad Sci USA 95:3902–3907

Mackenzie IC (1969) Ordered structure of the stratum corneum of mammalian skin. Nature 222:881–882

Mackenzie IC (1975) Spatial distribution of mitosis in mouse epidermis. Anat Rec 181:705–710

Mackenzie IC, Mackenzie SL, Rittman GA (1989) Isolation of subpopulations of murine epidermal cells using monoclonal antibodies against differentiation-related cell surface molecules. Differentiation 41:127–138

Miller DG, Adam MA, Miller D (1990) Gene transfer by retrovirus vectors occurs only in cells that are actively replicating at the time of infection. Mol Cell Biol 10:4329–4342

Morgan JR, Barrandon Y, Green H, Mulligan RC (1987) Expression of an exogenous growth hormone gene by transplantable human epidermal cells. Science 237:1476–1479

Morris RJ, Fischer SM, Klein-Szanto AJP, Slaga TJ (1990) Subpopulations of primary adult murine epidermal basal cells sedimented on density gradients. Cell Tissue Kinet 23:587–602

Orlic D, Anderson D, Bodine DM (1994) Biological properties of subpopulations of pluripotent hematopoietic stem cells enriched by elutriation and flow cytometry. Blood Cells 20:107–117

Potten CS (1974) The epidermal proliferative unit: the possible role of the central basal cell. Cell Tissue Kinet 7:77–88

Potten CS (1981) Cell replacement in epidermis (keratopoiesis) via discrete units of proliferation. Int Rev Cytol 69:271–318

Potten CS (1997) Stem Cells. Academic Press, London

Potten CS, Hendry HH (1973) Clonogenic cells and stem cells in the epidermis. Int J Radiat Biol 24:537–540

Potten CS, Lord BI (1983) Stem Cells: Their Identification and Characterization. Churchill Livingstone, London, UK

Potten CS, Morris RJ (1988) Epithelial stem cells in vivo. J Cell Sci 10:45–62

Sanes JR (1989) Analyzing cell lineage with a recombinant retrovirus. Trends Neurosci 12:21–28

Seitz CS, Giudice GJ, Balding SD, Marinkovich MP, Khavari PA (1999) BP180 gene delivery in junctional epidermolysis bullosa. Gene Therapy 6:42–47

Spangrude GJ, Heinfeld S, Weissman IL (1988) Purification and characterization of mouse hematopoietic stem cells. Science 241:58–62

Vogt PM, Thompson S, Andree C, Liu P, Brewing K, Hatzis D, Brown H, Mulligan RC, Eriksson E (1994) Genetically modified keratinocytes transplanted to wounds reconstitute the epidermis. Proc Natl Acad Sci USA 91:9307–9311

3   Relevant Animal Models for Skin Gene Therapy

M. J. Arin, T. Cao, T. R. Berton, Z. Zhou, X. J. Wang, D. R. Roop

Introduction

In recent years, animal models for various human diseases have been established and have greatly enhanced our understanding of how genetic defects lead to clinical disease. The use of transgenic mouse technology enables us to assess the consequences of overexpressing a gene of interest, e.g. oncogenes and growth factors or introducing mutant genes into the mouse genome. On the other hand, gene knockout technology is widely used to functionally analyze genes that are expressed in specific tissues and to assess the consequences of deleting certain genes of interest in vivo. The use of tissue specific promoters has enabled us to target genes specifically to tissues of interest or perturb normal gene expression at specific sites, thus yielding important information about physiological and pathological processes. Several transgenic and knockout mouse models have been established for genetic skin diseases and, given the marked similarities between mouse and human skin, have provided insights into the function and regulation of components of the epidermis and dermis in vivo. In several cases, this led to the identification of the genetic basis of specific hereditary skin disorders. The development of mouse models that harbor the same mutations found in man will provide a useful tool in assessing gene therapy approaches. Given its accessibility and its ease of handling, the skin will be an important tissue for the application of this technology.

Inherited skin disorders, where the underlying gene defect has been identified, are optimal candidate diseases for gene therapy. In recessive disorders, where two mutant copies are required to elicit the mutant phenotype, the introduction of one normal allele into skin cells would mimic the heterozygous "carrier" state, and is expected to result in a corrected phenotype. However, the treatment of dominant diseases is technically more challenging since the mutant allele must either be corrected or its expression inhibited. Critical for permanent or long-term expression of the corrected cells is the requirement to target gene therapy approaches to the stem cell population in the basal compartment of the epidermis. Technical advances have been made in recent years to optimize and enhance the efficacy of gene transfer into keratinocytes, improve the methods for transplanting ex vivo modified cells back to the host organism and transduce mouse skin in vivo. In this chapter, we will review the status of existing transgenic mouse models for inherited skin diseases and describe strategies for generating new mouse models which mimic the human diseases at the genetic level.

Dominant Diseases

Epidermolysis Bullosa Simplex

Epidermolysis bullosa (EB) is a group of hereditary mechanobullous disorders with at least eleven distinct forms, seven of which are dominantly inherited. The epidermolysis bullosa simplex (EBS) subtype is characterized by intraepidermal blistering and the majority of cases are due to dominant keratin mutations. The estimated incidence for EBS is 10 per one million births in the US with a considerable perinatal mortality due to electrolyte imbalance, marked protein loss and sepsis (Marinkovich et al. 1999). The four most common EBS types, which are all inherited in a dominant fashion, include the generalized forms Koebner and Dowling-Meara, the localized form Weber–Cockayne and the Ogna variety that is found in Norwegian kindreds. The most severe form of EBS, epidermolysis bullosa herpetiformis or Dowling-Meara (EBS-DM) presents at birth with generalized blistering (Anton-Lamprecht and Schnyder 1982). Blisters occur characteristically in groups on the trunk and extremities, including palms and soles and usually heal without scarring. Development of hyperkeratoses starts later in childhood. Interfamiliar phenotypic variations are not uncommon and have also been described among members of the same family. Blistering occurs within the epidermis and is due to the lysis of basal keratinocytes which show clumps of the intermediate filament (IF) network upon ultrastructural examination. EBS was linked to the type I keratin gene cluster on chromosome 17 (Bonifas et al. 1991) and the type II keratin gene cluster on chromosome 12 (Ryynanen et al. 1991). Mutations have been identified in the basally expressed keratins K5 and K14, and are mostly found in the conserved parts of the rod domain (Corden and McLean 1996, Irvine and McLean 1999). Interestingly, the more severe forms of EBS are caused by point mutations located at the beginning and end of the rod domain, whereas milder forms have been associated with mutations in less conserved regions either within or outside the rod domain (Corden and McLean 1996). Approximately 70% of the reported mutations in the Dowling-Meara form occur at the same mutational "hot spot", codon 125, which encodes a higly conserved arginine at the beginning of the rod domain of K14.

Mouse Models for Epidermolysis Bullosa Simplex

Transgenic Mice for Epidermolysis Bullosa Simplex

To date, two transgenic mouse models have been developed for EBS. The first model was generated by introducing a dominant negative mutant form of K14 into the germline of mice by a standard approach of injecting this DNA into fertilized embryos, followed by transplantation into pseudopregnant recipients (Vassar et al. 1991). Although the phenotype exhibited by these transgenic mice provided the first evidence suggesting that EBS may be caused by mutations in the K14 gene, this model is not identical to the human disease. First, the dominant negative mutation created a truncated from of the K14 protein, missing all of the C-terminus and approximately 30% of the rod domain. Second, these mice contain both wild type alleles, therefore the mutant protein must compete with the wild type K14 protein produced from both alleles. Third, with this approach the transgene integrates at random sites, thus, due to effects of surrounding sequences, transgene expression levels vary as does phenotypic severity.

Epidermolysis Bullosa Simplex Knockout Mice

The second transgenic model of EBS was created by targeted disruption of the K14 gene in mouse embryonic stem (ES) cells, yielding a recessive or null phenotype (Lloyd et al. 1995). These mice exhibited a severe EBS phenotype, which is in contrast to the few cases of recessive (null) EBS in humans that have been reported to date (Chan et al. 1994, Rugg et al. 1994, Jonkman et al. 1996). Clinically, these patients were diagnosed as Koebner, a less severe form than Dowling-Meara. An additional consideration from the point of view of developing a gene therapy approach is the increased technical challenge of correcting a dominantly inherited disease vs. a recessive disease. Thus, given that EBS-DM patients have the dominant form of the disease that occurs as a result of single point mutations at codon 125 (Corden and McLean 1996), there is an obvious need to produce a transgenic model with exactly the same mutation.

Mice Mimicking Epidermolysis Bullosa Simplex at the Genetic Level

To date, no mouse model exists that mimics EBS at the genetic level. As a prerequisite for valid gene therapy approaches, the need exists for a mouse model that harbors the same point mutation found in the majority of EBS patients. We are currently introducing a single point mutation into the germline of mice at the same position that has been found to be a "hot spot" in humans (Fig. 3.1). Mouse K14 codon 131, which is equivalent to human position 125 coding for a highly conserved arginine residue at the beginning of the rod domain, is altered by exchanging one nucleotide. This changes the basic amino acid arginine to

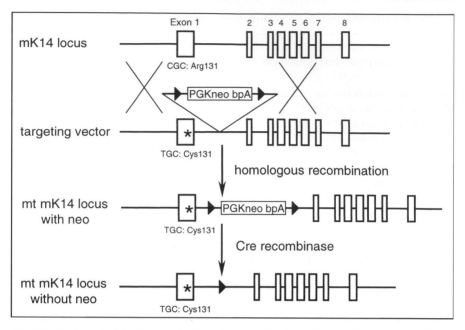

Fig. 3.1. Strategy to introduce a single point mutation into the germline of mice. Shown is the wild-type K14 locus, the targeting construct and the targeted locus after homologous recombination (mt mK14 locus). Note that only one loxP site along with the point mutation remains in the genome after Cre-mediated excision of the selection cassette. (*mK14*, mouse keratin 14; *PGKneobpA*, neomycin resistance gene; loxP sites are denoted by *arrows*)

cysteine, that carries a sulfhydryl group in its side chain. Using a knock-in/replacement strategy, the targeting construct is introduced into mouse ES cells, which serve to generate chimeric mice. Mice heterozygous for the point mutation will serve as a model for testing gene therapy approaches (see below).

Gene Therapy Approaches

EBS is a severe blistering disease due to dominant mutations in one of the basally expressed keratins K5 and K14. Interestingly, a mosaic form as seen in epidermolytic hyperkeratosis (EHK), due to postzygotic mutations, has never been described in EBS patients (Fuchs et al. 1994). This led to the hypothesis that, in the basal compartment, wild type stem cells must have a growth advantage over defective stem cells expressing a mutant keratin. Thus, a possible gene therapy approach would be to correct the point mutation in the defective stem cells through homologous recombination with the wild type gene ex vivo and graft the corrected stem cells back to the mouse from which the epidermal stem cells were originally obtained. Homologous recombination in primary keratinocytes occurs at a low frequency, however the enormous proliferative potential of stem cells should compensate for this potential drawback. The grafting could be done selectively in areas prone to blistering and it is anticipated that the corrected stem cells repopulate the area and dilute out the defective stem cells over time. Crucial at this step is the identification of stem cells and the selection of these cells versus transit amplifying cells that have limited growth potential and are thus not valuable for any long-lasting gene therapy approach. Progress has recently been made in this respect and several approaches have been proposed including selection of stem cells based on surface integrin patterns. We have been able to select for epidermal stem cells through rapid adhesion to collagen type IV, demonstrated the feasibility of genetically modifying a stem cell population and have observed long-term expression of a recombinant gene in organotypic culture (Bickenbach and Roop 1999).

Epidermolytic Hyperkeratosis

Epidermolytic hyperkeratosis (EHK; Bullous Congenital Ichthyosiform Erythroderma) is inherited in an autosomal dominant mode, the incidence is 1 in 200 000 to 300 000 newborns with up to 50% of the reported cases arising sporadically (Marinkovich et al. 1999). Affected children present at birth with erythroderma, blistering and peeling. Erythroderma and blistering diminish during the first year of life and hyperkeratoses develop, predominantly over the flexural areas of the extremities. The perinatal mortality and childhood morbidity is increased due to epidermal erosions and infections. The histopathological findings consist of hyperkeratosis and parakeratosis, lysis of the suprabasal keratinocytes and perinuclear vacuolar degeneration. The basal cell layer appears histologically normal, but exhibits hyperproliferation. The transit time for keratinocytes to move from the basal layer to the corneal layer is remarkably shortened in EHK and takes only about four days, instead of four weeks as in normal skin (Frost and Van Scott 1966).

Mutations have been identified in keratins K1 and K10 that cause clumping of keratin filaments in the cytoplasm of keratinocytes in the suprabasal layer of the epidermis. One particular arginine codon in exon 1 of the keratin 10 gene is most often affected in severe cases of EHK and seems to be a "hot spot" due to CpG methylation and deamination (Rothnagel et al. 1993). Interestingly, this is the same arginine residue that has been found to be mutated in K14 in the Dowling-Meara form of epidermolysis bullosa simplex (EBS-DM), the most severe form of EBS. An association between the localization of the mutation and the severity of the phenotype has been suggested, following the observation that mutations within the initiation and termination motifs of K1 and K10 lead to a more severe phenotype than mutations located within the rod domain. Clearly, mutations in the highly conserved regions of the rod domain are more disruptive to filament assembly and stability. However, to date clear genotype-phenotype correlations have not been established for the keratin diseases. Mosaic forms of the disease have been described, where individuals with sporadic, postzygotic mutations showed patchy or linear lesions of the skin. In case of germ-line involvement, these individuals can give rise to offspring with generalized EHK (Paller et al. 1994).

Mouse Models for Epidermolytic Hyperkeratosis

Transgenic Mice for Epidermolytic Hyperkeratosis

The generation of transgenic mice expressing a truncated hybrid K10/K14, that showed phenotypic features similar to the human disease EHK, was an early in-dication that the suprabasal keratins K1 and K10 were involved in this disease (Fuchs et al. 1992). By fusing the human K10 promoter and the amino-terminal non-helical domain of K10 to the previously used truncated, dominant-negative K14 construct, lacking 135 amino acids from the C-terminus (Vassar et al. 1991), transgenic animals were established that showed phenotypic and histo-logical features similar to those seen in the human disease. Generally, the pheno-type of the animals was more severe than usually seen in EHK patients and the variation between phenotypes was due to differences of the expression levels of the dominant-negative transgene.

To assess the consequences of K1 mutations on skin biology, a second mouse model was established when we introduced a dominant negative mutant form of human keratin 1 (HK1) into the germline of mice (Bickenbach et al. 1996). The transgene lacked 60 amino acids from the 2B segment of HK1. The phenotype resembled closely the human course of the disease with blistering and erythro-derma at birth and hyperkeratotic lesions developing later. Histological and ul-trastructural examination of neonatal mice homozygous for the mutation showed thickening of the epidermis and collapse of the IF network in suprabasal keratinocytes. The blisters diminished with hair growth suggesting a stabilizing role of the hair follicles. Adult mice showed predominantly thick hyperkeratoses resembling the clinical findings in adult EHK patients.

The third animal model was created by targeted disruption of K10 in mouse embryonic stem cells (Porter et al. 1996). By deleting exons 3–7 from the mouse keratin 10 gene, heterozygous mice were obtained that appeared normal at birth, but became hyperkeratotic with the onset of hair growth. It was only in the homozygous animals, that a severe blistering phenotype was observed at birth, and these animals died shortly thereafter. The deletion in the keratin 10 gene did not result in the complete ablation of the K10 protein, but created a trun-cated form of K10 that acted in a dominant negative fashion. Severe cytolysis was noted in the upper spinous and granular cells, which coincided with upregu-lation of K6/K16. The authors speculated that the poor IF forming properties of K6/K16 rather than or in addition to disruption of the K1/K10 network might be the underlying cause in EHK (Porter et al. 1996).

Mouse Model for EHK with the Same Point Mutation as Found in Humans

Since the majority of EHK patients have the dominant form of the disease that occurs as a result of single nucleotide mutations, it is desirable to generate a mouse model that mimics the human skin disorder at the genetic level. More than half of the reported mutations to date are located at codon 156 in exon 1 of the keratin 10 gene and these "hot spot" mutations have been associated with a severe phenotype. We are currently introducing the exact same nucleotide exchange (CGC-TGC) as identified in the majority of EHK patients into the germline of mice. By using ES cell technology, a targeting construct harboring the desired point mutation and a selection cassette are introduced into ES cells. Positive stem cell clones can be transiently transfected with an expression vector for CRE recombinase, which recognizes and excises sequences flanked by loxP sites and thus the selection cassette can be removed, leaving only the point mutation and one loxP site in the genome. These clones are injected into blastocysts and subsequently transplanted into pseudopregnant foster mice which will give birth to chimeric animals that consist of a mixture of cells derived from the blastocyst as well as from the manipulated ES cells. Heterozygous mice will be obtained by crossing chimeras to wild type mice of the same strain from which the blastocysts were obtained. Heterozygous mice, which carry the mutation on one allele will be used to test different gene therapy approaches (see below).

Gene Therapy Approaches

Unlike in EBS, EHK is caused by mutations in suprabasal keratins and the mutant allele is not expressed in the basal layer. Therefore, a correction of the mutation in basal cells would not be translated into a growth advantage of corrected stem cells over defective stem cells in the basal compartment. Consequently, any genetic modification of stem cells in EHK has to include a selection marker to specifically select modified stem cells, and allow ablation of defective stem cells. A possible selection marker is the multi-drug-resistance (MDR) gene. It has been used for selection of hemopoietic stem cells (Licht et al. 1997) and it has been shown that it can be efficiently introduced into keratinocytes (Pfutzner et al. 1999). Stem cells from the mouse model, heterozygous for the dominant K10 point mutation, will be isolated, corrected through homologous recombination and transduced by a retroviral vector containing the MDR resistance gene. Both procedures will be performed ex vivo. We will attempt to replace the mutant allele with a wild type allele through a classical replacement targeting strategy. Alternatively, we will determine whether chimeric DNA/RNA oligonucleotides can be used to efficiently correct the mutant K10 allele in epidermal stem cells (Cole-Strauss et al. 1996). If either approach is successful, the corrected and drug-resistant stem cells will be transplanted back to the mouse from which they were originally derived and the mouse will be treated topically with colchicine. The corrected stem cells would be expected to repopulate the epidermis while at the same time the defective stem cells would be ablated through the treatment with colchicine.

Another approach includes the use of ribozymes to inhibit the expression of the mutant K10 allele. Ribozymes have been shown to efficiently suppress the expression of targeted genes in transgenic mice with reduction of the target mRNA by 50–90% (L'Huillier et al. 1996, Lieber and Kay 1996, Lewin et al. 1998). One potential problem is the similarity between the mutant and the wild type K10 transcripts, which only differ by one nucleotide and are both likely to be degraded to a similar extent by the ribozyme. If this proves to be the case, it may be possible to modify a wild type K10 construct in such a way that it is resistant to ribozyme degradation (Millington-Ward et al. 1997). Thus, the ribozyme would inhibit expression of both the endogenous mutant and wild type alleles, but not interfere with expression of the modified wild type K10 construct. Introduction of appropriate selection cassettes and subsequent selection yields clones of epidermal stem cells that could be used for autologous transplantation to the same mouse from which the original stem cells were derived. Subsequent treatment with colchicine would yield a uniform population of wild type stem cells that would be expected to repopulate the epidermis.

Recessive Diseases

Lamellar Ichthyosis

The autosomal recessive congenital ichthyoses are a clinically heterogeneous group and comprise lamellar ichthyosis (LI) and congenital ichthyosiform erythroderma (CIE) (Williams and Elias 1985). The inheritance pattern is recessive, though some cases of dominant inheritance have been described (Traupe et al. 1984). LI presents at birth with erythema and a collodion-like membrane. Later in life large, thick brown scales develop that cover the entire body. Palmar and plantar hyperkeratoses are often present and eclabium and ectropium are complicating associated features, the latter being a cause of blindness. Histopathology shows acanthosis, hypergranulosis and hyperkeratosis of the epidermis.

Transglutaminases are calcium-dependent enzymes that catalyze ε-(γ-glutamyl)-lysine crosslinking of proteins in the process of cornified cell envelope (CE) formation in terminally differentiating keratinocytes (Greenberg et al. 1991). The keratinocyte specific transglutaminase 1 (TGase 1) is a membrane-bound isoform that catalyzes crosslinking of involucrin, loricrin, small proline-rich proteins and other components, to form a protein complex which builds the CE on the inner side of the plasma membrane (Ishida-Yamamoto et al. 1997). Moreover, it has been shown that membrane-bound TGase 1 is involved in the formation of the lipid envelope by attaching omega-hydroxyceramides to involucrin in the CE (Nemes et al. 1999). LI was linked to the transglutaminase gene locus on chromosome 14q11 (Polakowska et al. 1991) and mutations in the TGase 1 gene were identified in LI patients (Huber et al. 1995, Russell et al. 1995, Laiho et al. 1997, Hennies et al. 1998). A second type of LI was mapped to chromosome 2q33–q35 and was designated type 2 lamellar ichthyosis (Parmentier et al. 1996).

Mouse Models for Lamellar Ichthyosis

Mice deficient for TGase 1 were generated by targeted disruption of the TGase 1 gene in mouse ES cells (Matsuki et al. 1998). Homozygous knockout mice showed erythrodermic skin with severe disruption of the barrier function at birth and died a few hours thereafter. The phenotypic appearance with shiny, erythematous skin, covered by a translucent membrane was reminiscent of collodion babies with LI. Histologically, the stratum corneum was found to be defective as a result of lacking TGase 1 function. This model demonstrates the role of TGase 1 in development, maturation and integrity of the stratum corneum. However, the severe phenotype and high perinatal mortality do not make this model suitable for gene therapy approaches.

Dystrophic Epidermolysis Bullosa

The group of dystrophic forms of epidermolysis bullosa (DEB) encompasses disorders with the characteristic features of skin blistering and fragility of mucous membranes (Tidman and Eady 1985). The disease gene has been shown to be the gene for type VII collagen (COL7A1) on chromosome 3p21 (Uitto and Christiano 1992), in both autosomal dominant and recessive forms of DEB, and genotype-phenotype correlations have been implicated. According to these findings, most dominant forms are caused by missense mutations, whereas the recessive forms are the result of nonsense mutations, frame-shift and splice-site mutations, leading to truncation of the collagen VII protein (Jarvikallio et al. 1997). These truncation mutations have been identified either on both alleles in a homozygous state, or more frequently as a compound heterozygous state, and most of the truncated transcripts are degraded leading to a complete lack of a functional protein (Christiano et al. 1997). In the dominant forms, the anchoring fibrils are reduced in number and often structurally altered, whereas in the recessive forms, the fibrils are entirely absent (Bruckner-Tuderman 1999).

The most severe form of autosomal recessive dystrophic EB (RDEB), the Hallopeau-Siemens form, presents with generalized blisters at birth that heal by scar formation (Fine et al. 1991). The scarring can lead to hand and feet deformities and might even progress to flexion contracture of an entire extremity. Mucosa, scalp, nails and teeth are also involved in most cases. Patients with the Hallopeau-Siemens form have a high risk of developing squamous cell carcinomas in areas of scar formation. Ultrastructurally, cleavage occurs beneath the lamina densa and anchoring fibrils that attach the papillary dermis to the basement membrane are absent (Anton-Lamprecht and Schnyder 1979). Premature termination codon mutations on both alleles that lead to a complete lack of collagen

VII are the cause of the Hallopeau-Siemens form (Uitto and Christiano 1994, Hovnanian et al. 1997).

Mouse Models for Dystrophic Epidermolysis Bullosa

A severe congenital mechanobullous disorder with dermolytic blistering and recessive inheritance has been described in sheep (Bruckner-Tuderman et al. 1991). The affected animals exhibited blisters of skin, oral mucosa, tongue, and esophagus at birth, and ultrastructurally sublaminal blister formation was demonstrated. Complete absence of collagen type VII was noted in the skin of affected sheep. Based on genetic, clinical, ultrastructural, and immunohistochemical findings, the sheep disease was found to correspond to the severe mutilating subtype of RDEB in humans.

A xenograft model for RDEB was established by grafting human full-thickness DEB skin on the dorsum of severe combined immunodeficiency (SCID) mice (Kim et al. 1992). Blisters could be induced in these grafts with minor trauma and showed a sublamina densa separation and absence of collagen type VII.

Just recently, a mouse model for the recessive form of DEB has been generated through targeted disruption of exons 46–69 of the COL7A1 in mouse ES cells (Heinonen et al. 1999). The resultant protein lacked most of domain 1 of the collagen VII molecule. Heterozygous animals were phenotypically normal, whereas homozygous null mice exhibited extensive blistering at birth and died within the first two weeks. Electron microscopy revealed subepidermal blistering and absence of the anchoring fibrils. This model recapitulates the genetic, phenotypic and ultrastructural characteristics of the human disease, however, due to the early mortality and severe phenotype of the null mice, it is not a suitable model to test gene therapy approaches.

Development of an Inducible, Epidermal Specific Knockout System as a Model for Recessive Skin Diseases

The introduction of a somatic mutation in a given gene, in a specific tissue and at a given time is desirable when creating a mouse model for a human disease, especially when germline mutations are lethal during development or shortly after birth. To overcome these limitations, a conditional gene targeting strategy, which uses tissue-specific and inducible expression of the bacteriophage P1 Cre recombinase, has recently been developed (Gu et al. 1994, Barlow et al. 1997). Cre recombinase recognizes loxP (locus of crossover of bacteriophage P1) sites, which consist of two repetitive sequences of 13 bp each and a 8 bp center piece. In animal cells, it has been shown to efficiently excise a DNA segment that is flanked by two loxP sites in the same orientation (Sauer and Henderson 1989). Placing the Cre gene under a tissue specific promotor allows excision of the target DNA in a spatially controlled manner.

However, most keratin-based expression vectors, which direct transgene expression to epidermal stem cells, are also expressed in other epithelial tissues. Therefore, constitutive expression of Cre recombinase with these vectors may also induce embryonic lethality as a result of a deletion of the gene in other epithelial tissues. The combination of the tissue specificity with the temporal control of the expression of Cre would overcome this problem. This inducible, tissue specific knockout system utilizes tissue-specific and inducible expression of Cre recombinase, which is fused with a mutant form of the ligand binding domain of the human progesterone receptor (PR1) that binds progesterone antagonists but not progesterone. The fusion protein will be sequestered in the cytoplasm until a progesterone antagonist induces translocation of the fusion protein to the nucleus (Kellendonk et al. 1996). Two lines of mice are required in this system, each containing half of the knockout components: the tissue specific CrePR1 and the loxP flanked target gene. These two lines will then be crossed to generate bigenic mice containing both components. By applying a progesterone antagonist such as RU486 or its analogue ZK98.734 (ZK), an inducible tissue-specific knockout of the target gene will be achieved. Unlike other inducible reagents, RU486 does not have toxic effects even in long-term medical use up to 20 mg/kg in humans (Handerson 1987). To target Cre expression to the proliferative basal compartment of the epidermis, where keratinocyte stem cells are located, the Cre transgene is placed under the control of the K14 promotor (Fig. 3.2). Because epidermal stem cells renew this epithelium throughout the life of the organism, once RU486-induced excision occurs in an epidermal stem cell, a focal clone of cells that persist without the targeted gene for the remainder of the life of the mouse is expected. To confirm this, we performed the following experiments. K14.PR1 transgenic mice were crossed with a reporter construct strain in which a loxP flanked ("floxed") neomycin resistance minigene is located between the ROSA26 promotor and the bacterial lacZ gene. Upon RU486 mediated activation of the Cre recombinase in K14.CrePR1/ROSA26 bigenic mice (Vegeto et al. 1992), the neomycin resistance minigene is excised and the ROSA26 promotor drives the expression of the lacZ gene. The presence of β-galactosidase in the epidermis and hair follicles can be detected by a simple staining procedure using X-Gal as a substrate. Bigenic mice were treated with either RU486 or ethanol (vehicle alone) once a day for 5 days. A small area of the treated backskin was biopsied 24 hours after the last RU486 treatment and stained with X-Gal. The skin sections showed that the β-galactosidase expression was only seen in bigenic mouse skin treated with RU486 (Fig. 3.3), and was still focally detected in the epidermis and in hair follicles four months after the last application of RU486. This test system shows the feasibility of inducing a focal knockout of a target gene in stem cells of the epidermis and hair follicles in

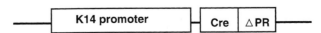

Fig. 3.2. Structure of the transgene under the control of the K14 promotor containing Cre recombinase fused to a mutant form of the ligand binding domain of the human progesterone receptor (PR1)

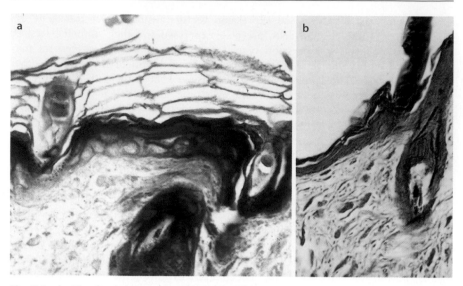

Fig. 3.3 a, b. The β-gal expression in K14.CrePR1/ROSA26 bigenic skin after RU486 treatment. **a** The β-gal activity (*blue*) in RU486-treated bigenic skin is detected in the epidermis and hair follicles. This same X-Gal staining pattern was also seen four months after the last RU486 application (data not shown). **b** Absence of β-gal activity in bigenic mice treated with the vehicle only

vivo, and should allow the development of viable mouse models of recessive skin disorders such as LI and RDEB.

Gene Therapy Approaches for Recessive Diseases

In contrast to dominant skin diseases, where one mutant allele is sufficient to cause the disease phenotype, recessive diseases are caused by two mutant alleles. Like in LI, where patients lack TGase 1 activity or dystrophic EB with loss of normal collagen type VII, one approach would be to introduce the wild type gene into keratinocytes. Several vectors for gene delivery have been developed, including adenovirus, adenovirus-associated, retroviral and lentiviral vectors. However, the time-dependent loss of virally delivered, promotor-driven transgene expression constitutes a major challenge in therapeutic cutaneous gene delivery (Hoeben et al. 1991, Taichman 1998). This is most likely due to either a failure of the viral vectors to integrate into the host cell genome or a failure to transduce stem cells. Retroviral vectors are very efficient regarding gene transfer and integration and are therefore the most frequently used vectors. Retroviral vectors require replicating cells for transduction (Miller et al. 1990), which is a potential problem regarding the slow-cycling stem cell population and consequently with respect to long-term expression. However, proliferation of stem cells has been achieved in response to wounding (Ghazizadeh et al. 1999) and transduction with retroviral vectors under these conditions resulted in long-term expression in vivo (see below). Alternative non-viral approaches for direct delivery of DNA to the skin are extremely inefficient and short-lived (Hengge et al. 1995).

A human skin/immunodeficient mouse xenograft model was used to correct TGase 1 deficiency in keratinocytes of LI patients in an ex vivo approach (Choate et al. 1996). The full-length TGase 1 cDNA was introduced into TGase 1 deficient keratinocytes by retroviral delivery in vitro and corrected keratinocytes were used to regenerate human epidermis on immunodeficient mice. Grafting of corrected keratinocytes, that exhibited restoration of normal TGase1 function, resulted in normalization of epidermal architecture and barrier function and was indistinguishable from normal epidermis. However, the effect was short-lived, suggesting that stem cells had not been successfully transduced.

One drawback of grafting ex vivo modified keratinocytes is that it requires full thickness excision at the graft site which may result in scarring. An in vivo approach with direct gene transfer to epidermal keratinocytes may overcome this limitation. Several methods of direct gene transfer to the epidermis have been tested such as intradermal injection of purified DNA or topical application of liposomes containing the gene to be delivered, however none of these methods showed sustained gene expression (Alexander and Akhurst 1995, Hengge et al. 1995, Vogel et al. 1996). Long-term transduction of mouse keratinocytes by a retroviral vector has been achieved in vivo just recently and resulted in sustained gene expression in the mouse epidermis (Ghazizadeh et al. 1999). Targeting of stem cells was achieved by dermabrasion to remove interfollicular epidermis and allow re-epithelialization from proliferating stem cells located in the hair follicles. A retroviral vector, carrying a lacZ reporter gene was injected directly into the epidermis, in the plane between the scab and the re-epithelializing surface. Transduction of hyperplastic epidermis resulted in stable gene transfer to keratinocytes of follicular and interfollicular epidermis. β-galactosidase expression was observed throughout the epidermis and lasted up to 16 weeks after transduction. However, long-term expression was only observed in immunodeficient mice. The loss of transgene expression in immunocompetent mice was attributed to immunological responses against the transgene products. This raises the question of whether an immune response will also occur when wild type proteins are expressed in keratinocytes of patients with recessive skin disorders.

Acknowledgements. This work was supported in part by grants from the National Institutes of Health [CA 52607, HD 25479, and AR 62228 (to DRR)]. MJA was partially supported by a fellowship from the Deutsche Forschungsgemeinschaft (Ar 291/1–1).

References

Alexander MY, Akhurst RJ (1995) Liposome-mediated gene transfer and expression via the skin. Hum Mol Genet 4:2279–2285

Anton-Lamprecht I, Schnyder UW (1979) Ultrastructure of epidermolyses with junctional blister formation. Dermatologica 159:377–382

Anton-Lamprecht I, Schnyder UW (1982) Epidermolysis bullosa herpetiformis Dowling-Meara. Report of a case and pathomorphogenesis. Dermatologica 164:221–235

Barlow C, Schroeder M, Lekstrom-Himes J, Kylefjord H, Deng CX, Wynshaw-Boris A, Spiegelman BM, Xanthopoulos KG (1997) Targeted expression of Cre recombinase to adipose tissue of transgenic mice directs adipose-specific excision of loxP-flanked gene segments. Nucleic Acids Res 25:2543–2545

Bickenbach JR, Roop DR (1999) Transduction of a preselected population of human epidermal stem cells: consequences for gene therapy. Proc Assoc Am Physicians 111:184–189

Bickenbach JR, Longley MA, Bundman DS, Dominey AM, Bowden PE, Rothnagel JA, Roop DR (1996) A transgenic mouse model that recapitulates the clinical features of both neonatal and adult forms of the skin disease epidermolytic hyperkeratosis. Differentiation 61:129–139

Bonifas JM, Rothman AL, Epstein EHJ (1991) Epidermolysis bullosa simplex: evidence in two families for keratin gene abnormalities. Science 254:1202–1205

Bruckner-Tuderman L (1999) Hereditary skin diseases of anchoring fibrils. J Dermatol Sci 20:122–133

Bruckner-Tuderman L, Guscetti F, Ehrensperger F (1991) Animal model for dermolytic mechanobullous disease: sheep with recessive dystrophic epidermolysis bullosa lack collagen VII. J Invest Dermatol 96:452–458

Chan Y, Anton-Lamprecht I, Yu QC, Jackel A, Zabel B, Ernst JP, Fuchs E (1994) A human keratin 14 "knockout": the absence of K14 leads to severe epidermolysis bullosa simplex and a function for an intermediate filament protein. Genes Dev 8:2574–2587

Choate KA, Medalie DA, Morgan JR, Khavari PA (1996) Corrective gene transfer in the human skin disorder lamellar ichthyosis. Nat Med 2:1263–1267

Christiano AM, Amano S, Eichenfield LF, Burgeson RE, Uitto J (1997) Premature termination codon mutations in the type VII collagen gene in recessive dystrophic epidermolysis bullosa result in nonsense-mediated mRNA decay and absence of functional protein. J Invest Dermatol 109:390–394

Cole-Strauss A, Yoon K, Xiang Y, Byrne BC, Rice MC, Gryn J, Holloman WK, Kmiec EB (1996) Correction of the mutation responsible for sickle cell anemia by an RNA-DNA oligonucleotide. Science 273:1386–1389

Corden LD, McLean WH (1996) Human keratin diseases: hereditary fragility of specific epithelial tissues. Exp Dermatol 5:297–307

Fine JD, Johnson LB, Wright JT (1991) Inherited blistering diseases of the skin. Pediatrician 18:175–187

Frost P, Van Scott EJ (1966) Ichthyosiform dermatoses. Classification based on anatomic and biometric observations. Arch Dermatol 94:113–126

Fuchs E, Esteves RA, Coulombe PA (1992) Transgenic mice expressing a mutant keratin 10 gene reveal the likely genetic basis for epidermolytic hyperkeratosis. Proc Natl Acad Sci USA 89:6906–6910

Fuchs E, Chan Y, Paller A, Yu Q (1994) Cracks in the foundation: keratin filaments and genetic disease. Trends Cell Biol 4:321–326

Ghazizadeh S, Harrington R, Taichman L (1999) In vivo transduction of mouse epidermis with recombinant retroviral vectors: implications for cutaneous gene therapy. Gene Ther 6:1267–1275

Greenberg CS, Birckbichler PJ, Rice RH (1991) Transglutaminases: multifunctional cross-linking enzymes that stabilize tissues. FASEB J 5:3071–3077

Gu H, Marth JD, Orban PC, Mossmann H, Rajewsky K (1994) Deletion of a DNA polymerase beta gene segment in T cells using cell type-specific gene targeting. Science 265:103–106

Handerson D (1987) Pharmacology and clinical uses of inhibitors of hormone secretion and action. Furr F, Wakeling A (eds), Bailliere Tindall, London, pp. 184–210

Heinonen S, Mannikko M, Klement JF, Whitaker-Menezes D, Murphy GF, Uitto J (1999) Targeted inactivation of the type VII collagen gene (Col7a1) in mice results in severe blistering phenotype: a model for recessive dystrophic epidermolysis bullosa. J Cell Sci 112:3641–3648

Hengge UR, Chan EF, Foster RA, Walker PS, Vogel JC (1995) Cytokine gene expression in epidermis with biological effects following injection of naked DNA. Nat Genet 10:161–166

Hennies HC, Kuster W, Wiebe V, Krebsova A, Reis A (1998) Genotype/phenotype correlation in autosomal recessive lamellar ichthyosis. Am J Hum Genet 62:1052–1061

Hoeben RC, Migchielsen AA, van der Jagt RC, van Ormondt H, van der Eb AJ (1991) Inactivation of the Moloney murine leukemia virus long terminal repeat in murine fibroblast cell lines is associated with methylation and dependent on its chromosomal position. J Virol 65:904–912

Hovnanian A, Rochat A, Bodemer C, Petit E, Rivers CA, Prost C, Fraitag S, Christiano AM, Uitto J, Lathrop M, Barrandon Y, de Prost Y (1997) Characterization of 18 new mutations in COL7A1 in recessive dystrophic epidermolysis bullosa provides evidence for distinct molecular mechanisms underlying defective anchoring fibril formation. Am J Hum Genet 61:599–610

Huber M, Rettler I, Bernasconi K, Frenk E, Lavrijsen SP, Ponec M, Bon A, Lautenschlager S, Schorderet DF, Hohl D (1995) Mutations of keratinocyte transglutaminase in lamellar ichthyosis. Science 267:525–528

Irvine AD, McLean WH (1999) Human keratin diseases: the increasing spectrum of disease and subtlety of the phenotype-genotype correlation. Br J Dermatol 140:815–828

Ishida-Yamamoto A, Kartasova T, Matsuo S, Kuroki T, Iizuka H (1997) Involucrin and SPRR are synthesized sequentially in differentiating cultured epidermal cells. J Invest Dermatol 108:12–16

Jarvikallio A, Pulkkinen L, Uitto J (1997) Molecular basis of dystrophic epidermolysis bullosa: mutations in the type VII collagen gene (COL7A1). Hum Mutat 10:338–347

Jonkman MF, Heeres K, Pas HH, van Luyn MJ, Elema JD, Corden LD, Smith FJ, McLean WH, Ramaekers FC, Scheffer H (1996) Effects of keratin 14 ablation on the clinical and cellular phenotype in a kindred with recessive epidermolysis bullosa simplex. J Invest Dermatol 107:764–769

Kellendonk C, Tronche F, Monaghan AP, Angrand PO, Stewart F, Schutz G (1996) Regulation of Cre recombinase activity by the synthetic steroid RU 486. Nucleic Acids Res 24:1404–1411

Kim YH, Woodley DT, Wynn KC, Giomi W, Bauer EA (1992) Recessive dystrophic epidermolysis bullosa phenotype is preserved in xenografts using SCID mice: development of an experimental in vivo model. J Invest Dermatol 98:191–197

L'Huillier PJ, Soulier S, Stinnakre MG, Lepourry L, Davis SR, Mercier JC, Vilotte JL (1996) Efficient and specific ribozyme-mediated reduction of bovine alpha-lactalbumin expression in double transgenic mice. Proc Natl Acad Sci USA 93:6698–6703

Laiho E, Ignatius J, Mikkola H, Yee VC, Teller DC, Niemi KM, Saarialho-Kere U, Kere J, Palotie A (1997) Transglutaminase 1 mutations in autosomal recessive congenital ichthyosis: private and recurrent mutations in an isolated population. Am J Hum Genet 61:529–538

Lewin AS, Drenser KA, Hauswirth WW, Nishikawa S, Yasumura D, Flannery JG, LaVail MM (1998) Ribozyme rescue of photoreceptor cells in a transgenic rat model of autosomal dominant retinitis pigmentosa. Nat Med 4:967–971

Licht T, Herrmann F, Gottesman MM, Pastan I (1997) In vivo drug-selectable genes: a new concept in gene therapy. Stem Cells 15:104–111

Lieber A, Kay MA (1996) Adenovirus-mediated expression of ribozymes in mice. J Virol 70:3153–3158

Lloyd C, Yu QC, Cheng J, Turksen K, Degenstein L, Hutton E, Fuchs E (1995) The basal keratin network of stratified squamous epithelia: defining K15 function in the absence of K14. J Cell Biol 129:1329–1344

Marinkovich MP, Herron GS, Khavari PA, Bauer EA (1999) Hereditary epidermolysis bullosa. In: Dermatology in General Medicine. Friedberg EM, Eisen AZ, Wolff K, Austen KF, Goldsmith LA, Katz SI, Fitzpatrick TB (eds) McGraw-Hill, New York, pp 690–702

Matsuki M, Yamashita F, Ishida-Yamamoto A, Yamada K, Kinoshita C, Fushiki S, Ueda E, Morishima Y, Tabata K, Yasuno H, Hashida M, Iizuka H, Ikawa M, Okabe M, Kondoh G, Kinoshita T, Takeda J, Yamanishi K (1998) Defective stratum corneum and early neonatal death in mice lacking the gene for transglutaminase 1 (keratinocyte transglutaminase). Proc Natl Acad Sci USA 95:1044–1049

Miller DG, Adam MA, Miller AD (1990) Gene transfer by retrovirus vectors occurs only in cells that are actively replicating at the time of infection. Mol Cell Biol 10:4239–4242

Millington-Ward S, O'Neill B, Tuohy G, Al-Jandal N, Kiang AS, Kenna PF, Palfi A, Hayden P, Mansergh F, Kennan A, Humphries P, Farrar GJ (1997) Stratagems in vitro for gene therapies directed to dominant mutations. Hum Mol Genet 6:1415–1426

Nemes Z, Marekov LN, Fesus L, Steinert PM (1999) A novel function for transglutaminase 1: attachment of long-chain omega- hydroxyceramides to involucrin by ester bond formation. Proc Natl Acad Sci USA 96:8402–8407

Paller AS, Syder AJ, Chan YM, Yu QC, Hutton E, Tadini G, Fuchs E (1994) Genetic and clinical mosaicism in a type of epidermal nevus. N Engl J Med 331:1408–1415

Parmentier L, Lakhdar H, Blanchet-Bardon C, Marchand S, Dubertret L, Weissenbach J (1996) Mapping of a second locus for lamellar ichthyosis to chromosome 2q33–35. Hum Mol Genet 5:555–559

Pfutzner W, Hengge UR, Joari MA, Foster RA, Vogel JC (1999) Selection of keratinocytes transduced with the multidrug resistance gene in an in vitro skin model presents a strategy for enhancing gene expression in vivo. Hum Gene Ther 10:2811–2821

Polakowska RR, Eddy RL, Shows TB, Goldsmith LA (1991) Epidermal type I transglutaminase (TGM1) is assigned to human chromosome 14. Cytogenet Cell Genet 56:105–107

Porter RM, Leitgeb S, Melton DW, Swensson O, Eady RA, Magin TM (1996) Gene targeting at the mouse cytokeratin 10 locus: severe skin fragility and changes of cytokeratin expression in the epidermis. J Cell Biol 132:925–936

Rothnagel JA, Fisher MP, Axtell SM, Pittelkow MR, Anton-Lamprecht I, Huber M, Hohl D, Roop DR (1993) A mutational hot spot in keratin 10 (KRT 10) in patients with epidermolytic hyperkeratosis. Hum Mol Genet 2:2147–2150

Rugg EL, McLean WH, Lane EB, Pitera R, McMillan JR, Dopping-Hepenstal PJ, Navsaria HA, Leigh IM, Eady RA (1994) A functional "knockout" of human keratin 14. Genes Dev 8:2563–2573

Russell LJ, Digiovanna JJ, Rogers GR, Steinert PM, Hashem N, Compton JG, Bale SJ (1995) Mutations in the gene for transglutaminase 1 in autosomal recessive lamellar ichthyosis. Nat Genet 9:279–283

Ryynanen M, Knowlton RG, Uitto J (1991) Mapping of epidermolysis bullosa simplex mutation to chromosome 12. Am J Hum Genet 49:978–984

Sauer B, Henderson N (1989) Cre-stimulated recombination at loxP-containing DNA sequences placed into the mammalian genome. Nucleic Acids Res 17:147–161

Taichman LB (1998) Gene therapy. Periodontal Clin Investig 20:7–9

Tidman MJ, Eady RA (1985) Evaluation of anchoring fibrils and other components of the dermal-epidermal junction in dystrophic epidermolysis bullosa by a quantitative ultrastructural technique. J Invest Dermatol 84:374–377

Traupe H, Kolde G, Happle R (1984) Autosomal dominant lamellar ichthyosis: a new skin disorder. Clin Genet 26:457–461

Uitto J, Christiano AM (1992) Molecular genetics of the cutaneous basement membrane zone. Perspectives on epidermolysis bullosa and other blistering skin diseases. J Clin Invest 90:687–692

Uitto J, Christiano AM (1994) Molecular basis for the dystrophic forms of epidermolysis bullosa: mutations in the type VII collagen gene. Arch Dermatol Res 287:16–22

Vassar R, Coulombe PA, Degenstein L, Albers K, Fuchs E (1991) Mutant keratin expression in transgenic mice causes marked abnormalities resembling a human genetic skin disease. Cell 64:365–380

Vegeto E, Allan GF, Schrader WT, Tsai MJ, McDonnell DP, O'Malley BW (1992) The mechanism of RU486 antagonism is dependent on the conformation of the carboxy-terminal tail of the human progesterone receptor. Cell 69:703–713

Vogel JC, Walker PS, Hengge UR (1996) Gene therapy for skin diseases. Adv Dermatol 11:383–398

Williams ML, Elias PM (1985) Heterogeneity in autosomal recessive ichthyosis. Clinical and biochemical differentiation of lamellar ichthyosis and nonbullous congenital ichthyosiform erythroderma. Arch Dermatol 121:477–488

4   Nonviral Gene Transfer into the Skin

B. Volc-Platzer, U. R. Hengge, A. Udvardi

Introduction

Corrective gene therapy requires efficient devices for the delivery of genes and gene sequences into target cells. In addition to viral systems which may represent the gene delivery system(s) of choice for one or another specific indication in the near future, there is a considerable need for alternative systems that can be easily produced and applied, similar to low-molecular substances or proteins. But there is still an urgent need to improve the low gene transfer rates that have not been overcome so far with nonviral gene transfer systems. For in vivo application plasmid DNA has to fulfill several requirements that allow transcription in the nucleus and its translation in the cytoplasm. Some of these requirements are common for both viral and nonviral gene delivery systems, such as binding to the cell surface, penetration of the cell (by fusion and/or by endocytosis), release from the endosome(s), transfer to the nuclear membrane, penetration of the nucleus, expression of the encoded gene of interest via the cell's specific transcription mechanisms.

Methods of nonviral nucleic acid delivery to the skin are based on the epicutaneous and intracutaneous application of plasmid DNA. Nucleic acid(s) may be applied as

- Naked DNA (Chen and Okayama 1987, Wolff et al. 1990, Hengge et al. 1995)
- By physical methods such as
  - Microinjection for targeting of single cells (Cappecchi 1980)
  - Electroporation (Neumann et al. 1982)
  - Particle bombardment (Sanford 1988)
- By (bio)chemical techniques such as
  - The classical nucleic acid precipitation (Graham and van der Eb 1973)
  - Complexing of DNA with lipids (DNA/lipid complexes=lipoplexes; Felgner et al. 1987 and 1997)
  - Complexing of DNA with polycationic polymers (polyplexes; Boussif et al. 1995, Felgner et al. 1997)
  - Complexing of DNA with peptide ligands for receptor-mediated endocytosis (Wagner et al. 1990 and 1994), with additional coupling to adenovirus for further enhancement of transfection efficiency (Curiel 1994).

Nonviral gene delivery systems, in particular naked DNA and biochemical vector systems may be applied to the epidermis by leaving the skin barrier intact, e.g. by epicutaneous application, as well as by penetrating the cutaneous barrier, i.e. by intracutaneous and subcutaneous injection.

Naked Plasmid DNA

The direct injection of DNA dissolved in saline was initially tested in muscle tissue (Wolff et al. 1990, Acsadi et al. 1991, Jiao et al. 1992). Direct injection of the dystrophin gene in animal models of Duchenne's muscle dystrophy, however, did not lead to sufficient and sustained gene expression so that the disease could be cured or, at least, ameliorated for a prolonged time (Acsadi et al. 1991, Danko et al. 1994).

Naked plasmid DNA was introduced into the skin by direct injection (Hengge et al. 1995, Ciernik et al. 1996, Eriksson et al. 1998). Injection of plasmids encoding the beta-galactosidase (β-Gal) reporter gene under the control of the cytomegalovirus (CMV) promoter into the superficial dermis of pig skin led to the visible expression of the encoded protein mainly in the *Stratum spinosum* or middle layer of the epidermis overlying the injection site. Unexpectedly, very little reporter gene expression was seen in the injected connective tissue (Hengge et al. 1995). The expression of the reporter gene could be demonstrated for three days, whereas the protein was visualized for up to three weeks (Hengge et al. 1995). When naked DNA was topically applied to mouse skin under certain conditions (Yu et al. 1999), the reporter gene activity was comparable with that produced by intradermal injection.

Whereas it has been convincingly shown that keratinocytes and other cellular constituents of the skin are capable of taking up DNA, the possible mechanism(s) of uptake of foreign DNA is (are) still unclear. It may well be that DNA is not actively taken up by the target cells but is rather passively transferred together with other molecules.

Injection of naked DNA as well as epicutaneous application resulted in an at least transient expression of the encoded protein(s), comparable to what has been described for muscle tissue (Wolff et al. 1990). However, naked plasmid DNA encoding for reporter genes or cytokines (Hengge et al. 1995) is not integrated in the host genome and is not stably maintained extrachromosomally. Therefore, expression of exogeneous DNA in the skin is not as long lasting as in muscle tissue (Wolff et al. 1992), and this technique of nonviral gene delivery to the skin may be useful if transient expression is required.

The i.m. injection of genes encoding various viral antigens, provoked cellular and humoral immune responses in various animal models (Ulmer et al. 1993, Wang et al. 1993). Injecting DNA directly into the skin has yielded an effective immune response (Raz et al. 1994) which is comparable to the protective immune responses generated by genetic immunization through other routes (Tang et al. 1992, Fynan et al. 1993). Whether genetic immunization of the skin results in T helper 2 (Th$_2$) or Th$_1$ immune responses or whether CD8 positive cytotoxic T cells are being induced, appears to be a question of the technique (injection of naked DNA versus bombardement of DNA-coated microprojectiles), the amount of DNA used, and the site of immunization (Barry and Johnston 1997).

Physical Gene Transfer – Microinjection of Naked DNA, Electroporation, Gene Gun

Microinjection is the injection of genes and oligonucleotides directly into the nucleus. Occasionally, there occurs an integration of the foreign genetic sequence into the host genome (Cappecchi 1980). This technique is useful for functional in vitro experiments in single cells or cell lines and to generate transgenic animals but it will probably never gain importance as a widely used technique in gene therapy.

Electroporation or electrotransfection are commonly used laboratory techniques (Neumann et al. 1982). Electroporation is based on the formation of transient hydrophilic pores in the cell membrane induced by an electric field. The efficiency of gene transfer is dependent on the number of generated pores.

Any mammalian cell can be transfected by electroporation (Potter 1988), but the technical requirements have to be established for each cell type (Sukharev et al. 1992). More recently, skin-depth targeting has been achieved by varying electrical fields and subsequent pressure from caliper-type electrodes on topically applied naked DNA encoding the *lacZ* gene (Zhang et a 1996).

Particle bombardment or ballistic gene transfer is based on the use of small particles, usually gold particles, which are coated with DNA and transferred via a gene gun. Initially, this technology was developed for gene transfer into plants and plant cells. The high velocity of the microparticles may be achieved by high voltage (McCabe et al. 1988, Sanford 1988) or high pressure via helium gas (Williams et al. 1991, Fitzpatrick-McElligott 1992).

Numerous cells can be transfected by particle bombardment, including primary cells such as monocytes, lymphocytes and fibroblasts as well as cultured cells (Burkholder et al. 1993). Successful in vivo ballistic gene transfer could be demonstrated in various animals, e.g. mice, rats, hamsters, rhesus monkeys (Yang 1992, Cheng et al. 1993). Expression of the transgene is usually limited, lasting from a few days only up to 4 weeks (Udvardi et al. 1999). According to the technical circumstances, the areas beneath the bombarded surface can be reached via the gene gun. Therefore, efficient expression of the transfected gene can be achieved only in and near the surface of a transfected tissue. However, depending on the indication and/or the purpose of the gene transfer the depth reached in the targeted tissue(s) may well be sufficient, e.g. for enhancement of wound healing (Eming et al. 1999).

The gene gun is an additional technique supplementing the armamentarium for genetic immunization (DNA vaccination). Particle bombardment of various target tissues that led to antigen expression was used for vaccination in animal models (Tang et al. 1992, Eisenbraun et al. 1993, Fynan et al. 1993, Robinson et al. 1993, Wang et al. 1993). Particle bombardement of the skin results in substantial expression of encoded antigens in the epidermal layer and, moreover, in detectable expression in dendritic cells derived from the skin in draining lymph nodes (Condon et al. 1996). Although it has been initially described that gene gun administration favors Th_2 cell/B cell responses (Fynan et al. 1993, Pertmer et al. 1996, Feltquate et al. 1997) further possibilities have only recently been explored. It has been shown that cutaneous gene gun immunization induces considerable augmentation of gene expression by dendritic cells in the draining lymph node thus enhancing antigen presentation and priming of antigen-specific cytotoxic T lymphocytes (Porgador et al. 1998). Finally, modifications of the vaccination schedule, coprecipitation of a GM-CSF encoding plasmid and coinjection of immunostimulatory CpG motifs together with plasmids encoding immunodominant listerial antigens resulted in DNA vaccination against listeriosis (Fensterle et al. 1999).

Other devices for injecting foreign DNA into the skin and keratinocytes, respectively, include air propulsion systems ("jet injectors") commonly used for delivering corticosteroids or local anesthetic solutions (Sawamura et al. 1999) and systems for microseeding of cells or tattooing (Eriksson et al. 1998).

(Bio)Chemical Gene Transfer (Precipitation, Lipofection, Polyfection, Receptor-Mediated Endocytosis)

Precipitation of Nucleic Acid(s)

The precipitation of nucleic acids is the oldest method to transfer nucleic acid(s) into eukaryotic cells (Graham and van der Eb 1973). This method was developed to test the infectivity of purified adenovirus DNA. In the following years, the original transfection protocol that was based on the coprecipitation of DNA and $CaPO_4$ (Chen and Okayama 1987) has been repeatedly modified, e.g with the polycation DEAE-dextran (McCutchan and Pagano 1968, Holter et al. 1989, Ishikawa and Homey 1992) or with other cations such as polylysine and polybrene (Kawai and Nishizawa 1984).

Subsequent to the uptake by endocytosis, a large amount of the ingested DNA is split into small fragments of 100 bp within endosomal compartments. Thereafter, DNA fragments are transported into the lysosomes. The majority of transfected DNA is lysed, and only a small fraction is further transported to the nucleus. It is possible that the transfer to the nucleus is mediated via a vesicular transport mechanism that may result in the fusion with the nuclear membrane (Orrantia and Chang 1990). Only about 5% of endocytosed nucleic acid-$CaPO_4$-complexes reach the nucleus. The optimal transfection efficiency of 50% transfected cells can only be reached in cell lines whereas primary cells are generally resistant to $CaPO_4$ coprecipitation. Successful transduction is dependent on the cell type and size of the preformed complexes. Since nucleic acids transfected by

$CaPO_4$ coprecipitation usually do not integrate in the host genome, the transfection is only transient. In principal, this method is used for in vitro gene transfer but not for systemic or local gene therapy. Recently, $CaPO_4$ coprecipitation has gained attention for optimizing adenoviral gene delivery into the airway epithelium (Walters and Welsh 1999). However, $CaPO_4$ – mediated transfection is not applicable to primary human keratinocytes, since high concentrations of Ca^{2+} ions trigger terminal differentiation.

Lipofection

Lipid molecules have a polar and a non-polar portion, and each molecule contains two hydrophobic chains. In aqueous solutions lipids form a double layer (lamellae, bilayers) of about 4 nm in thickness. The hydrophilic parts of the lamellae point to the aqueous phase whereas the hydrophobic portions point inwards. For thermodynamic reasons, the lipid molecules form spherical conformations, i.e. liposomes. Liposomes may consist of one bilayer only, i.e. unilamellar liposomes, or may consist of several layers, i.e. multilamellar liposomes. The size of the various liposomes varies between 20 nm and 100 μm. The most useful and efficient liposomes for the transport of therapeutic substances (that have been tested for medical purposes) are multilamellar and between 80 and 200 nm in size (Felgner et al. 1996). Liposomes which are bigger than 5 μm are usually unstable, and may lead to obstruction of small capillaries.

According to their charge, two groups of liposomes are used for the transfer of nucleic acids, i.e. cationic liposomes which are positively charged, and anionic liposomes which are negatively charged and pH-sensitive. Cationic liposomes form complexes with the negatively charged DNA because of the electrostatic interaction. The DNA is not found in the lumen of the liposomes, but the lipids form particle-like complexes via condensation of the DNA. Numerous nucleic acid molecules participate in the formation of DNA/lipid complexes. When anionic liposomes are used, the DNA is "trapped" in their aqueous interior. The membrane of this second type of liposomes is pH-sensitive, i.e. the liposomes are destabilized at low pH.

The first and probably best known cationic lipid which has been used for gene transfer is DOTMA (Felgner et al. 1987, Felgner and Ringold 1989). A neutral phospholipid, e.g. DOPE, is added to form the DNA/DOTMA complex in order to stabilize the complex and to facilitate the transfer through the cytosol. During the past few years several other cationic lipids have also been used as transfer systems, i.e. DMRIE (Felgner et al. 1996), DOTAP (McLachlan et al. 1994), and DC-CHOL (Gao and Huang 1991) are among the best known and most widely used cationic lipids. Combinations of various cationic lipids with different co-lipids (e.g. monooleoglycerids or cholesterol) display variable transfer efficiencies in different cell types. Optimal mixtures and formulations are still largely empirical, and a systematic approach has not yet been established. Moreover, the mechanism of internalization of cationic lipids is not fully understood. According to their positive charge, they bind strongly and efficiently to the surface of cells. A possible mechanism is the fusion of the liposome membrane and the plasma membrane (Felgner et al. 1987). The main mechanism of uptake, however, appears to be via endocytosis. The release of the DNA from the endosomes is primarily based on the low pH in the endosome (pH 5,0–6,5). In addition, the endosomal membrane is destabilized by the co-lipid, resulting in enhanced release of the nucleic acid. All these processes have to be completed before entering the lysosomes where the subsequent degradation of the transferred nucleic acid occurs. pH-sensitive, anionic lipids are more rapidly released than cationic lipids (but this seems to be their only advantage over cationic lipids; Legendre and Szoka 1992). To improve the endosomal lysis process several techniques have been developed. Adenoviral capsids were included that are known to have an endosomolytic activity, in particular the penton protein (Blumenthal et al. 1986, Seth 1994).

It has been reported that pH-sensitive lipids were also successfully used for DNA transfer (Wang and Huang 1987 and 1989). These liposomes consisted of DOPE and palmitoylhomocystein, free fatty acids or diacylsuccinylglycerol. However, according to the negative charge of these types of liposomes, they contained only small amounts of DNA and were less efficient than cationic lipids. Newly developed pH-sensitive cationic lipids combine the advantages of more efficient endosomolysis with a more efficient DNA loading. The results of gene transfer were superior to those achieved with DOTMA (Budker et al. 1996).

Gene expression due to lipid-mediated gene transfer persists for several days up to one month. Transferred plasmid DNA persists episomally in the nucleus with subsequent stepwise elimination of the DNA. To maintain the plasmid DNA in the episomal form in the nucleus, genetic sequences are introduced into the plasmid which function as origin of replication in eukaryotic cells. However, the isolation of these genomic sequences of eukaryotic cells has not been established so far, except for a few sequences of eukaryotic viruses (HSV, EBV, papovaviruses). Prolongation of gene expression could be achieved for up to three months by using plasmids that contained the replication origin of the human BK virus (papovavirus) following intravenous delivery in a liposome formulation. Expression of the transfected gene was detected in the lungs, liver, spleen, heart, and gut (Thierry et al. 1995).

Various types of liposomes have been used for gene delivery to murine skin. Recent studies have reported promising results with cationic liposomes for topical transfection with reporter gene expression in the dermis, epidermis and hair follicles (Alexander and Akhurst 1995, Yu et al. 1999). Another group of lipids exists which comprises lipopolyamines, that do not require co-lipids and are therefore applicable for DNA transfer (Behr et al. 1989). A synthetic lipopolyamine such as DPPES (dipalmitoyl phosphatidylethanolamine spermine) has been shown simple to prepare, non-toxic, and this transfection mixture resulted in a 20–30% transfection efficiency of primary human keratinocytes (Staedel et al. 1994). Another possibility to transfect cultured primary human keratinocytes is the poly-L-mediated gene transfer (Nead and McCance 1995). The transfection efficiency with the latter method has been reported to approach 20% cells.

However, it appears that non-cationic liposomes are favoured by some investigators over certain cationic complexes because they appear to inhibit the efficiency of cutaneous gene transfer. DNA complexed to cationic lipids may be sequestered in the lamellar bodies of the epidermis, and – thus trapped – may not be further available for gene expression (Menon et al. 1992). Moreover, optimal gene expression in the skin may be limited by toxic effects of cationic liposomes, which seems to be a dose-dependent phenomenon (Hofland et al. 1996).

Li and Hoffman (1995) and Niemiec et al. (1997) have used non-cationic complexes to target hair follicle epithelium and to express the delivered gene. Expression of the transgene was limited to areas of skin treated with non-cationic liposomes, and significant levels of the encoded protein were detectable for at least 5 days (Niemiec et al. 1997). Recently, liposome-mediated (DMRIE/DOPE) gene transfer has resulted in sustained production of interferon alpha, and the expression correlated with induced regression of human basal cell carcinoma (Hottiger et al. 1999).

Another interesting application of cutaneous gene delivery is the ex vivo transfection of primary keratinocytes and the subsequent transplantation onto the stroma of the host. Two models, in which gene transfer into keratinocytes has been achieved with cationic liposomes, have provided evidence that the transfected and transplanted keratinocytes express the foreign functional gene, albeit for a short period only (Jensen et al. 1994). More recently, the use of epidermal specific promoters has allowed the expression of a stably transfected gene encoding VEGF (vascular endothelial growth factor) at high levels in grafted pig epidermis for more than 4 weeks (Del Rio et al. 1999).

Although synthetic delivery systems have been somewhat behind viral vectors, the importance of nonviral gene transfer is increasingly being recognized. Whereas cationic liposome-based delivery systems are being evaluated in phase II and phase III clinical trials for the treatment of human cancer (Nabel et al. 1993) and cystic fibrosis, the cationic polymer-based systems have been associated with the generation of receptor-mediated gene delivery systems.

Polyfection and Receptor-Mediated Targeting/ Receptor-Mediated Endocytosis

To improve the efficiency of DNA uptake into target cells, the DNA can be attached to a domain capable of binding to a cell surface receptor. Receptor-mediated gene delivery constructs consist of a receptor-binding ligand conjugated to a DNA-binding moiety, usually high molecular weight poly-L-lysine. These constructs are capable of delivering DNA molecules to cells expressing the appropriate receptor. The molecular constructs complex with the plasmid DNA through electrostatic interactions between positively charged lysine residues and negatively charged phosphate backbones of the nucleic acids. They can form highly condensed structures that allow internalization and protection of the packaged DNA from nucleases. After uptake into endosomes DNA/complexes are still contained within a membrane vesicle.

Many different ligands including transferrin (Wagner et al. 1991), and asialo-glycoprotein (Chowdhury et al. 1993) beside several others have been employed for targeting. Histone and nonhistone proteins have been used as DNA-binding elements (Böttger et al. 1988, Yin and Cheng 1994). One of the great advantages of these receptor-targeting delivery systems using plasmid DNA is the lack of size restrictions of the coding insert.

To overcome the initial disadvantage of low transfection efficiency that occurred due to the rapid transport of nucleic acid into the lysosomes with its subsequent degradation, inactivated adenoviral capsids have been added to the artificial particles for ligand-mediated transfection (Cotten et al. 1993). For this purpose, the DNA has been complexed on the surface of adenovirus capsids via covalent binding with polylysine or biotinylation of the virus surface and binding of the DNA via streptavidin (Cristiano et al. 1993, Curiel 1994, Fisher and Wilson 1994). It is still not clear which domains of the penton protein are responsible for endosomolysis. The hemeagglutinin protein of the influenza virus has a comparable activity in the endosome but does not improve the transfer efficiency as well as the adenovirus particles (Wagner et al. 1992a). Another possibility to enhance the transfer efficiency is the addition of weak basic compounds such as chloroquine or colchicine (Cotten et al. 1990), because both substances improve the release of nucleic acids from the endosome. However, according to their toxic side effects it does not appear realistic to use these drugs for in vivo gene transfer.

The transferrinfection or AVET (adenovirus-enhanced transferrinfection) can be used to introduce a multiplicity of DNA plasmid copies per cell into both quiescent and dividing cells from primary cell cultures (Wagner et al. 1992b). Recently, its application has been documented in an uncontrolled, open label, multicenter phase I melanoma vaccine trial (Schreiber et al. 1999) with autologous tumor cells. The same system is currently being used in another comparable melanoma vaccine trial with allogeneic interleukin 2 – transfected cancer cells (A. Schneeberger, personal communication).

However, transferrinfection augmented by adenovirus has not yet been widely investigated for in vivo transfer into the skin. Preliminary data from our own observations in the hairless mouse model did not yield a high transfection efficiency upon intracutaneous or epicutaneous application (Udvardi et al. 1999).

One of the most intriguing options for the future appears to be the use of integrin-binding peptides in the receptor-targeted delivery systems (Hart et al. 1995, Harbottle et al. 1998), which may allow a tissue- or site-specific application of this nonviral gene delivery system without affecting other organs.

Outlook and Future Directions

As the transfer of genes is not trivial, different and specific steps have to be mastered in order to make it efficient. Genetic treatments have to be safe and should not remain on the high technical level of an experimental treatment but rather allow the application by a specialized medical doctor in a particular field of medicine. The ideal genetic treatment would be based on:

- Stability of the formulation in the different compartments and microenvironments of the body, e.g. in the circulation after i.v. application

- No or only low immunogenicity in order to avoid sensitization and allow repeated treatments of the recipient
- Cell- or organ-specific adhesion due to cell-specific receptor binding
- Rapid and unimpaired release from the endosome or circumvention of the endosome
- Highly efficient transfer into the nucleus = "nuclear targeting" or "nuclear localization"
- Modulation of the expression of the transferred genes, e.g. via cell-specific promoters
- Persistence of the transferred genes within the nucleus
- Targeted integration in the host genome

At present, the techniques of nonviral gene transfer are constantly being refined. However, the application of techniques such as the microinjection will probably remain restricted to research. Other techniques which target more cells or an entire organ will be applicable for therapeutic gene transfer as well. Precipitation techniques and even more electroporation may be the preferred techniques for ex vivo gene transfer. Particle bombardment and application of vaccination devices for transfer of plasmid DNA may be used for ex vivo as well as for in vivo applications. Clinical studies, however, are currently performed with lipoplexes, polyplexes or oligoplexes ("prospective genetic drugs"), to explore the alternatives to viral vector systems. Beyond the increasing possibilities to enhance the specificity and the transfection efficiency, biosafety considerations and safety precautions are less problematic in non-viral gene transfer.

Acknowledgement: This work was supported in part by grants from the Austrian Ministry of Education, Science and Cultural Affairs.

References

Acsadi G, Dickson GD, Love DR, Walsh FS, Gurusinghe A, Wolff JA, Davies KE (1991) Human dystrophin expression in mdx mice after intramuscular injection of DNA constructs. Nature 352:815–818

Alexander MY, Akhurst RJ (1995) Liposome-mediated gene transfer and expression via the skin. Hum Mol Genet 4:2279–2285

Barry MA, Johnston SA (1997) Biological features of genetic immunization. Vaccine 15:788–791

Behr JP, Demeneix B, Loeffler JP, Perez-Mutul J (1989) Efficient gene transfer into mammalian primary endocrine cells with lipopolyamine-coated DNA. Proc Natl Acad Sci USA 86:6982–6989

Blumenthal R, Seth P, Willingham MC, Pastan I (1986) pH-dependent lysis of liposomes by adenovirus. Biochemistry 25:2231–2237

Böttger M, Vogel F, Platzer M, Kiessling U, Grade K, Strauss M (1988) Condensation of vector DNA by the chromosomal protein HMG 1 results in efficient transfection. Biophys Acta 950:221–228

Boussif O, Lezoualch F, Zanta MA, Mergny MD, Scherman D, Demeneix B, Behr JP (1995) A versatile vector for gene and oligonucleotide transfer into cells in culture and in vivo: polyethylenimine. Proc Natl Acad Sci USA 92:7297–7301

Budker V, Gurevich V, Hagstrom JE, Bortzov F, Wolff JA (1996) pH sensitive, cationic liposomes: a new synthetic virus-like vector. Nat Biotechnol 14:760–764

Burkholder JK, Decker J, Yang NS (1993) Transgene expression in lymphocyte and macrophage primary cultures after particle bombardment. J Immunol Methods 165:149–156

Cappecchi MR (1980) High efficiency transformation by direct microinjection of DNA into cultured mammalian cells. Cell 22:479–488

Chen C and Okayama H (1987) High-efficiency transformation of mammalian cells by plasmid DNA. Mol Cell Biol 7:2745–2752

Cheng L, Ziegelhoffer PR, Yang NS (1993) A novel approach for studying in vivo transgene activity in mammalian systems. Proc Natl Acad Sci USA 90:4455–4459

Chowdhury NR, Wu CH, Wu GY, Yerneni PC, Bommineni VR, Chowdhury JR (1993) Fate of DNA targeted to the liver by asialoglycoprotein receptor mediated endocytosis in vivo. Prolonged persistence in cytoplasmic vesicles after partial hepatectomy. J Biol Chem 268:11 265–11 271

Ciernik IF, Krayenbühl BH, Carbone DP (1996) Puncture-mediated gene transfer to the skin. Hum Gene Ther 7:893–899

Condon C, Watkins SC, Celluzzi CM, Thompson K, Falo LD Jr (1996) DNA-based immunization by in vivo transfection of dendritic cells. Nat Med 2:1122–1128

Cotten M, Langle-Rouault F, Kirlappos H, Wagner E, Mechtler K, Zenke M, Beug H, Birnstiel ML (1990) Transferrin-polycation-mediated introduction of DNA into human leukemic cells: stimulation by agents that affect the survival of transfected DNA or modulate transferrin receptor levels. Proc Natl Acad Sci USA 87:4033–4037

Cotten M, Wagner E, Zatloukal K, Birnstiel ML (1993) Chicken adenovirus (CELO-virus) particles augment receptor mediated DNA delivery to mammalian cells and yield exceptional levels of stable transformants. J Virol 67:3777–3785

Cristiano JR, Smith LC, Kay MA, Brinkley BR, Woo S (1993) Hepatic gene therapy: efficient gene delivery and expression in primary hepatocytes utilizing a conjugated adenovirus-DNA complex. Proc Natl Acad Sci USA 90:11 548–11 552

Curiel DT (1994) High-efficiency gene transfer employing adenovirus-polylysine-DNA complexes. Nat Immun 13:141–164

Danko I, Fritz JD, Latendresse JS, Herweiler H, Schultz E, Wolff JA (1994) Dystrophin expression improves myofiber survival in mdx muscle following intramuscular plasmid DNA expression. Hum Mol Genet 2:2055–2061

Del Rio M, Larcher F, Meana A, Segovia JC, Alvarez A, Jorcano JL (1999) Nonviral transfer of genes to pig primary keratinocytes. Induction of angiogenesis by composite grafts of modified keratinocytes overexpressing VEGF driven by a keratin promoter. Gene Ther 6:1734–1741

Eisenbraun MD, Fuller DH, Haynes JR (1993) Examination of parameters affecting the elicitation of humoral immune response by particle bombardment-mediated genetic immunization. DNA Cell Biol 12:791–797

Eming SA, Whitsitt JS, He L, Krieg T, Morgan JR, Davidson JM (1999) Particle-mediated gene transfer of PDGF isoforms promotes wound repair. J Invest Dermatol 112:297–302

Eriksson E, Yao F, Svensjö T, Winkler T, Slama J, Macklin MD, Andree C, McGregor M, Hinshaw V, Swain W (1998) In vivo gene transfer to skin and wound by microseeding. J Surg Res 78:85–91

Felgner JH, Ringold GM (1989) Cationic liposome-mediated transfection. Nature 337:387–388

Felgner JH, Gadek TR, Holm M, Roman R, Chan HW, Wenz M, Northrop JP, Ringold GM, Danielsen M (1987) Lipofection: a highly efficient, lipid-mediated DNA-transfection procedure. Proc Natl Acad Sci USA 84:7413–7417

Felgner JH, Kumar R, Sridhar CN, Wheeler CJ, Tsai YJ, Border R, Ramsey P, Martin M, Felgner PL (1996) Enhanced gene delivery and mechanism studies with a novel series of cationic lipid formulations. J Biol Chem 269:2550–2561

Felgner PL, Barenholz Y, Behr JP, Cheng SH, Cullis PR, Huang L, Jessee J, Seymour LW, Szoka FC, Thierry AR, Wagner E, Wu G (1997) Nomenclature for synthetic gene delivery systems. Hum Gene Ther 8:511–512

Feltquate DM, Heaney S, Webster RG, Robinson HL (1997) Different T helper cell types and antibody isotypes generated by saline and gene gun DNA immunization. J Immunol 158:2278–2284

Fensterle J, Grode L, Hess J, Kaufmann SHE (1999) Effective DNA vaccination against listeriosis by prime/boost inoculation with the gene gun. J Immunol 163:4510–4518

Fisher KJ, Wilson JM (1994) Biochemical and functional analysis of an adenovirus based ligand complex for gene transfer. Biochem J 299:49–58

Fitzpatrick-McElligott S (1992) Gene transfer to tumor infiltrating lymphocytes and other mammalian somatic cells by microprojectile bombardement. Biotechnology 10:1036–1046

Fynan EF, Webster RG, Fuller DH, Haynes JR, Santoro JC (1993) DNA vaccines: protective immunizations by parenteral, mucosal, and gene-gun inoculations. Proc Natl Acad Sci USA 90:11 478–11 482

Gao XA, Huang L (1991) A novel cationic liposome reagent for efficient transfection of mammalian cells. Biochem Biophys Res Commun 179:280–285

Graham FL, van der Eb AJ (1973) A new technique for the assay of infectivity of human adenovirus 5 DNA. Virology 52:456–467

Harbottle RP, Cooper RG, Hart SL, Fadhoff A, McKay T, Knight AM, Wagner E, Miller AD, Cuoteille C (1998) An RGD-oligolysine peptide: a prototype construct for integrin-mediated gene delivery. Hum Gene Ther 9:1037–1047

Hart SL, Harbottle RP, Cooper R, Miller A, Williamson R, Coutelle C (1995) Gene delivery and expression mediated by an integrin-binding peptide. Gene Ther 2:552–554

Hengge UR, Chan EF, Foster RA, Walker PS, Vogel JC (1995) Cytokine gene expression in epidermis with biological effects following injection of naked DNA. Nat Genet 10:161–166

Hofland HEJ, Shephard L, Sullivan SM (1996) Formation of stable cationic lipid/DNA complexes for gene transfer. Proc Natl Acad Sci USA 93:7305–7309

Holter W, Fordis CM, Howard BH (1989) Efficient gene transfer by sequential treatment of mammalian cells with DEAE-dextran and deoxyribonucleic acid. Exp Cell Res 184:546–551

Hottiger MO, Dam TN, Nickoloff BJ, Johnson TM, Nabel GJ (1999) Liposome-mediated gene transfer into human basal cell carcinoma. Gene Ther 6:1929–1935

Ishikawa Y, Homcy CJ (1992) High efficiency gene transfer into mammalian cells by a double transfection protocol. Nucleic Acids Res 20:4367

Jiao S, Williams P, Berg RK, Hodgeman BA, Liu L, Repetto G, Wolff JA (1992) Direct gene transfer into non-human primate myofibers in vivo. Hum Gene Ther 3:21–33

Jensen UB, Jensen TG, Jensen PKA, Rygaard J, Hansen BS, Fogh J, Kolvraa S, Bolund L (1994) Gene transfer into cultured human epidermis and its transplantation onto immunodeficient mice: an experimental model for somatic gene therapy. J Invest Dermatol 103:391–394

Kawai S, Nishizawa M (1984) New procedure for DNA transfection with polycation and dimethyl sulfoxide. Mol Cell Biol 4:1172–1174

Legendre JY, Szoka FC (1992) Delivery of plasmid DNA into mammalian cell lines using pH-sensitive liposomes: comparison with cationic liposomes. Pharm Res 9:1235–1242

Li L, Hoffmann RM (1995) The feasibility of targeted selective gene therapy of the hair follicle. Nat Med 1:705–706

McCabe D, Swain W, Martinell P, Christou B (1988) Stable transformation of soy bean (glycine max) by particle acceleration. Biotechnology 6:923–926

McCutchan JH, Pagano JS (1968) Enhancement of the infectivity of Simian virus 40 desoxyribonucleic acid with diethyl-amino-ethyl-dextran. J Natl Cancer Inst 41:351–356

McLachlan G, Davidson H, Davison D, Dickinson P, Dorin J, Porteous D (1994) DOTAP as a vehicle for efficient gene delivery in vitro and in vivo. Biochemia 11:19–21

Menon GK, Ghadially R, Williams ML, Elias PM (1992) Lamellar bodies as delivery systems of hydrolytic enzymes: implications for normal and abnormal desquamation. Br J Dermatol 126:337 345

Nabel GJ, Nabel GE, Yang ZY, Fox BA, Plautz GE, Gao X, Huang L, Shu S, Gordon D, Chang AE (1993) Direct gene transfer with DNA-liposome complexes in melanoma:

expression, biologic activity and lack of toxicity in humans. Proc Natl Acad Sci USA 90:11 307–11 311

Nead MA, McCance DJ (1995) Poly-L-ornithine-mediated transfection of human keratinocytes. J Invest Dermatol 105:668–671

Neumann E, Schafer-Rider M, Wang Y, Hofschneider PH (1982) Gene transfer to mouse melanoma cells by electroporation in high electric fields. EMBO J 1:841–845

Nimiec SM, Latta JM, Ramachandran C, Weiner ND, Roessler BJ (1997) Perifollicular transgenic expression of human interleukin-1 receptor antagonist protein following topical application of novel liposome-plasmid DNA formulations in vivo. J Pharmaceut Sci 86:701–708

Orrantia E, Chang PL (1990) Intracellular distribution of DNA internalized through calcium phosphate precipitation. Exp Cell Res 190:170–174

Pertmer TM, Roberts TR, Haynes JR (1996) Influenza virus nucleoprotein-specific immunoglobulin G subclass and cytokine responses elicited by DNA vaccination are dependent on the route of vector DNA delivery. J Virol 70:6119–6125

Porgador A, Irvine KR, Iwasaki A, Barber BH, Restifo NP, Germain RN (1998) Predominant role for directly transfected dendritic cells in antigen presentation to CD8+ T cells after gene gun immunization. J Exp Med 188:1075–1082

Potter H (1988) Electroporation in biology: methods, applications and instrumentations. Anal Biochem 174:361–373

Raz E, Carlson DA, Parker SE, Parr TB, Abai AM, Aichinger G, Baird AM, Rhodes GH (1994) Intradermal gene immunization: the possible role of DNA uptake in the induction of cellular immunity to viruses. Proc Natl Acad Sci USA 91:9519–9523

Robinson HL, Hunt LA, Webster RG (1993) Protection against a lethal influenza virus challenge by immunization with a hemagglutinin-expressing plasmid DNA. Vaccine 11:957–960

Sanford J (1988) The biolistic process. Trends Biotechnol 6:299–302

Sawamura D, Ina S, Itai K, Meng X, Kon A, Tamai K, Hanada K, Hashimoto I (1999) In vivo gene introduction into keratinocytes using jet injection. Gene Ther 6:1785–1787

Schreiber S, Kämpgen E, Wagner E, Pirkhammer D, Trcka J, Korschan H, Lindemann A, Dorffner R, Kittler H, Kasteliz F, Kupcu Z, Sinski A, Zatloukal K, Buschle M, Schmidt W, Birnstiel M, Kempe RE, Voigt T, Weber HA, Pehamberger H, Mertelsmann R, Bröcker EB, Wolff K, Stingl G (1999) Immunotherapy of metastatic malignant melanoma by a vaccine consisting of autologous interleukin 2-transfected cancer cells: outcome of a phase I study. Hum Gene Ther 10:983–993

Seth P (1994) Adenovirus-dependent release of choline from plasma membrane vesicles at an acidic pH is mediated by the penton base protein. J Virol 68:1204–1206

Staedel C, Remy J-S, Hua Z, Broker TR, Chow LT, Behr J-P (1994) High-efficiency transfection of primary human keratinocytes with positively charged lipopolyamine:DNA complexes. J Invest Dermatol 102:768–772

Sukharev SI, Klenchin VA, Serow SM, Chernomordik LV, Chizmadzhev JA (1992) Electroporation and electrophoretic DNA transfer into cells. The effect of DNA interaction with electropores. Biophys J 63:1320–1327

Tang DC, DeVit M, Johnston SA (1992) Genetic immunization is a simple method for eliciting an immune response. Nature 356:152–154

Thierry AR, Lunardi-Iskandar Y, Bryant JL, Rabinovich P, Gallo RC, Mahan LC (1995) Systemic gene therapy: biodistribution and long term expression of a transgene in mice. Proc Natl Acad Sci USA 92:9742–9746

Udvardi A, Kufferath I, Grutsch H, Zatloukal K, Volc-Platzer B (1999) Uptake of exogenous DNA via the skin. J Mol Med 77:744–750

Ulmer JB, Donnelley JJ, Parker SE, Rhodes GH, Felgner PL, Dwarki VJ, Gromkowski SH, Deck RR, Dewitt CM, Friedman A, Hawe LA, Leander KR, Martinez D, Perry HC, Shiver JW, Montgomery DL, Liu MA (1993) Heterologous protection against influenza by injection of DNA encoding a viral protein. Science 259:1745–1749

Wagner E, Zenke M, Cotten M, Beug H, Birnstiel ML (1990) Transferrin-polycation conjugates as carriers for DNA uptake into cells. Proc Natl Acad Sci USA 87:3410–3414

Wagner E, Cotten M, Foisner R, Birnstiel ML (1991) Transferrin-polycation DNA complexes: the effect of polycations on the structure of the complex and DNA delivery to cells. Proc Natl Acad Sci USA 88:4255–4259

Wagner E, Plank C, Zatloukal K, Cotten M, Birnstiel ML (1992a) Influenza virus hemagglutinin HA-2 N-terminal fusogenic peptides augment gene transfer by transferrin-polylysine-DNA complexes: toward a synthetic virus-like gene transfer vehicle. Proc Natl Acad Sci USA 89:7934–7938

Wagner E, Zatloukal K, Cotten M, Kirlappos H, Mechtler K, Curiel D, Birnstiel ML (1992b) Coupling of adenovirus to transferrin-polylysine/DNA complexes greatly enhances receptor-mediated gene delivery and expression of transfected genes. Proc Natl Acad Sci USA 89:6099–6103

Wagner E, Curiel D, Cotten M (1994) Delivery of drugs, proteins and genes into cells using transferrin as a ligand for receptor-mediated endocytosis. Adv Drug Delivery Rev 14:113–135

Walters RW, Welsh MJ (1999) Mechanism by which calcium phosphate coprecipitation enhances adenovirus-mediated gene transfer. Gene Ther 6:1845–1850

Wang CY, Huang L (1987) pH-sensitive immunoliposomes mediate target-cell specific delivery and controlled expression of a foreign gene in mouse. Proc Natl Acad Sci USA 84:7851–7855

Wang CY, Huang L (1989) Highly efficient DNA delivery mediated by pH-sensitive immunoliposomes. Biochemistry 28:9508–9514

Wang B, Ugen KE, Srikantan V, Agadjanyan MG, Dang K, Refaeli J, Sato AL, Boyer J, Williams WV, Weiner DB (1993) Gene inoculation generates immune responses against human immunodeficiency virus type I. Proc Natl Acad Sci USA 90:4156–4160

Williams RS, Johnston SA, Riedy M, DeVit MJ, McElligott SG, Sanford JC (1991) Introduction of foreign genes into tissues of living mice by DNA-coated micro projectiles. Proc Natl Acad Sci USA 88:2726–2730

Wolff JA, Malone RW, Williams P, Chong W, Acsadi G, Jani A, Felgner PL (1990) Direct gene transfer into mouse muscle in vivo. Science 247:1465–1468

Wolff JA, Ludtke JJ, Acsadi G, Williams P, Jani A (1992) Long-term persistence of plasmid DNA and foreign gene expression in mouse muscle. Hum Mol Genet 1:363–369

Yang N (1992) Gene transfer into mammalian somatic cells in vivo. Crit Rev Biotechnol 12:335–356

Yin W, Cheng PW (1994) Lectin conjugate-directed gene transfer to airway epithelial cells. Biochem Biophys Res Commun 205:826–833

Yu WH, Kashani-Sabet M, Liggitt D, Moore D, Heath TD, Debs RJ (1999) Topical gene delivery to murine skin. J Invest Dermatol 112:370–375

Zhang L, Li L, Hoffmann GA, Hoffmann RM (1996) Depth-targeted efficient gene delivery and expression in the skin by pulsed electric fields: an approach to gene therapy of skin aging and other diseases. Biochem Biophys Res Comm 220:633–636

5   Safety and Pharmacokinetics of Naked Plasmid DNA: Studies on Dissemination and Ectopic Expression

U. R. Hengge, B. Dexling, A. Udvardi, B. Volc-Platzer, A. Mirmohammdsadegh

Introduction

Gene therapy is a new field of biotechnology attempting to treat diseases with DNA. Naked i.e. uncoated plasmid DNA is a large, highly negatively charged molecule that usually belongs to the nucleus or the mitochondria. Naked plasmid DNA does not exhibit various limitations that characterize viral vectors such as the elicitation of adverse immune responses, promotor shutdown and insertional mutagenesis. On the other hand, expression is generally transient in the range of a few of days in skin and up to one year in skeletal muscle. In addition, at this point it remains elusive, why keratinocytes (and various other cells) take up DNA and translate it into the corresponding protein.

Plasmid DNA has rapidly become a popular vector in gene therapy. Early gene transfer experiments using plasmid DNA were performed using the gene gun, where DNA coated onto fine gold particles was accelerated to target a variety of mammalian tissues and cells *in vitro* and *in vivo* (for review see Hengge and Schadendorf 2000). Subsequently the direct injection of naked plasmid DNA was established for muscle and skin eliminating the need of expensive technical devices (Wolff et al. 1990, Hengge et al. 1995, 1996, and 1998). In the meantime, various other tissues such as thyroid (Sikes et al. 1994), synovial cells (Yovandich et al. 1995) and stomach (Takehara et al. 1996) have been directly injected with plasmid DNA. In addition, the intratracheal delivery as an aerosol has been shown to transfect airway epithelia using naked DNA (Stribling et al. 1992, Meyer et al. 1995).

This review will discuss the safety of naked plasmid DNA. It will focus on its pharmacokinetics, distribution and ectopic expression following various routes of application.

Clinically Documented Safety of DNA Application in Humans

Since the first therapeutic experiments in the late 80ies more than 250 additional clinical gene therapy trials were approved and more than 4000 patients were treated worldwide for cancer or infection (Marcel et al. 1997). Currently, clinical trials of naked DNA against influenza, malaria and HIV are being conducted (Donnelly et al. 1995, Wang et al. 1998, Calarota et al. 1998). Intramuscular DNA vaccination against *Plasmodium falciparum* (Malaria) has been performed in volunteers (Wang et al. 1998). Plasmid was administered three times in monthly intervals into the *M. deltoideus*. Four groups of four volunteers each received 20 µg, 100 µg, 500 µg or 2500 µg of plasmid DNA. While the goal of the study was to evaluate the induction of specific cytotoxic T lymphocytes (CTL) following three immunizations, no significant toxicity except erythema at the application site and mild fever has been observed (Wang et al. 1998).

In a phase-I-study by MacGregor et al. the immunization of HIV-patients with intramuscular application of an expression plasmid was performed harboring a modified env- and rev-gene under the control of the CMV-promoter (MacGregor et al. 1998). Patients received 30 µg, 100 µg and 300 µg plasmid DNA (5 patients each). Significant side effects were not detected. In another phase-I-study by Calarota et al. HIV-patients received intramuscular injections in the *M. deltoideus* on days 0, 60 and 180 of 100 µg plasmid DNA (Calarota et al. 1998). The plasmid contained the CMV immediate-early promotor and the HIV-genes nef, rev or tat. No relevant toxicity has been seen.

DNA has also been administered for anti-tumor vaccination. In that regard, various clinical trials have been performed against colon carcinoma (Conry et al. 1996), melanoma (Klatzmann et al. 1998, Schreiber et al. 1999, Sun et al. 1998), head and neck squamous cell cancer (Wollenberg et al. 1999) and against B cell lymphoma (Syrengelas et al. 1996). Conry et al. vaccinated patients with metastasized colorectal carcinoma using a carcinoembryonal antigen (CEA) expression plasmid (Conry et al. 1996). The vaccination was performed at a dose between 100–3000 µg with a vector being derived from pcDNA$_3$. This vector served to construct the pVAX-1 vector, that has been designed following the safety recommendations of the FDA (Food and Drug Administration), USA, Center for Biologics, Evaluation and Research (CBER) (Docket No. 96N-0400) and is now commercially available (Invitrogen, Catalogue-No.: V260–20). It does not contain the ampicillin resistance gene that created two problems. First, since the plasmid preparations may contain minute amounts of ampicillin following the culture of *E. coli* in the presence of the antibiotic, it may lead to immediate-type allergies upon injection into patients. Second, the bacterial ampicillin gene contains intrinsic immunostimulatory sequences, that may lead to more severe inflammatory reactions. Therefore, in the pVAX-1, the ampicillin has been replaced by the mammalian kanamycin resistance gene.

Furthermore, in a phase-I-study, idiotype vaccination in patients with follicular cell lymphoma is being evaluated with intramuscular injection into the *M. deltoideus* (Hawkins et al. 1997). The vector contains the RSV-LTR-promotor and the ampicillin resistance gene (Hawkins et al. 1997). In another ongoing phase-I-study, patients with head and neck carcinomas are treated by intratumoral injection of an IL-2-expressing plasmid using DOTMA-Chol (Wollenberg et al. 1999). Doses range from 300–2400 µg/injection. Safety data are not yet available.

For therapeutic purposes, thrombangitis obliterans has been successfully treated with two intramuscular administrations of 2000 µg and 4000 µg of a VEGF-expressing plasmid at four-weekly intervals leading to new vessel formation (Isner et al. 1998), although the results have recently been questioned. Aside from some tenderness at the injection site in 6 patients, no significant side effects were noted (Isner et al. 1998). The same group used plasmid DNA for the therapy of myocardial ischemia without significant side effects (Losordo et al. 1998).

Specific Safety Analysis of Plasmid DNA

From a safety standpoint the intravenous route of plasmid delivery represents the greatest potential for the detection of systemic distribution and manifestation of toxicity. The earliest study addressing the overall safety of injected DNA analyzed its potential transforming ability following its injection into mammals (Gosse et al. 1965). In addition, intravenous injection of DNA was used to study the pathophysiological mechanism of systemic lupus erythematosus, an autoimmune disease (Emlen et al. 1988). These studies showed that DNA was rapidly removed from the circulation and that the liver played a major role for this observed clearance.

With regard to gene therapy, the intravenous injection of DNA complexed to cationic lipids was performed by Nabel et al. in mice, rats and rabbits (Nabel et al. 1992). Neither organ damage nor localization to the gonads was seen as evidenced by PCR following the injection of an allogeneic MHC expression plasmid. However, the potential integration of plasmid DNA into the host genome has just recently been analyzed (Schubbert et al. 1997, Martin et al. 1999) and was shown to concur with mathematical models of plasmid integration (Ledley and Ledley 1994). When injected plasmid DNA copies were quantified at 30 and 60 days following intramuscular injections in mice using PCR-based methods, about 1500 copies per 150000 genomes (10 fg per µg genomic DNA) were detected. The time after injection (i.e. 30 or 60 days) was no predictor of the plasmid copy number associated with the genomic DNA, since between 3 and 30 copies always remained associated with the genomic DNA. However, the researchers could not determine whether the plasmid sequences were covalently linked to (i.e. integrated) or simply accidently associated with the genomic DNA. Even in the worst case scenario, if all detectable 30 copies were integrated, the calculated rate of mutations would still be 3000 times less than the spontaneous mutation rate for mammalian genomes (Martin et al. 1999). This level of integration was not considered to pose a safety concern, if it should occur.

When different application routes (intravenous, intramuscular and intradermal) were compared, significant clinical or histological toxicity has not been detected (Wolff et al. 1992b, Davis et al. 1993, Parker et al. 1995, Hartikka et al. 1996, Winegar et al. 1996, Torres et al. 1997). Davis et al. detected some degree of muscle fiber degeneration and regeneration following intramuscular application of reporter gene- and HBsAg-expressing plasmids (Davis et al. 1997). The observed muscle fiber degeneration was generally mild.

Fate of DNA Following Uptake via Mucosal Surfaces

Uptake of foreign DNA has also been investigated in the gastrointestinal system of the mouse (Schubbert et al. 1997). These experiments are particularly important, since DNA is constantly ingested with food and might be taken up by cells and become integrated at random into the cellular genome. The authors showed that unprotected M13 phage DNA was not completely degraded upon passage through the gastrointestinal tract of the mouse. After feeding between 10–15 ng of M13 phage DNA as double-stranded supercoiled circular or linearized DNA, the authors found M13 DNA sequences up to 900 bases in white blood cells as early as 2–4 hours after feeding in 1 of 1000 peripheral leukocytes. On a quantitative level, 3–4% of the ingested DNA was recovered in the feces, while in the blood stream the percentage was between 0.01% and 0.1%. In addition, M13 DNA could be demonstrated in columnar epithelial cells, leukocytes of the Peyer's patch, in liver cells, lymphocytes and splenocytes. These findings suggested transport of foreign DNA though the intestinal wall and Peyer's patches into blood leukocytes and several other tissues. When excessive amounts of DNA were fed, M13 DNA could even be recloned from spleen DNA into a lambda phage vector. Some of the isolated plaques were shown to contain mouse DNA, bacterial DNA and rearranged lambda DNA.

Pharmacokinetics and Distribution of Plasmid DNA Following Intravenous Injection

To evaluate the pharmacokinetics of DNA complexed to cationic lipids, mice were injected with 50 µg of supercoiled plasmid DNA complexed with DMRIE-DOPE (Lew et al. 1995). Pharmacokinetic data were obtained up to six months after injection. When DNA was isolated from blood between 1–6 minutes after injection, supercoiled plasmid was not present at any time point. Linear and relaxed circular plasmids were detected by Southern blot, but rapidly diminished within the first 30 minutes post-injection. The highest levels of residual plasmid were present in heart, kidney, liver, lung and spleen, which are highly vascularized. However, within one hour, plasmid DNA was also detected in bone marrow and muscles but was no longer detectable in the brain, large intestine, small intestine, ovaries and testes. Up to 24 hours, plasmid was retained in the lung, spleen, liver, heart, kidney, bone marrow and muscles as evidenced by Southern-blot. At seven days post-injection, there was no intact plasmid DNA in any tissue (Lew et al. 1995). Given the sensitivity of Southern blotting being in the range of about 1 pg/10 μg DNA, approximately 0.15 copies of plasmid per genome were detected in the experimental samples. In these experiments skin has not been examined.

While Southern blot analysis detected no intact plasmid in tissues beyond 24 hours, PCR results indicated the presence of plasmid DNA in all tissues at 7 and 28 days post-injection. At six months, plasmid DNA was exclusively detected in muscles in the femtogram range. The range of residual plasmid was low in brain, intestine and gonads (< 1 fg/μg sample) and about 64 fg/μg in the bone marrow, heart, liver, spleen and muscles, representing approximately 250–16000 copies/μg genomic DNA. By 28 days, bone marrow, heart, kidney, liver, lung, spleen and muscles still had the greatest amounts of amplifiable plasmid. Between day 7 and 28, there was a mean drop of about 128-fold in these tissues with considerable variability among animals. By day 28, the level of plasmid DNA was at or below the level of 100 fg/μg genomic DNA in all samples (Lew et al. 1995). However, on the protein level, the transgene could not be detected beyond one week. Only in muscular tissues, plasmid DNA could be detected for more than one year following direct intramuscular injection (Wolff et al. 1992 b, Davis et al. 1993).

In another study, the localization of radioactively labeled, naked plasmid DNA (45 μg/mouse equaling 1–3 μCi) and naked plasmid DNA complexed to cationic lipids was compared following intravenous injection into BALB/c mice. Various differences were observed (Osaka et al. 1996). Radioactively labeled naked DNA was detected 2 minutes after injection with the highest concentration being achieved in the liver >lung, spleen and kidney. 24 hours after injection, the accumulation was highest in the liver and spleen followed by kidney, lung and blood. The radioactivity measured in skin samples at 24 hours after injection was about 0.6–1.6% dose equivalents per gram tissue, an activity comparable to the level obtained in brain, eye, intestinal mucosa, and salivary glands. Interestingly, the plasmid was not expressed in any of the above mentioned tissues at 24 hours. In contrast, when DNA was complexed to lipids, it accumulated in the lungs to a very high extent. The DNA was expressed as early as 1.5 hours in the lung with all organs being positive at 24 hours after injection.

This study concluded, that the use of cationic lipids significantly altered the normal biodistribution of plasmid DNA and its expression pattern. While plasmid complexed to cationic lipids accumulated in tissues containing abundant reticulo-endothelial system (RES) cells such as the liver and lungs, naked plasmid showed higher levels in blood up to 20 minutes after injection suggesting that naked plasmid DNA is less prone to entrapment by the RES. In that regard, cationic lipids are thought to facilitate transfection by the efficient capture of negatively charged DNA (condensation), increase cellular uptake due to the interaction of positively charged complexes with negatively charged biological surface molecules leading to efficient membrane fusion. The observed high levels of radioactivity in bone (cortical, marrow and growth plate) in both groups may represent the uptake of the ^{33}P-labeled DNA by the cellular components of the bone marrow such as macrophages and may as well reflect the deposition of phosphate in the bone matrix following degradation of DNA (Osaka et al. 1996). Both studies demonstrated that intravenously administered supercoiled plasmid DNA was immediately subjected to degradation, probably by nucleases present in serum.

Pharmacokinetics and Distribution of Plasmid DNA Following Intramuscular Injection

When muscle was directly injected with plasmid DNA, *in vivo* light microscopical studies showed that the plasmid was distributed throughout the muscle and was able to diffuse through the extracellular matrix, cross the external lamina and enter myofibers. Furthermore, it was shown by electron microscopy, that colloidal gold conjugated to plasmid DNA traversed the external lamina and entered T-tubules in caveolae, while gold particles complexed to other highly negatively charged molecules such as polylysine, polyethylenglycol or polyglutamate primarily remained outside the myofibers. This evidence suggested that specific DNA uptake mechanisms exist in muscle and that transient membrane disruptions induced by needle injection are not responsible for the uptake of DNA.

The pharmacokinetics and distribution of plasmid DNA were analyzed in rabbits by quantitative PCR and in situ hybridization techniques (Winegar et al. 1996). Following the injection of either 100 μg or 400 μg of plasmid DNA into the posterolateral muscle of the hind leg, sampling was performed between 4 hours and 24 days. Interestingly, plasmid was mainly found in the skin and muscle at the injection site and in plasma. For example, 4 hours after the injection of the higher dose, the plasmid was detected at the injection site at a mean copy number of 10^6 in muscles and 4×10^4 in skin per μg tissue, respectively. The plasmid copy number in muscle declined rapidly during the first 24 hours and was undetectable at 7 and 24 days after injection, respectively. In contrast, the decline was slower in skin overlaying the muscular injection site where the plasmid was still detectable at 28 days. In contrast to the findings by Lew et al. (Lew et al. 1995), where DNA/cationic lipid complexes were injected intravenously, plasmid DNA was undetectable by PCR in most of the tissues and fluids examined such as spleen, liver, jejunum, brain, lymph nodes and gonads at a detection limit of 10 copies/μg of tissue. By in situ hybridization, the plasmid was detected in muscle, mainly in the perimysium and to a lesser degree in the endomysium and within the muscle fiber during the first week after injection. As a limitation of this study, an accurate estimation of the copy number of plasmid in a given amount of tissue could not be performed, since DNA was extracted as opposed to the preparation and analysis of tissue homogenates. Furthermore, no analysis of expression was performed. Although initially higher levels of plasmid DNA were achieved in muscle as opposed to skin, the plasmid copy number fell more rapidly and dropped earlier below the detection level in muscles than in skin. One explanation is, that plasmid in the skin may be compartmentalized and retained in the connective tissue, thereby decreasing the rate of clearance.

In accordance with other studies (Nabel et al. 1992, Lew et al. 1995), there was no evidence of uptake by the testes and ovaries.

Other investigators have detected plasmid DNA in mouse muscle for several months after injection (Wolff et al. 1992a and b). More specifically, Wolff et al. demonstrated that intramuscularly injected plasmid DNA did not integrate into the host genome and was maintained in an episomal state (Wolff et al. 1990, Wolff et al. 1992b). The differences in the detectability of plasmid DNA across various studies using intramuscular injection may be due to the coadministration and timing of bupivacaine that leads to muscle fiber destruction and may alter the plasmid distribution and/or persistence (Wells 1993). In addition, species-related effects must be considered. For example, rabbits have a much larger posterolateral muscle than mice. Consequently, it is more difficult to sample the entire muscle. Moreover, because whole tissue homogenates rather than isolated DNA were used, fewer cell equivalents were analyzed in each PCR reaction. Therefore, this procedure used proportionally less DNA per amount of tissue leading to a decreased sensitivity.

Pharmacokinetics and Distribution of Plasmid DNA Following Intranasal Inhalation

The intratracheal gene delivery has been assessed in terms of plasmid DNA expression and pharmacokinetics in mouse airways (Meyer et al. 1995). Transgene expression was detected up to 28 days after administration with a peak at day 2. When DNA was complexed to cationic lipids (e.g. DOTMA-DOPE), plasmid was retained for extended periods of time, whereas the length of expression remained unaffected. This study also determined that expression was independent of the buffer used, gender, age and strain of mice. Even the addition of carrier DNA did not affect the level of expression. When the structure of the DNA was analyzed with respect to expression, only supercoiled circular, but not linearized plasmid was expressed. Surprisingly, naked DNA was found to be equally effective in transfecting mouse airway epithelia as DNA complexed to cationic lipids by some groups (Meyer et al. 1995), but not by others (Yoshimura et al. 1992).

In terms of plasmid distribution, up to 30% of iodinated plasmid accumulated in the lungs at 5 min after instillation followed by trachea, head and stomach. At 20 min and 9 hours, only about 8 and 2% were detected in the lungs, respectively. For comparison, when DNA was complexed to cationic lipids, pulmonary accumulation peaked at 20 min with 44% of plasmid being detected. The accumulation in stomach was thought to be due to plasmid clearance from the airways with subsequent swallowing of the DNA by the animal. In conclusion, while both naked and cationic lipid bound DNA lead to comparable expression, the pharmacokinetics of DNA complexed to lipids is delayed.

Pharmacokinetics and Distribution
of Plasmid DNA Following Intradermal Injection

In order to assess the safety of naked plasmid DNA in an animal model relevant for skin gene therapy, we analyzed if intracutaneously injected plasmid DNA was transported to other organs and if ectopic expression occurred. Therefore, intradermal injections of a "superdose" of 2 mg CMV:β-Gal plasmid DNA were performed into the right hind leg of four 30 kg minipigs (Dexling et al. 1999).

To minimize the risk of cross-sample contamination, each tissue was processed in the tube in which it was frozen. Tissue sample preparation, PCR reaction setup, PCR amplification, and PCR analysis were each performed in separate laboratories. Following DNA and RNA extraction by the cesium chloride method, PCR analysis was performed to detect DNA (Hengge et al. 1995). In addition, expression was analyzed following DNAse treatment of the extracted RNA prior to amplification by RT-PCR. Positive controls were performed using β-actin primers. Following euthanasia of the animals at several time points (day 1 (n = 1), day 3 (n = 2) and day 11 (n = 1)), various organs were analyzed for the presence of DNA and their potential expression. The PCR results are depicted in Fig. 5.1. Following three days after injection, DNA could be recovered from all organs analyzed except spinal cord and bone marrow. By day 11, DNA could still

Tissue	day 1	day 3	day 11
Injection site	+	ND	+
3cm away	+	+	+
10cm away	+	ND	+
Draining lymph node	+	+	+
Muscle	ND	+	+
Ovary	ND	+	-
Heart	ND	+	+
Uterus	ND	+	+
Diaphragm	ND	+	+
Brain	ND	+	-
Thyroid	ND	+	-
Kidney	ND	+	-
Liver	ND	+	-
Intestine	ND	+	-
Stomach	ND	+	-
Spleen	ND	+	-
Lung	ND	+	-
Spinal cord	ND	-	-
Bone marrow	ND	-	-

2 to 10 independent samples were analyzed per time point and tissue; ND: not determined

Fig. 5.1. Distribution of β-Gal plasmid DNA following intradermal injection

Tissue	day 1	day 3	day 11
Injection site	+	ND	+
3cm away	+	+	+
10cm away	+	ND	+
Draining lymph node	+	+	-
Muscle	ND	+	-
Ovary	ND	+	-
Heart	ND	-	-
Brain	ND	-	-
Thyroid	ND	-	ND
Kidney	ND	-	ND
Liver	ND	-	ND
Intestine	ND	-	-
Stomach	ND	-	-
Spleen	ND	-	-
Lung	ND	-	-
Uterus	ND	-	-
Diaphragm	ND	-	-
Spinal cord	ND	-	-
Bone marrow	ND	-	-

Fig. 5.2. Ectopic RNA expression in various tissues following intradermal DNA injection

2 to 3 independent samples were analyzed per time point and tissue; ND: not determined

be recovered from skin (injection site, and at 3 and 10 cm distance, respectively), draining lymph nodes, and muscular tissues (skeletal muscle, heart, uterus, diaphragm) (Fig. 5.1). Integration into the host genome was not detected at any time point (Hengge et al. 1995). When these samples were analyzed for expression, RNA was found at day 3 in skin, draining lymph node, muscle and ovary, whereas at day 11 it was only expressed at the injection site and at 3 and 10 cm around it, respectively (Fig. 5.2).

Our experiments confirmed the transient presence of plasmid DNA in tissues, probably due to the degradation (nucleases) and loss of DNA from the constantly renewing epidermis. Udvardi et al. investigated the presence and expression of naked plasmid DNA after epicutaneous and intracutaneous application using PCR (Udvardi et al. 1999). Following epicutaneous application to intact mouse skin, the DNA could be detected for up to one week in contrast to 48 hours when DNA was applied to healing wounds. The plasmid DNA was only expressed after intracutaneous injection or particle bombardment, but not after epicutaneous administration (Udvardi et al. 1999).

Taken together, these results show that plasmid DNA is transported to almost all organs in a relevant large animal model with skin similar to humans. The transport mechanisms for plasmid dissemination are not entirely clear, but transport via dendritic cells, blood and lymph fluid is suspected. Topically applied naked DNA is not routinely transcribed. As expected, naked plasmid DNA is almost entirely degraded at later time points following various different application modalities to the skin. However, the relatively short time frame of uptake and expression is suitable to elicit important biological responses such as seen in genetic vaccination.

Inhibition of Plasmid Accumulation Points to Potential Mechanisms of Uptake

To gain information on the potential mechanism of DNA uptake, the physical, chemical and pharmacokinetic characteristics of radioactively labeled plasmid DNA (0.1 mg/kg) complexed to cationic liposomes were investigated following intravenous injection in mice (Mahato et al. 1995). Such labeled DNA was predominantly taken up by liver non-parenchymal cells. Hepatic uptake could be inhibited by the administration of dextran sulfate but not by polycytidine or polyinosine (poly-I). Since only negatively charged dextran sulfate, a non-specific inhibitor of phagocytosis, significantly inhibited the hepatic uptake of DNA-liposome complexes up to 40–50%, a receptor-mediated uptake by Kupffer cells has been suggested. However, hepatic uptake did not occur via scavenger receptors since polyinosine, a well-known ligand for the scavenger receptors, did not inhibit uptake of DNA-liposome complexes. These results were essentially confirmed by Osaka et al. (Osaka et al. 1996).

On the other hand, scavenger receptors on parenchymal cells were identified to be involved in uptake of naked DNA due to uptake inhibition by poly-I. These findings were explained by the positive ζ(zeta)-potential for DNA complexed to liposomes in contrast to the negative ζ-potential for naked plasmid DNA, thus suggesting different physicochemical properties of the resulting preparations. It was further concluded that the ζ-potential seems to influence the lung and spleen accumulation of plasmid/liposome-complexes. Besides the ζ-potential, the size of DNA/liposome complexes (600–1200 nm) was considerably larger than naked plasmid DNA and, thus, could also influence the nature of uptake. Recently, targeting of DNA complexed to glycosylated polylysines ("glycoplexes") has been systematically analyzed in airway epithelial cells (Fajac et al. 1999). Interestingly, the level of uptake did not correlate with the level of DNA expression. Therefore, the transfection of epithelial cells is not solely determined by lectin targeting, but also by intracellular routing of DNA.

Degradation and Excretion of Plasmid DNA

In a study by Kawabata et al., the half-life of naked plasmid DNA was calculated in the order of 10 minutes (Kawabata et al. 1995). Interestingly, after intravenous injection the naked plasmid, DNA was degraded at a significantly faster rate than observed in whole blood, suggesting that plasmid DNA in vivo is degraded in additional compartments than blood. The degradation products of naked plasmid DNA were found up to 6% in the urine as opposed to a maximum of 1% when DNA was complexed to liposomes.

Contribution of Nucleases to DNA Degradation

Despite certain advantages for gene therapy with naked DNA, there are fundamental problems associated with the unprotected character of plasmid DNA. In particular, the reduction of genome equivalents will translate into a loss of gene expression. In that regard a recent paper analyzed the existence of nucleases in various tissues (Barry et al. 1999). Calcium-dependent endonucleases have been identified to be responsible for the degradation of DNA in spleen, liver, kidney and skin of mice. It was found, that within 90 minutes after injection, the endonucleases in skin and muscle led to the degradation of 99% of the injected naked DNA. In contrast, skeletal or cardiac muscle had low levels of acidic endonuclease activity. The activity of the calcium-dependent nuclease was especially high in blood, whereas the acidic endonuclease was – as expected – not active in blood because of its high pH. Despite the massive destruction, tissue nuclease levels did not determine the transfection efficiency in skin and muscle.

Besides the destruction of plasmid DNA, nucleases might play a different, yet important role in the process of genetic immunization by cleaving large plasmids into small oligonucleotides that can be easily taken up by various types of immune cells and stimulate the elicitation of CpG-depending immune responses (Krieg et al. 1995). Therefore, it was concluded that for genetic immunization to be successful, the right balance between the nuclease effects of DNA destruction (immunostimulatory fragments) and sufficient expression of the gene of interest has to be reached. While most of the exogenous DNA is rapidly destroyed by nucleases, especially in muscle and skin, this degradation did not appear to determine the transfection efficiency. Rather, cell- and tissue-specific uptake and expression and perhaps more subtle nuclease effects may act in concert (Barry et al. 1999).

These results contribute to the understanding of DNA distribution and longevity of expression. From a safety standpoint, skin gene therapy with naked plasmid DNA can be considered safe due to the rapid biodegradation of plasmid DNA and the (only) transient expression of foreign gene exclusively in tissues, that are known to take up DNA.

Acknowledgements. The support of Dr. Jonathan Vogel, Dermatology Branch, NIH, is gratefully acknowledged. In addition, the expert veterinarian treatment of Dr. Victoria Hamshire and Melissa Williams were invaluable throughout the entire study. The expert editorial skills of Nicole C. Bartosch for the entire book are gratefully acknowledged.

References

Barry ME, Pinto-Gonzalez D, Orson FM, McKenzie GJ, Petry GR, Barry MA (1999) Role of endogenous endonucleases and tissue site in transfection and CpG-mediated immune activation after naked DNA injection. Hum Gene Ther 10:2461–2480

Calarota S, Bratt G, Nordlund S, Hinkula J, Leandersson AC, Sandstrom E, Wahren B (1998) Cellular cytotoxic response induced by DNA vaccination in HIV-1-infected patients. Lancet 351:1320-1325

Conry RM, Widera G, LoBuglio AF, Fuller JT, Moore SE, Barlow DL, Turner J, Yang NS, Curiel DT (1996) Phase Ia trial of a polynucleotide anti-tumor immunization to a human carcinoembryonic antigen in patients with metastatic colorectal cancer. Hum Gene Ther 7:755-772

Davis HL, Whalen RG, Demeneix BA (1993) Direct gene transfer into skeletal muscle in vivo: factors affecting efficiency of transfer and stability of expression. Hum Gene Ther 4:151–159

Davis HL, Millan CL, Watkins SC (1997) Immune-mediated destruction of transfected muscle fibers after direct gene transfer with antigen-expressing plasmid DNA. Gene Ther 4:181–188

Dexling B, Mirmohammadsadegh A, Hengge UR (1999) Ectopic expression of naked plasmid DNA. J Invest Dermatol 113:445

Donnelly JJ, Friedman A, Martinez D, Montgomery DL, Shiver JW, Motzel SL, Ulmer JB, Liu MA (1995) Preclinical efficacy of a prototype DNA vaccine: enhanced protection against antigenic drift in influenza virus. Nat Med 1:583-587

Emlen W, Rifai A, Magilavy D, Mannik M (1988) Hepatic binding of DNA is mediated by a receptor on nonparenchymal cells. Am J Pathol 133:54–60

Fajac I, Briand P, Monsigny M, Midoux P (1999) Sugar-mediated uptake of glycosylated polylysines and gene transfer into normal and cystic fibrosis airway epithelial cells. Hum Gene Ther 10:395–406

Gosse C, Le Pecq JB, Defrance P, Paoletti C (1965) Initial degradation of deoxyribonucleic acid after injection in mammals. Cancer Res 25:877–883

Hartikka J, Sawdey M, Cornefert-Jensen F, Margalith M, Barnhart K, Nolasco M, Vahlsing HL, Meek J, Marquet M, Hobart P, Norman J, Manthorpe M (1996) An improved plasmid DNA expression vector for direct injection into skeletal muscle. Hum Gene Ther 7:1205–1217

Hawkins R, Russell SJ, Marcus R, Ashworth LJ, Brissnik J, Zhang J, Winter G, Bleehen NM, Shaw MM, Williamson L, Ouwehand W, Stevenson F, Hamblin T, Oscier D, Zhu D, King C, Kumar S, Thompsett A, Stevenson GT (1997) A pilot study of idiotypic vaccination for follicular B-cell lymphoma using a genetic approach. Hum Gene Ther 8:1287–1299

Hengge UR, Schadendorf D (2000) Modification of melanoma cells via ballistic gene delivery for vaccination. In: Lasic, Templeton (eds) Gene Therapy: Therapeutic mechanisms and strategies. Marcel Dekker, New York, pp 165–180

Hengge UR, Chan EF, Foster RA, Walker PS, Vogel JC (1995) Cytokine gene expression in epidermis with biological effects following injection of naked DNA. Nat Genet 10:161–166

Hengge UR, Walker PS, Vogel JC (1996) Expression of naked DNA in human, pig and mouse skin. J Clin Invest 97:2911–2916

Hengge UR, Pfützner W, Williams M, Goos M, Vogel JC (1998) Efficient expression of naked plasmid DNA in mucosal epithelium: prospective for the treatment of skin lesions. J Invest Dermatol 111:605–608

Isner JM, Baumgartner I, Rauh G, Schainfeld R, Blair R, Manor O, Razvi S, Symes JF (1998) Treatment of thromboangiitis obliterans (Buerger's disease) by intramuscular gene transfer of vascular endothelial growth factor: preliminary clinical results. J Vasc Surg 28:964–973

Kawabata K, Takakura Y, Hashida M (1995) The fate of plasmid DNA after intravenous injection in mice: involvement of scavenger receptors in its hepatic uptake. Pharm Res 12:825–830

Klatzmann D, Cherin P, Bensimon G, Boyer O, Coutellier A, Charlotte F, Boccaccio C, Salzmann JL, Herson S (1998) A phase I/II dose-escalation study of herpes simplex virus type 1 thymidine kinase "suicide, gene therapy for metastatic melanoma. Study Group on Gene Therapy of Metastatic Melanoma. Hum Gene Ther 9:2585–2594

Krieg AM, Yi AK, Matson S, Waldschmidt TJ, Bishop GA, Teasdale R, Koretzky GA, Klinman DM (1995) CpG motifs in bacterial DNA trigger direct B-cell activation. Nature 374:546–549

Ledley TS and Ledley FD (1994) Multicompartment, numerical model of cellular events in the pharmacokinetics of gene therapies. Hum Gene Ther 5:679–691

Lew D, Parker SE, Latimer T, Abai AM, Kuwahara-Rundell A, Doh SG, Yang ZY, Laface D, Gromkowski SH, Nabel GJ, Manthorpe M, Norman J (1995) Cancer gene therapy using plasmid DNA: pharmacokinetic study of DNA following injection in mice. Gene Ther 6:553–564

Losordo DW, Vale PR, Symes JF, Dunnington CH, Esakof DD, Maysky M, Ashare AB, Lathi K, Isner JM (1998) Gene therapy for myocardial angiogenesis: initial clinical results with direct myocardial injection of phVEGF165 as sole therapy for myocardial ischemia. Circulation 98:2800–2804

MacGregor RR, Boyer JD, Ugen KE, Lacy KE, Gluckman SJ, Bagarazzi ML, Chattergoon MA, Baine Y, Higgins TJ, Ciccarelli RB, Coney LR, Ginsberg RS, Weiner DB (1998) First human trial of a DNA-based vaccine for treatment of human immunodeficiency virus type 1 infection: safety and host response. J Infect Dis 178:92–100

Mahato RI, Kawabata K, Nomura T, Takakura Y, Hashida M (1995) Physicochemical and pharmacokinetic characteristics of plasmid DNA/cationic liposome complexes. J Pharm Sci 84:1267–1271

Martin T, Parker SE, Hedstrom R, Le T, Hoffman SL, Norman J, Hobart P, Lew D (1999) Plasmid DNA malaria vaccine: the potential for genomic integration after intramuscular injection. Hum Gene Ther 10:759–768

Meyer KB, Thompson MM, Levy MY, Barron LG, Szoka FC Jr (1995) Intratracheal gene delivery to the mouse airway: characterization of plasmid DNA expression and pharmacokinetics. Gene Ther 2:450–460

Nabel EG, Gordon D, Yang ZY, Xu L, San H, Plautz GE, Wu BY, Gao X, Huang L and Nabel GJ (1992) Gene transfer in vivo with DNA-liposome complexes: lack of autoimmunity and gonadal localization. Hum Gene Ther 3:649–656

Osaka G, Carey K, Cuthbertson A, Godowski P, Patapoff T, Ryan A, Gadek T, Mordenti J (1996) Pharmacokinetics, tissue distribution, and expression efficiency of plasmid [33P] DNA following intravenous administration of DNA/cationic lipid complexes in mice: use of a novel radionuclide approach. J Pharm Sci 85:612–618

Parker SE, Vahlsing HL, Serfilippi LM, Franklin CL, Doh SG, Gromkowski SH, Lew D, Manthorpe M, Norman J (1995) Cancer gene therapy using plasmid DNA: safety evaluation in rodents and non-human primates. Hum Gene Ther 6:575–590

Schreiber S, Kämpgen E, Wagner E, Pirkhammer D, Trcka J, Korschan H, Lindemann A, Dorffner R, Kittler H, Kasteliz F, Kupcu Z, Sinski A, Zatloukal K, Buschle M, Schmidt W, Birnstiel M, Kempe RE, Voigt T, Weber HA, Pehamberger H, Mertelsmann R, Bröcker EB, Wolff K, Stingl G (1999) Immunotherapy of metastatic malignant melanoma by a vaccine consisting of autologous interleukin 2-transfected cancer cells: outcome of a phase I study. Hum Gene Ther 10:983–993

Schubbert R, Renz D, Schmitz B, Doerfler W (1997) Foreign (M13) DNA ingested by mice reaches peripheral leukocytes, spleen, and liver via the intestinal wall mucosa and can be covalently linked to mouse DNA. Proc Natl Acad Sci USA U S A 94:961–966

Sikes ML, O'Malley BW Jr, Finegold MJ, Ledley FD (1994) In vivo gene transfer into rabbit thyroid follicular cells by direct DNA injection. Hum Gene Ther 5:837–844

Stribling R, Brunette E, Liggitt D, Gaensler K, Debs R (1992) Aerosol gene delivery in vivo. Proc Natl Acad Sci USA U S A 89:11 277–11 281

Sun Y, Jurgovsky K, Moller P, Alijagic S, Dorbic T, Georgieva J, Wittig B, Schadendorf D (1998) Vaccination with IL-12 gene-modified autologous melanoma cells: preclinical results and a first clinical phase I study. Gene Ther 5:481–490

Syrengelas AD, Chen TT, Levy R (1996) DNA immunization induces protective immunity against B-cell lymphoma. Nat Med 2:1038–1041

Takehara T, Hayashi N, Yamamoto M, Miyamoto Y, Fusamoto H, Kamada T (1996) *In vivo* gene transfer and expression in rat stomach by submucosal injection of plasmid DNA. Hum Gene Ther 7:589–593

Torres CA, Iwasaki A, Barber BH, Robinson HL (1997) Differential dependence on target site tissue for gene gun and intramuscular DNA immunizations. J Immunol 158:4529–4532

Udvardi A, Kufferath I, Grutsch H, Zatloukal K, Volc-Platzer B (1999) Uptake of exogenous DNA via the skin. J Mol Med (1999) 77:744 –750

Wang R, Doolan DL, Le TP, Hedstrom RC, Coonan KM, Charoenvit Y, Jones TR, Hobart P, Margalith M, Ng J, Weiss WR, Sedegah M, de Taisne C, Norman JA, Hoffman SL (1998) Induction of antigen-specific cytotoxic T lymphocytes in humans by a malaria DNA vaccine. Science 282:476–480

Wells D (1993) Improved gene transfer by direct plasmid injection associated with regeneration in mouse skeletal muscle. FEBS Lett 332:179–182

Winegar RA, Monforte JA, Suing KD, O'Loughlin KG, Rudd CJ, MacGregor JT (1996) Determination of tissue distribution of an intramuscular plasmid vaccine using PCR and in situ DNA hybridization. Hum Gene Ther 7:2185–2194

Wolff JA, Malone RW, Williams P, Chong W, Acsadi G, Jani A, Felgner PL (1990) Direct gene transfer into mouse muscle *in vivo*. Science 247:1465–1468

Wolff JA, Dowty ME, Jiao S, Repetto G, Berg RK, Ludtke JJ, Williams P, Slautterback DB (1992a) Expression of naked plasmids by cultured myotubes and entry of plasmids into T tubules and caveolae of mammalian skeletal muscle. J Cell Sci 103:1249–1259

Wolff JA, Ludtke JJ, Acsadi G, Williams P, Jani A (1992b) Long-term persistence of plasmid DNA and foreign gene expression in mouse muscle. Hum Mol Genet 1:363–369

Wollenberg B, Kastenbauer, Mundl H, Schaumberg J, Mayer A, Andratschke M, Lang S, Pauli C, Zeidler R, Ihrler S, Lohrs, Naujoks K, Rollston R (1999) Gene Therapy – Phase I trial for primary untreated head and neck squamous cell cancer UICC Stage II–IV with a single intratumoral injection of hIL-2 plasmids formulated in DOTMA/Chol. Hum Gene Ther 10:141–147

Yoshimura K, Rosenfeld MA, Nakamura H, Scherer EM, Pavirani A, Lecocq JP, Crystal RG (1992) Expression of the human cystic fibrosis transmembrane conductance regulator gene in the mouse lung after in vivo intratracheal plasmid-mediated gene transfer. Nucleic Acids Res 20:3233–3240

Yovandich J, O'Malley B Jr, Sikes M, Ledley FD (1995) Gene transfer to synovial cells by intra-articular administration of plasmid DNA. Hum Gene Ther 65:603–610

6 Uptake of DNA by Keratinocytes

U. R. HENGGE, E. TSCHAKARJAN,
A. MIRMOHAMMDSADEGH, M. GOOS, H. E. MEYER

Introduction

For genes to be expressed in skin and other tissues, a variety of different events have to occur. First, following intradermal injection of naked plasmid DNA, it has to be transported to the cells that potentially take it up. Most likely, physical pressure and the concentration gradient play an important role. Secondly, when plasmid DNA reaches the basal membrane, it has to overcome this adhesion structure. Thirdly, transport within the epidermis has to occur and plasmid DNA has to reach the keratinocyte cell membrane. At the cell membrane, uptake into the cytoplasm may occur. When inside the cell, the majority of the plasmid will be degraded in endosomal and lysosomal compartments. However, a proportion of the DNA will be released from the acidic compartments and arrive at the nuclear membrane, where some of it may be internalized into the nucleus for transcription to occur. All these steps are prerequisites before DNA can be transcribed. Whereas many of the mentioned processes are only incompletely understood, more detailed information exists on the various uptake mechanisms.

Mechanisms of Endocytosis

All eukaryotic cells possess one or multiple forms of endocytosis (Mukherjee et al. 1997; Fig. 6.1). Its major function is the maintenance of cellular homeostasis through uptake, secretion and transmission of metabolic and proliferative signals. Most information is available on receptor-mediated endocytosis, where specificity is maintained by receptor-ligand interactions such as the epithelial and keratinocyte growth factor receptor (Marchese et al. 1998, Smith and Wu 1999). Other endocytosis mechanisms are less specific such as phagocytosis, pinocytosis and uptake through caveolae (potocytosis) or clathrin-coated pits (Fig. 6.1).

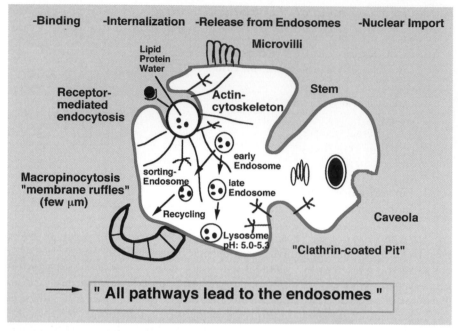

Fig. 6.1. Cellular uptake mechanisms

Receptor-Mediated Endocytosis

In receptor-mediated endocytosis, the receptor-ligand complex is internalized upon binding of the ligand to its respective receptor. Inside the cytoplasm, the complex is packaged and transported as a clathrin-coated vesicle to the endosomes, where disassembly occurs (Pisharee and Payne 1998). The structure of the clathrin-coated vesicle is composed of the triskelion (three 192 kD and three 30 kD proteins) and the adaptins that are required for intracellular delivery to certain organelles. Together with accessory proteins these proteins form the characteristic polyhedral structure of clathrin-coated vesicles (Hirst and Robinson 1998, Pisharee and Payne 1998). Recently, the ubiquitin-proteasome system has been identified as a regulator of endocytosis (Stous and Govers 1999).

Phagocytosis and Pinocytosis

Phagocytosis and pinocytosis are alternative endocytosis mechanisms in response to particulate stimuli (Kwiatkowska and Sobota 1999). Phagocytic leukocytes such as macrophages, neutrophils and monocytes utilize conserved programs of signaling and motility to engulf foreign pathogens of up to 1 or 2 μm (Gottlieb et al. 1993, Greenberg 1999). Upon particle binding to scavenger receptors, receptor clustering occurs which is followed by the activation of protein kinases. For Fc (IgG)-receptor mediated phagocytosis, the recruitment of cytosolic tyrosine kinases, most notably Syk, has been shown (Hunter et al. 1999). As a consequence, actin filaments assemble enabling pseudopod extension. This process is controlled by several GTPases, including Rac-1, ARF6 and Cdc42.

Caveolae and Potocytosis

Potocytosis characterizes the uptake of small molecules via caveolae (Anderson 1998). Caveolae were first identified in 1955. They are rod-like invaginations of the plasma membrane with a diameter of 50–100 nm (Chang et al. 1994). They occur in most cell types and are not continuously coated. Caveolae are very dynamic structures and fulfill a variety of different functions (Anderson 1998). These functions include signal transduction (Lisanti et al. 1994), potocytosis and transcytosis (Anderson 1998), and receptor-mediated endocytosis (Schnitzer et al. 1994). However, little is known about the regulation of invagination and sprouting of caveolae. In contrast to receptor-mediated endocytosis with clathrin-coated pits, potocytosis can be inhibited by cholesterin-binding drugs such as filipin (Schnitzer et al. 1994), cytochalasin D (Parton et al. 1994) and inhibitors of protein kinase C (Smart et al. 1994).

Caveolae are characterized by caveolins 1–3, 20–25 kD proteins, which contain hair pin structures in their hydrophobic region within the plasma membrane, whereas the amino- and carboxy-domains remain intracytoplasmatic (Rothberg et al. 1992). Within the caveolae, a variety of different proteins such as phosphotyrosine kinase, glycolipids, inositol triphosphate and glycosylphosphatidylinositol (GPI)-anchored proteins have been described (Fujimoto et al. 1993, Fiedler et al. 1994, Mayor et al. 1994, Schnitzer et al. 1995).

Caveolae have been proposed as a mechanism for uptake of small molecules of less than 2000 kD. Perhaps DNA, with a diameter of 2 nm can be considered such a small molecule. If the plasmid DNA enters cells in a circular form, the smallest possible cross-sectional diameter would be about 2 nm×4 nm.

Alternatively, McNeil and Steinhardt have suggested that cells undergo transient membrane microdisruptions (McNeil and Steinhardt 1997). They have shown that a variety of cells such as gastric epithelial cells or skin epidermal cells take up fluorescent dextran or horseradish peroxidase into the cytoplasm. In that regard, plasmid DNA could enter epithelial cells via such membrane disruptions. The decreased expression by myotubes exposed to naked DNA at 4 °C could result from a decrease in transient membrane disruptions as a result of reduced membrane fluidity. The entry of DNA into T-tubules of muscle and caveolae at 4 °C indicated that this distribution was energy-independent (Wolff et al. 1992). In contrast to plasmid DNA uptake, oligonucleotides are likely taken up by endocytosis (Loke et al. 1989, Shoji et al. 1991, Zhao et al. 1993).

Mechanisms of DNA Uptake by Keratinocytes

Various mechanisms such as receptor-mediated endocytosis or uptake by caveolae (called potocytosis) have been implicated in DNA uptake (Wolff et al. 1992, Anderson 1998). More specifically, uptake in muscle cells has been shown to depend on their differentiation state with small myotubes exhibiting the highest uptake. Uptake was also temperature-dependent with higher uptake (and expression) occurring at 37 than at 4 °C (Dowty et al. 1995). The presence of plasmid DNA in the majority of mouse myofibers suggested that access of the plasmid DNA to the myofiber was not the rate-limiting step for expression since only a proportion of cells expressed the marker gene. However, in primate muscles, the injected plasmid DNA was located more within the perimysial than within the endomysial space. This difference is likely due to the primate perimysium being thicker than the mouse perimysium (Jiao et al. 1992, Dowty et al. 1995). This also helps to explain the lower DNA expression following injection of primate muscle. The demonstration that transfected myofibers occur at sites distant from the injected area indicated transport of DNA within myofibers.

Generally it seems unlikely, that there is a special uptake mechanism for DNA. More likely, the DNA may use an existing pathway of another molecule. Active uptake of naked plasmid DNA by mammalian cells has never been described, but it is known that gram-positive bacteria are transformed by the transport of single-stranded DNA through a protein pore in the bacterial membrane (Lacks and Greenberg 1976). Moreover, gram-positive bacteria such as hemophilus have specific membrane receptors that enable double-stranded DNA to enter small surface vesicles.

In summary, the mechanism by which keratinocytes internalize plasmid DNA is unknown, but a protein-mediated transport has been suggested (Noonberg et al. 1993, Brandt et al. 1998, Laktionov et al. 1999, White et al. 1999 a). It has also been hypothesized how DNA fragments are involved in the pathogenesis of lupus erythematosus, a systemic autoimmune disease (Bennett et al. 1987, Hefeneider et al. 1990). In lupus erythematosus patients, a variety of autoantibodies against nuclear constituents and cell membrane surface molecules can be detected. A putative 30 kD DNA-binding protein has been identified on white blood cells i.e. T lymphocytes, B lymphocytes, monocytes and neutrophils and may serve as a target in lupus patients (Bennett et al. 1987, Hefeneider et al. 1990). Binding occurred with a saturable ligand receptor kinetics and a K_d of 10^{-9}. In addition, gene therapy has exploited basic principles by targeting DNA to certain tissues (e.g. liver or lung) via scavenger receptors such as the asialoglycoprotein receptor or glycoproteins for targeting to lectins present on epithelial cells (Fajac et al. 1999, Smith and Wu 1999).

DNA-Binding Proteins of the Cell Membrane

DNA-binding proteins have been described on various cell membranes (Bennett et al. 1985, Hefeneider et al. 1990, Schubbert et al. 1997). In that regard oligonucleotide-binding and plasmid DNA-binding proteins have to be distinguished.

On human lymphocytes, Gasparro et al. have described three DNA-binding proteins (28 kD, 59 kD and 79 kD) following hybridization with ^{32}P-labeled calf thymus DNA (Gasparro et al. 1990). On skeletal muscle of rabbits, Hagstrom et al. have identified three DNA-binding proteins as 28 kD, 60 kD and 95 kD using a ^{32}P-labeled double-stranded linearized pBluescript probe (Hagstrom et al. 1996, Levy et al. 1996).

On the other hand, oligonucleotide-binding proteins have been identified on plasma membranes. These oligonucleotide-binding proteins have been characterized as 75 kD and 90 kD in size and named nucleic acid-binding protein-1 (Loke et al. 1989, Yakubov et al. 1989). Additional oligonucleotide-binding proteins have been identified in K562 leukemia-cells (137–147 kD and 79–85 kD) and, more recently, in kidney tubuli with a molecular weight of 97 kD (Beltinger et al. 1995, Hanss et al. 1998). In addition, oligonucleotides have been demonstrated to bind to the EGF- and VEGF-receptor, and to other heparin-binding proteins such as acid and basic fibroblast growth factor (FGF) and platelet-derived growth factor (PDGF) (Guvakova et al. 1995). Recently, the leukocyte integrin Mac-1 (CD11b/CD18) has been identified to bind phosphodiester and phosphorothioate oligodeoxynucleotides (Benimetskaya et al. 1997).

Demonstration of Oligonucleotide Uptake in Keratinocyte Cultures

To expand on the reported data of oligonucleotide uptake between 20mer and 40mer phosphodiester and phosphorothioate oligonucleotides that have been shown to localize in a perinuclear and nucleolar distribution (Noonberg et al. 1993, Laktionov et al. 1999, White et al. 1999a and b), we generated DNA fragments of 120 bp, 262 bp and 664 bp from the expression vector pcDNA$_3$, that were FITC-labeled.

Primary human keratinocytes were shown to readily take up oligonucleotides up to 664 base pairs without the presence of cationic lipids (Tschakarjan et al. 1999). As has been described, they localized to the nucleus and nucleolus following three hours incubation at a concentration of 4 μM. The uptake and internalization was temperature-dependent. This is in line with other reports, where in HaCaT cells uptake was reduced at 4 °C (Noonberg et al. 1993, Brandt et al. 1998). In accordance with the literature, the uptake was time-dependent, the transfection rate being 5% after 1 hour, whereas after 3 hours up to 20% of cultured keratinocytes contained labeled oligonucleotides. Other investigators have shown that oligonucleotides known to readily enter cultured keratinocytes had a decreased ability to penetrate the skin under iontophoretic conditions (Brandt et al. 1998). When uptake was studied after enzymatic digestion with trypsin, almost no uptake was seen. Following keratinocyte culture, a transfection rate of close to 20% could again be demonstrated suggesting a protein-mediated uptake mechanism. Various factors have been identified to increase oligonucleotide delivery to keratinocytes such as liposomal encapsulation (2.3-fold), low confluence (3.3-fold) and release from M-phase arrest (Noonberg et al. 1993, White et al. 1999b). Interestingly, oligonucleotide uptake in HaCaT cells was only detected at about 1% by White et al. (1999b), but up to 15% by other investigators (Laktionov et al. 1999). Collectively, these results showed that oligonucleotide uptake is fast, irreversible, saturable and temperature-dependent (Laktionov et al. 1999). High-affinity, cell-specific interactions were detected with membrane proteins of 61–63 and 35 kD, respectively. Uptake was considerably reduced following trypsinization and pretreatment with polyanions or unlabeled oligonucleotides, suggesting a specific interaction.

The interaction of oligonucleotides with various barrier fluid proteins occurring in tear and saliva revealed binding to lactoferrin, lysozyme and immunoglobulins A and G (Laktionov et al. 1997). Binding was likely interfering with the stability and permeation of biological barriers.

Flow cytometric analysis of keratinocyte uptake of FITC-oligonucleotides has shown two different populations of cells (Wingens et al. 1998). A bright population of highly fluorescent small cells and a dim population of less fluorescent but larger cells have been characterized. The heterogeneity of uptake between these two populations was not a result from differences in cell cycle. In contrast to other investigators, the magnitude of fluorescence was seen intracytoplasmatically (Wingens et al. 1998).

The in vivo uptake of FITC-labeled oligonucleotides has also been investigated with regard to differentiation in a 3-dimensional skin model (Giachetti and Chin 1996). Whereas in culture about 9% of keratinocytes showed nuclear staining, up to 95% of granular cells accumulated oligonucleotides in the 3-dimensional model, where keratinocytes had the ability to undergo differentiation. Interestingly, basal keratinocytes were only FITC-positive in 3% and revealed a membrane staining pattern. 75% of the differentiating cells with accumulating oligonucleotides were viable. A recent study from White et al. has shown that a high concentration of phosphorothioate anti-sense oligonucleotide (10–50 µM) was found in the nuclei of basal and suprabasal cells 1–2 hours after intradermal injection into athymic mice as evidenced by live confocal microscopy (White et al. 1999a). Single FITC-labeled nucleotides did not accumulate in a nuclear pattern, therefore making a premature degradation unlikely. Upon topical application, most FITC-staining was seen in the stratum corneum. Following tape-stripping, as little as 5 µM anti-sense oligonucleotide was required to yield nuclear staining.

Uptake of Plasmid DNA

Uptake and expression of plasmid DNA has been demonstrated in the skin following intradermal injection (Hengge et al. 1995, 1996, 1998) and recently also in hair follicles upon topical delivery (Fan et al. 1999). While amounts of the expressed transgene seemed smaller than in interfollicular keratinocytes, the generation of humoral and cellular immune responses was possible (Fan et al. 1999). Our latest results showed an important tropism of adeno-associated virus vectors for hair follicle keratinocytes (Hengge and Goos 2000).

To elucidate the mechanism of internalization, the existence of plasmid DNA-binding proteins of the keratinocyte membrane was investigated. Therefore, membrane proteins were prepared from epidermal lysates and reacted with labeled DNA in Southwestern blot assays. For hybridization, a digoxigenin-labeled calf thymus DNA probe was used. Membrane preparations from lymphocytes and skeletal muscle were used as positive controls. Using this technique, we were able to characterize three membrane proteins with DNA-binding ability. These proteins were found to have a molecular weight of 78 kD, 80 kD and 98 kD (Tschakarjan et al. 1999; Fig. 6.2). In porcine mucosa, three additional proteins were found of 65 kD, 120 kD and 130 kD in size. These proteins bound ultrasound-treated calf thymus DNA as well as double-stranded linearized pcDNA3. By two-dimensional gel electrophoresis two of the three proteins could again be demonstrated to bind DNA (Fig. 6.3). By mass spectrometry, these proteins were identified as ezrin (80 kD) and moesin (78 kD). In Western blots, ez-

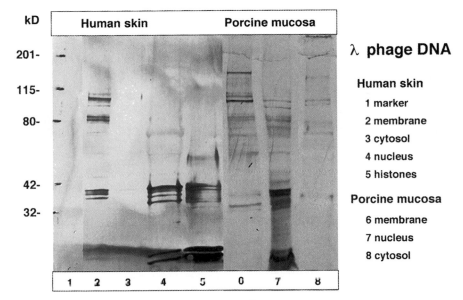

Fig. 6.2. DNA-binding proteins: South-Western Blot

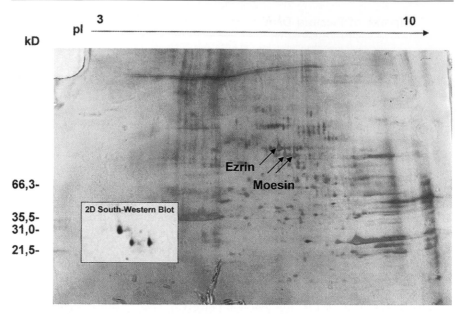

Fig. 6.3. DNA-binding proteins: 2D-gel electrophoresis

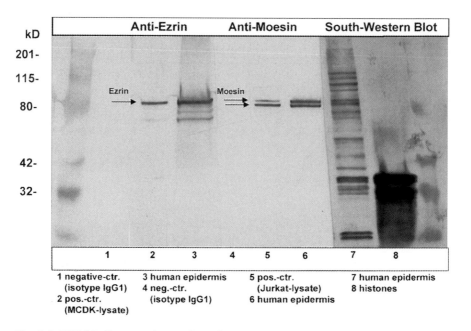

Fig. 6.4. DNA-binding proteins: Ezrin and moesin

rin and moesin were visualized to colocalize with the two DNA-binding membrane proteins seen in Southwestern technique (Fig. 6.4).

The response of keratinocytes to exogenous DNA is currently being investigated. Recent studies of the splenocyte response to exogenous DNA have demonstrated to stimulate splenocyte proliferation. The addition of monovalent Fab fragments of anti-mouse antibodies reduced the plasmid DNA-induced lymphocyte proliferation suggesting the involvement of immunoglobulin receptors (Rykova et al. 1999).

Ezrin and Moesin as Membrane–Cytoskeleton Linkers

Ezrin and moesin belong to a highly homologous family of proteins that connect the plasma membrane with the actin skeleton at specific locations (Lankes and Furthmayr 1991, Sato et al. 1992, Bretscher 1999). In addition, ezrin and moesin are involved in signal transduction (Bretscher 1999) and growth control (Fazioli et al. 1993, Gautreau et al. 1999). Although ezrin (and moesin) have no transmembrane portion, they are functionally associated with a variety of transmembrane receptors such as ICAM-1 and -2, CD44, CD43 and the EGF-receptor (Yonemura et al. 1998).

Whereas the members of the band 4.1-family of cytoskeletal proteins (talin, merlin, radixin, moesin and ezrin) contain a high degree of homology in the amino-terminal portion, ezrin, moesin and radixin are highly homologous in the entire sequence (Sato et al. 1992, Majander-Nordenswan et al. 1998). They contain a homologous amino-terminus, followed by an α-helix (Fig. 6.5). In the ezrin and radixin molecules a polyprolin stretch is inserted before the C-terminus. Whereas the C-terminus contains binding sites for F-actin (Sato et al. 1992), the amino-terminus is used to interact with transmembrane receptors such as CD44 through a 357 amino acid binding protein, named EBP50 (ezrin-, radixin-, moesin-binding phosphoprotein-50) (Reczek et al. 1997, Reczek and Bretscher 1998) that has been found in polarized epithelia. This protein was found to co-localize with ezrin in apical microvilli of epithelial cells (Reczek and Bretscher 1998). It was found to bind to the 30 carboxy-terminal amino acids of the N-terminus of ezrin, radixin and moesin. Binding sites at the N-terminus (EBP50) that are expected to interact with the intracytoplasmic portions of various transmembrane receptors have not yet been characterized. The N-terminus of ezrin contains a multivalent binding site shown to interact with EBP50, Rho-GDI, with the C-terminus of ezrin and the cytoplasmic part of CD44. However, there exist no sequence homologies among the binding partners.

Besides binding to actin, a homotypic binding of the C-terminus to the N-terminus has been described for moesin and ezrin masking the binding site for actin (Gary and Bretscher 1993, Matsui et al. 1998, Oshiro et al. 1998; Fig. 6.5). Following phosphorylation of ezrin, the homotypic head-to-tail-binding is resolved and the binding site for F-actin is exposed. Actin can bind the C-terminus of ezrin and contribute to the cell morphology. Following the phosphorylation of ezrin, actin and ezrin have been shown to accumulate at zones of membrane protrusion. In association with the enlargement of the cell surface, the endocytotic activity increases.

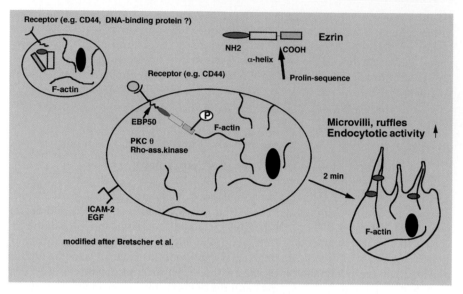

Fig. 6.5. Ezrin/Moesin – crosslinkers and signal transducers?

Ezrin and moesin are expressed in human lymphocytes, monocytes and neutrophils. However, moesin is the more abundant ERM protein in lymphocytes
with up to 0.5% of the entire cellular protein in lymphocytes and endothelial
cells. Moesin is the only ERM protein in platelets, liver and gut. From a functional standpoint, ezrin, radixin and moesin seem to be redundant since a moesin knockout mouse did not reveal any morphological or functional alterations
on the cellular and tissue level (Doi et al. 1999).

Ezrin and Signal Transduction via the EGF-receptor

In addition to the established role of ezrin as a membrane-actin-bridge protein,
several studies have analyzed the interaction of ezrin with second messengers. It
has been found, that ezrin serves as a target for several protein kinases
(Bretscher 1989, Bretscher and Aguado-Velasco 1998). For example in A431-cells,
two minutes following stimulation with EGF, causing transient phosphorylation
of tyrosine residues, a phenotypic change of the cell morphology with membrane ruffles and microvilli occurs (Bretscher 1989; Fig. 6.5). Phosphorylation
occurs on tyrosine 146 and 354 of ezrin by the EGF-receptor tyrosine kinase
(Krieg and Hunter 1992, Bretscher and Aguado-Velasco 1998, Marchese et al.
1998). In addition, recent data showed that the association of ERM-proteins with
transmembrane receptors such as CD44 is regulated through Rho-dependent
pathways (Hall 1990, Ridley and Hall 1992, Hirao et al. 1996, Mackay et al. 1997,
Takahashi et al. 1997, Matsui et al. 1998).

Following these results, the DNA-binding epitopes in the ezrin molecule need
to be characterized in order to elucidate the mechanism and biological function

of this newly recognized property of proteins commonly known as cytoskeleton-membrane linkers. In addition, the reaction of keratinocytes in response to uptake of exogenous DNA needs to be investigated.

Acknowledgements. The contribution of Kirsten Trappmann (Department of Dermatology, Venerology and Allergology, University of Essen) and Dorian Immler (Institute of Physiological Chemistry, University of Bochum) with regard to the identification of DNA-binding proteins of keratinocytes is gratefully acknowledged. We are grateful to Hagen Apel for expert photographical support.

References

Anderson RG (1998) The caveolae membrane system. Annu Rev Biochem 67:199–225

Beltinger C, Saragovi HU, Smith RM, LeSauteur L, Shah N, DeDionisio L, Christensen L, Raible A, Jarett L, Gewirtz AM (1995) Binding, uptake, and intracellular trafficking of phosphorothioate-modified oligodeoxynucleotides. J Clin Invest 95:1814–1823

Benimetskaya L, Loike JD, Khaled Z, Loike G, Silverstein SC, Cao L, Khoury JE, Cai TQ, Stein CA (1997) Mac-1 (CD11/CD18) is an oligodeoxynucleotide-binding protein. Nat Med 3:414–420

Bennett RM, Gabor GT, Merritt MM (1985) DNA binding to human leukocytes. Evidence for a receptor-mediated association, internalization, and degradation of DNA. J Clin Invest 76:2182–2190

Bennett RM, Kotzin BL, Merritt MJ (1987) DNA receptor dysfunction in systemic lupus erythematosus and kindred disorders. J Exp Med 166:850–863

Brandt RM, Haase K, Hannah TL, Iversen PL (1998) An experimental model for interpreting percutaneous penetration of oligonucleotides that incorporates the role of keratinocytes. J Invest Dermatol 111:1166–1171

Bretscher A (1989) Rapid phosphorylation and reorganization of ezrin and spectrin accompany morphological changes induced in A-431 cells by epidermal growth factor. J Cell Biol 108:921–930

Bretscher A (1999) Regulation of cortical structure by the ezrin-radixin-moesin protein family. Curr Opin Cell Biol 11:109–116

Bretscher MS, Aguado-Velasco C (1998) EGF induces recycling membrane to form ruffles. Curr Biol 8:721–724

Chang WJ, Ying YS, Rothberg KG, Hooper NM, Turner AJ, Gambliel HA, De Gunzburg J, Mumby SM, Gilman AG, Anderson RG (1994) Purification and characterization of smooth muscle cell caveolae. J Cell Biol 126:127–138

Doi Y, Itoh M, Yonemura S, Ishihara S, Takano H, Noda T, Tsukita S (1999) Normal development of mice and unimpaired cell adhesion/cell motility/actin-based cytoskeleton without compensatory up-regulation of ezrin or radixin in moesin gene knockout. J Biol Chem 22:2315–2321

Dowty ME, Williams P, Zhang G, Hagstrom JE, Wolff JA (1995) Plasmid DNA entry into postmitotic nuclei of primary rat myotubes. Proc Natl Acad Sci USA 92:4572–4576

Fajac I, Briand P, Monsigny M, Midoux P (1999) Sugar-mediated uptake of glycosylated polylysines and gene transfer into normal and cystic fibrosis airway epithelial cells. Hum Gene Ther 10:395–406

Fan H, Lin Q, Morrissey GR, Khavari PA (1999) Immunization via hair follicles by topical application of naked DNA to normal skin. Nat Biotechnol 17:870–872

Fazioli F, Wong WT, Ullrich SJ, Sakaguchi K, Appella E, Di Fiore PP (1993) The ezrin-like family of tyrosine kinase substrates: receptor-specific pattern of tyrosine phosphorylation and relationship to malignant transformation. Oncogene 8:1335–1345

Fiedler K, Parton RG, Kellner R, Etzold T, Simons K (1994) VIP36, a novel component of glycolipid rafts and exocytic carrier vesicles in epithelial cells. EMBO J 13:1729–1740

Fujimoto T, Miyawaki A, Mikoshiba K (1995) Inositol 1,4,5-triphosphate receptor-like protein in plasmalemmal caveolae is linked to actin filaments. J Cell Sci 108:7–15

Gary R, Bretscher A (1993) Heterotypic and homotypic associations between ezrin and moesin, two putative membrane-cytoskeletal linking proteins. Proc Natl Acad Sci USA 90:10 846–10 850

Gasparro FP, Dall'Amico R, O'Malley M, Heald PW, Edelson RL (1990) Cell membrane DNA: a new target for psoralen photoadduct formation. Photochem Photobiol 52:315–321

Gautreau A, Poullet P, Louvard D, Arpin M (1999) Ezrin, a plasma membrane-microfilament linker, signals cell survival through the phosphatidylinositol 3-kinase/Akt pathway. Proc Natl Acad Sci USA 96:7300–7305

Giachetti C, Chin DJ (1996) Increased oligonucleotide permeability in keratinocytes of artificial skin correlates with differentiation and altered membrane function. J Invest Dermatol 106:412–418

Greenberg S (1999) Modular components of phagocytosis. J Leukoc Biol 66:712–717

Gottlieb TA, Ivanov IE, Adesnik M, Sabatini DD (1993) Actin microfilaments play a critical role in endocytosis at the apical but not the basolateral surface of polarized epithelial cells. J Cell Biol 120:695–710

Guvakova MA, Yakubov LA, Vlodavsky I, Tonkinson JL, Stein CA (1995) Phosphorothioate oligodeoxynucleotides bind to basic fibroblast growth factor, inhibit its binding to cell surface receptors, and remove it from low affinity binding sites on extracellular matrix. J Biol Chem 270:2620–2627

Hagstrom JE, Sebestyen MG, Budker V, Ludtke JJ, Fritz JD, Wolff JA (1996) Complexes of non-cationic liposomes and histone H1 mediate efficient transfection of DNA without encapsulation. Biochem Biophys Acta 1284:47–55

Hall A (1990) The cellular functions of small GTP-binding proteins. Science 249:635–640

Hanss B, Leal-Pinto E, Bruggeman LA, Copeland TD, Klotman PE (1998) Identification and characterization of a cell membrane nucleic acid channel. Proc Natl Acad Sci USA 95:1921–1926

Hefeneider SH, Bennett RM, Pham TQ, Cornell K, McCoy SL, Heinrich MC (1990) Identification of a cell-surface DNA receptor and its association with systemic lupus erythematodes. J Invest Dermatol 94:79 S–84 S

Hengge UR, Goos M (2000) Adeno-associated virus expresses transgenes in hair follicles and epidermis. Mol Ther, in print

Hengge UR, Chan EF, Foster RA, Walker PS, Vogel JC (1995) Cytokine gene expression in epidermis with biological effects following injection of naked DNA. Nat Genet 10:161–166

Hengge UR, Walker PS, Vogel JC (1996) Expression of naked DNA in human, pig and mouse skin. J Clin Invest 97:2911–2916

Hengge UR, Pfützner W, Williams M, Goos M, Vogel JC (1998) Efficient expression of naked plasmid DNA in mucosal epithelium: prospective for the treatment of skin lesions. J Invest Dermatol 111:605–608

Hirao M, Sato N, Kondo T, Yonemura S, Monden M, Sasaki T, Takai Y, Tsukita Sh, Tsukita S (1996) Regulation mechanism of ERM (ezrin/radixin/moesin) protein/plasma membrane association; possible involvement of phosphatidylinositol turnover and rho-dependent signaling pathway. J Cell Biol 135:37–51

Hirst J, Robinson MS (1998) Clathrin and adaptors. Biochem Biophys Acta 1404:173–193

Hunter S, Sato N, Kim MK, Huang ZY, Chu DH, Park JG, Schreiber AD (1999) Structural requirements of Syk kinase for Fc gamma receptor-mediated phagocytosis. Exp Hematol 5:875–884

Jiao S, Williams P, Berg RK, Hodgeman BA, Liu L, Repetto G, Wolff JA (1992) Direct gene transfer into nonhuman primate myofibers in vivo. Hum Gene Ther 3:21–33

Krieg J, Hunter T (1992) Identification of the two major epidermal growth factor-induced tyrosine phosphorylation sites in the microvillar core protein ezrin. J Biol Chem 267:19 258–19 265

Kwiatkowska K, Sobota A (1999) Signaling pathways in phagocytosis. Bioassays 5:422–431

Lacks S, Greenberg B (1976) Single-strand breakage on binding of DNA to cells in the genetic transformation of Diplococcus pneumoniae. J Mol Biol 101:255–275

Laktionov PP, Rykova EYu, Krepkii DV, Bryksin AV, Vlassov VV (1997) Interaction of oligonucleotides with barrier fluid proteins. Biochemistry 62:613–618

Laktionov PP, Dazard JE, Vives E, Rykova EY, Piette J, Vlassov VV, Lebleu B (1999) Characterisation of membrane oligonucleotide-binding proteins and oligonucleotide uptake in keratinocytes. Nucleic Acids Res 27:2315–2324

Lankes WT, Furthmayr H (1991) Moesin: A member of the protein 4.1-talin-ezrin family of proteins. Proc Natl Acad Sci USA 88:8297–8301

Levy MY, Barron LG, Meyer KB, Szoka FC Jr (1996) Characterization of plasmid DNA transfer into mouse skeletal muscle: evaluation of uptake mechanism, expression and secretion of gene products into blood. Gene Ther 3:201–211

Lisanti MP, Tang ZL, Sargiacomo M (1993) Caveolin forms a hetero-oligomeric protein complex that interacts with an apical GPI-linked protein: implications for the biogenesis of caveolae. J Cell Biol 123:595–604

Loke SL, Stein CA, Zhang XH, Mori K, Nakanishi M, Subasinghe C, Cohen JS, Neckers LM (1989) Characterization of oligonucleotide transport into living cells. Proc Natl Acad Sci USA 86:3474–3478

Mackay DJG, Esch F, Furthmayr H, Hall A (1997) Rho- and Rac-dependent assembly of focal adhesion complexes and actin filaments in permeabilized fibroblasts: an essential role for ezrin/radixin/moesin proteins. J Cell Biol 138:927–938

Majander-Nordenswan P, Sainio M, Tuurunen O, Jääskeläinen J, Carpén O, Kere J, Vaheri A (1998) Genomic structure of the human ezrin gene. Hum Genet 103:662–665

Marchese C, Mancini P, Belleudi F, Felici A, Gradini R, Sansolini T, Frati L, Torrisi MR (1998) Receptor-mediated endocytosis of keratinocyte growth factor. J Cell Science 111:3517–3527

Matsui T, Maeda M, Doi Y, Yonemura S, Amano M, Kaibuchi K, Tsukita S, Tsukita Sh (1998) Rho-kinase phosphorylates COOH-terminal threonines of ezrin/radixin/moesin (ERM) proteins and regulates their head-to-tail association. J Cell Biol 140:647–657

Mayor S, Rothberg KG, Maxfield F (1994) Sequestration of GPI-anchored proteins in caveolae triggered by cross-linking. Science 264:1948–1951

McNeil PL, Steinhardt RA (1997) Loss, restoration, and maintenance of plasma membrane integrity. J Cell Biol 137:1–4

Mukherjee S, Gnosh RN, Maxfield FR (1997) Endocytosis. Physiological Reviews 77:759–790

Noonberg SB, Garovoy MR, Hunt CA (1993) Characteristics of oligonucleotide uptake in human keratinocyte cultures. J Invest Dermatol 101:727–731

Oshiro N, Fukata Y, Kaibuchi K (1998) Phosphorylation of moesin by rho-associated kinase (Rho-kinase) plays a crucial role in the formation of microvilli-like structures. J Biol Chem 25:34663–34666

Parton RG, Joggerst B, Simons K (1994) Regulated internalization of caveolae. J Cell Biol 127:1199–1215

Pisharee B and Payne GS (1998) Clathrin coats – threads laid bare. Cell 95:443–446

Reczek D, Bretscher A (1998) The carboxyl-terminal region of EBP50 binds to a site in the amino-terminal domain of ezrin that is masked in the dormant molecule. J Biol Chem 273:18452–18458

Reczek D, Berryman M, Bretscher A (1997) Identification of EBP50: A PDZ-containing phosphoprotein that associates with members of the ezrin-radixin-moesin family. J Cell Biol 139:169–179

Ridley AJ, Hall A (1992) The small GTP-binding protein rho regulates the assembly of focal adhesions and actin stress fibers in response to growth factors. Cell 70:389–399

Rothberg KG, Heuser JE, Donzell WC, Ying YS, Glenney JR, Anderson RGW (1992) Caveolin, a protein component of caveolae membrane coats. Cell 68:673–682

Rykova EY, Laktionov PP, Vlassov VV (1999) Activation of spleen lymphocytes by plasmid DNA. Vaccine 17:1193–1200

Sato N, Funayama N, Nagafuchi A, Yonemura S, Tsukita S, Tsukita S (1992) A gene family consisting of ezrin, radixin and moesin. Its specific localization at actin filament/plasma membrane association sites. J Cell Sci 103:131–143

Schnitzer JE, Oh P, Pinney E, Allard J (1994) Filipin-sensitive caveolae-mediated transport in endothelium: reduced transcytosis, scavenger endocytosis, and capillary permeability of select macromolecules. J Cell Biol 127:1217–1232

Schnitzer JE, Liu J, Oh P (1995) Endothelial caveolae have the molecular transport machinery for vesicle budding, docking, and fusion including VAMP, NSF, SNAP, annexins, and GTPases. J Biol Chem 270:14399–14404

Schubbert R, Renz D, Schmitz B, Doerfler W (1997) Foreign (M13) DNA ingested by mice reaches peripheral leukocytes, spleen, and liver via the intestinal wall mucosa and can be covalently linked to mouse DNA. Proc Natl Acad Sci USA 94:961–966

Shoji Y, Akhtar S, Periasamy A, Herman B, Juliano RL (1991) Mechanism of cellular uptake of modified oligodeoxynucleotides containing methylphosphonate linkages. Nucleic Acids Res 19:5543–5550

Smart EJ, Foster DC, Ying YS, Kamen BA, Anderson RG (1994) Protein kinase C activators inhibit receptor-mediated potocytosis by preventing internalization of caveolae. J Cell Biol 124:307–313

Smith RM, Wu GY (1999) Hepatocyte-directed gene delivery by receptor-mediated endocytosis. Semin Liver Dis 19:83–92

Stous GJ, Govers R (1999) The ubiquitin-proteasome system and endocytosis. J Cell Sci 112:1417–1423

Takahashi K, Sasaki T, Mammoto A, Takaishi K, Kameyama T, Tsukita S, Tsukita Sh, Takai Y (1997) Direct interaction of the Rho GDP dissociation inhibitor with ezrin/radixin/moesin initiates the activation of the Rho small G protein. J Biol Chem 272: 23371–23375

Tschakarjan E, Trappmann K, Immler D, Meyer HE, Mirmohammadsadegh A, Hengge UR (1999) Keratinocytes take up naked plasmid DNA: evidence for DNA-binding proteins in keratinocyte membranes. J Invest Dermatol 113:434

White PJ, Fogarty RD, Liepe IJ, Delaney PM, Werther GA, Wraight C (1999a) Live confocal microscopy of oligonucleotide uptake by keratinocytes in human skin grafts on nude mice. J Invest Dermatol 112:887–892

White PJ, Fogarty RD, McKean SC, Venables DJ, Werther GA, Wraight CJ (1999b) Oligonucleotide uptake in cultured keratinocytes: influence of confluence, cationic liposomes, and keratinocyte cell type. J Invest Dermatol 112:699–705

Wingens M, van Hooijdonk CA, de Jongh GJ, Schalkwijk J, van Erp PE (1998) Flow cytometric and microscopic characterization of the uptake and distribution of phosphorothioate oligonucleotides in human keratinocytes. Arch Dermatol Res 290:119–125

Wolff JA, Dowty ME, Jiao S, Repetto G, Berg RK, Ludtke JJ, Williams P, Slatterback DB (1992) Expression of naked plasmids by cultured myotubes and entry of plasmids into T tubules and caveolae of mammalian skeletal muscle. J Cell Sci 103:1249–1259

Yakubov LA, Deeva EA, Zarytova VF, Ivanova EM, Ryte AS, Yurchenko LV, Vlassov VV (1989) Mechanism of oligonucleotide uptake by cells: involvement of specific receptors? Proc Natl Acad Sci USA 86:6454–6458

Yonemura S, Hirao M, Doi Y, Takhashi N, Kondo T, Tsukita S, Tsukita Sh (1998) Ezrin/radixin/moesin (ERM) proteins bind to a positively charged amino acid cluster in the juxta-membrane cytoplasmic domain of CD44, CD43, and ICAM-2. J Cell Biol 140: 885–895

Zhao Q, Matson S, Herrera CJ, Fisher E, Yu H, Krieg AM (1993) Comparison of cellular binding and uptake of antisense phosphodiester, phosphorothioate, and mixed phosphorothioate and methylphosphonate oligonucleotides. Antisense Res Dev 3:53–66

Treatment of Skin Diseases

7 Gene Therapy of Inherited Skin Diseases

G. Meneguzzi, J. Vailly

Introduction

The notion of transferring a gene encoding a therapeutic protein and the design of vectors enabling the introduction of a curative transgene into eukaryotic cells emerged as soon as the first single-gene defects associated with inherited diseases were defined. The extraordinary progress of human genetics in the past ten years has fueled a tremendous interest in gene therapy. Seldom, the general public manifested such an attention to a field of scientific endeavor despite the limited improvement in medical therapies.

Gene transfer to keratinocytes constitutes an attractive strategy for the treatment of genetic disorders because of the ease with which the epidermal cells can be biopsied, expanded in culture, genetically manipulated, grafted back to the patients following well-established procedures used in the treatment of burn injuries and chronic ulcers.

The ultimate goal of gene therapy is to permanently introduce new genetic information into autologous somatic cells and express therapeutic gene products. Gene therapy of inherited skin diseases, however, faces impediments and limitations that, in the eyes of a number of scientists, clinicians and patients make progress uncertain (Hengge et al. 1999). For instance, the general problem of targeting the delivery vectors to a specific cell type and that of regulating the expression of the therapeutic genes remain unresolved. The immune response to specific recombinant polypeptides is another open question.

In this chapter, we shall review the recent progress in somatic gene therapy of genetic skin disorders. The aspects that need to be resolved by basic researchers and clinicians to achieve transfer of therapeutic genes will be emphasized.

Candidate Conditions for a Gene Therapy Approach

Remarkable progress has recently been achieved in elucidating the molecular basis of a variety of monogenic inherited skin diseases (Table 7.1). As a logical consequence, the diseased cells can potentially be cured by the delivery of a wild-type copy of the aberrant gene. Complementation of the two mutated alleles by addition of a normal gene sequence to the cells of affected individuals is theoretically feasible in recessive disorders, where expression, or re-expression of a functional protein is sufficient to restore a defective function. The possibility of manipulating certain functions of a cell or of a whole organ at the molecular level becomes problematic in dominant disorders. Under these conditions, the abnormal gene product thwarts the activity of the wild-type counterparts and also that of any protein synthesized by a curative transgene. As a consequence, in recessive diseases the addition of a functional or therapeutic gene increasing the amount of a curative polypeptide is expected to result in an immediate benefit. Conversely, in dominant conditions, only the inactivation of the mutant allele or the genetic correction of the faulty gene restoring the expression of a normal protein product can reverse the transdominant effect of the causative mutation. At present, the accurate repair of the genetic defects by gene targeting or by trans-splicing remains an ideal method which is, however, severely handicapped by an extremely low efficiency (Milich and Sullenger 1997, Yanez and Porter 1998).

As in other fields, the feasibility of gene therapy strategies for inherited skin diseases has been investigated in recessive conditions such as specific forms of epidermolysis bullosa (EB), ichthyosis, and xeroderma pigmentosum (XP). Dominant diseases, like epidermolytic hyperkeratosis and the simplex and dystrophic forms of epidermolysis bullosa remain at present less amenable to treatment by gene transfer (Table 7.2).

Table 7.1. Progress of gene therapy in specific inherited skin diseases

Condition	Selected genes	Animal model	Stem cell targeting	Reference
Dystrophic EB	Collagen type VII	Yes	No	Sawamura et al. 1999, Palazzi et al. 2000
Junctional EB	Laminin-5 ($\alpha3\ \beta3\ \gamma2$)	Yes	Yes	Gagnoux-Palacios et al. 1996, Dellambra et al. 1998, Vailly et al. 1998
	Collagen XVII	No	No	Seitz et al. 1999
	Integrin $\beta4$	No	No	Gagnoux-Palacios et al. 1997
Lamellar ichthyosis	Transglutaminase 1	Yes	No	Choate et al. 1996b
X-linked ichthyosis	Steroid sulfatase	Yes	No	Freiberg et al. 1997
Xeroderma pigm.	X-A, X-B, X-C groups	No	No	Zeng et al. 1997

EB, Inherited epidermolysis bullosa; Xeroderma pigm., xeroderma pigmentosum

Table 7.2. Selected dermatoses as candidates for skin gene therapy

Selected condition	Candidate genes	Inheritance	Reference
Junctional EB	Integrin $\alpha6$	AR	Ruzzi et al. 1997
Simplex EB	Keratins 5 & 14	AD	Coulombe et al. 1991
Simplex EB with MD	Plectin	AR	Smith et al. 1996
Epidermolytic hyperkeratosis	Keratins 1 & 10	AD	Cheng et al. 1992
Ichtyosis bullosa of Siemens	Keratin 2e	AD	Rothnagel et al. 1994
Epidermolytic PPK	Keratin 9	AD	Torchard et al. 1994
Non-epidermolytic PPK	Keratin 16	AD	Shamsher et al. 1995
Pachyonychia congenita	Keratin 6a & 16/17	AD	McLean et al. 1995
Vohwinkel's syndrome variant	Loricrin	AD	Maestrini et al. 1996
Vohwinkel's syndrome	Connexin26	AD/AR	Maestrini et al. 1999
Basal cell nevus syndrome	Patched	AD	Hahn et al. 1996
Striate PPK	Desmoglein 1	AD	Rickman et al. 1999
Darier's disease	ATP2A2	AD	Sakuntabhai et al. 1999
XP Group E	DDB2	AR	Cleaver et al. 1999
XP Group F	ERCC1	AR	Li et al. 1994
XP Group V	DNA polymerase eta	AR	Masutani et al. 1999

EB, Inherited epidermolysis bullosa; MD, muscular dystrophy; PPK, palmoplantar keratoderma; XP, xeroderma pigmentosum; AR, Autosomal recessive; AD, autosomal dominant

Gene Delivery

Gene therapy exploits the best available technology to optimize gene delivery.
Since keratinocytes and fibroblasts are easily expanded in tissue culture, efficient
gene transfer can be achieved using a range of procedures commonly utilized to
induce mammalian cells to take up and express functional recombinant genes.
These include physical DNA-mediated transfection including direct injection or
electroporation of pure plasmid DNA, the introduction of DNA complexed with
surface-receptors ligands, adenoviral particles, cationic liposomes or ballistic
microprojectiles. These methods are reviewed in chapter 4 of this book. The efficiency of physical transfection is low with a small percentage of targeted cells
both in vitro and in vivo, as demonstrated by the direct transfer of genes into
the integument of animals. Therefore, these procedures are more applicable to
basic studies of gene expression than to somatic gene therapy of inherited genodermatoses. Indeed, gene transfer has been proven to be of inferior efficiency
for a potential clinical use, and the integration of the newly introduced DNA
into the host genome was too infrequent to sustain appreciable stable expres-

sion. The population of transfected keratinocytes can, of course, be enriched using cotransfected selectable genes, but the clonogenic and differentiation potential of the selected cells is often compromised.

Because viruses provide a remarkable assortment of well characterized genetic elements designed to deliver and regulate expression of foreign genes in cells, viral vectors are very relevant to DNA transfer technology. The strong constitutive cytomegalovirus immediate early (the CMV-IE) promoter and retroviral promoters (the LTRs) are widely used to ensure high level expression of recombinant transgenes. Various viral systems have been adapted to develop high efficiency somatic gene transfer. These include vectors based on herpes virus, vaccinia and adeno-associated virus (Mulligan 1993) and more frequently replication-defective adenovirus or retroviruses (Strauss and Barranger 1997). Most of these systems have been designed and used for transient but highly efficient gene transfer. Retroviral vectors based on murine leukemia virus are currently used to achieve long-term phenotypic reversion of diseased cells. The recombinant retroviral particles infect a wide range of mammalian cell types including keratinocytes and permanently integrate into the host cell chromosomes where they are expressed at high efficiency. Since integration requires host cell division, retroviral vectors are conveniently used both to transfect cultured keratinocytes and to target proliferative cells in regenerating tissues in vivo (Ghazizadeh et al. 1999).

Gene Transfer Studies in Genetic Skin Disorders

Inherited Skin Diseases

Epidermolysis bullosa constitutes the prototype condition for genetic therapy because no beneficial treatment is available. The term epidermolysis bullosa encompasses a group of bullous disorders of the skin and mucous membranes characterized by blister formation following varying degrees of trauma. The major forms of epidermolysis bullosa have been classified in defined clinical subtypes according to the morphology and distribution of the lesions and the mode of inheritance (Fine et al. 2000). The genes involved in these disorders have been recently identified. Molecular genetic analysis disclosed that the heterogeneity of clinical phenotypes correlates with a variety of genetic defects altering the expression of the structural proteins connecting the cytoplasm of basal keratinocytes to the basement membrane zone of the dermal-epidermal junction and the papillary dermis (Pulkkinen and Uitto 1999) (Fig. 7.1).

The most recurrent subtypes of the epidermolytic forms of epidermolysis bullosa are autosomal dominant-inherited diseases characterized by an intraepidermal cleavage caused by mutations in the cytokeratin intermediate filaments. At present, the dominant negative nature of the genetic defects causing these ailments represents an overwhelming hurdle for any gene therapy approach. Conversely, cells from patients affected by junctional and recessive dystrophic epidermolysis bullosa provide an ideal scenario to evaluate the capacity of somatic gene

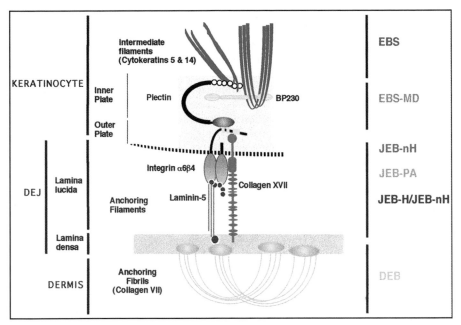

Fig. 7.1. Schematic representation of the basement membrane zone of the dermal-epidermal junction and related genodermatoses. The location of the major protein components of the hemidesmosome-anchoring filament complex and the anchoring fibrils is indicated as suggested by immunoelectron microscopy and recent progress in molecular biology. Hemidesmosomes link the epithelial intermediate filament network to the anchoring filaments of the dermal-epidermal junction (*DEJ*) that interact with the anchoring fibrils of the papillary dermis. Genetic mutations affecting cytokeratins 5 and 14 disrupt the intermediate filaments and are associated with epidermolysis bullosa simplex (*EBS*). Genetic alterations of plectin, which localizes in the inner plate of the hemidesmosome, result in epidermolysis bullosa simplex associated with muscular dystrophy. Integrin $\alpha_6\beta_4$, laminin-5 and collagen XVII are implicated in the junctional forms of epidermolysis bullosa (*JEB*), while genetic abnormalities of collagen VII result in the dystrophic forms (*DEB*) of the disease. *JEB-H,* Herlitz junctional EB; *JEB-nH,* non-Herlitz JEB; *JEB-PA,* JEB with pyloric atresia

therapy to re-express biologically-active adhesion proteins with multiple functional domains that assemble in supramolecular complexes. Such cell adhesion structures, besides providing the cohesion of the integument, mediate signaling between the epithelium and the mesenchyme (Borradori and Sonnenberg 1999).

Thus far, six distinct genes have been identified, resulting in junctional epidermolysis bullosa when mutated. The genes encode three components of the hemidesmosome-anchoring filament complex. Lack of expression of either the cell receptor integrin $\alpha_6\beta_4$ or its extracellular ligand, laminin-5, results in the absence of hemidesmosomes and accounts for the most severe forms of the condition (Aberdam et al. 1994, Vidal et al 1995). Altered expression of these two proteins and that of collagen XVII (McGrath et al. 1995) underlies the milder variants of the disease characterized by skin fragility and blistering that do not affect the patients' life span (Fine et al. 2000). The mild junctional forms of epidermolysis bullosa appear particularly suitable to the development of gene therapy strategies, because these conditions do not require treatment of the whole integument, and the curative polypeptides are encoded by relatively small cDNAs that are easily carried by viral vectors.

The initial efforts of genetic correction of epidermolysis bullosa were performed using immortalized keratinocytes obtained from patients with Herlitz disease. This devastating manifestation of the junctional form of the condition is associated with the absent expression of one of the three chains of laminin-5 (a_3, β_3 or γ_2). Transfer of a eukaryotic cassette expressing the laminin γ_2 chain into laminin γ_2-deficient immortalized keratinocytes led to the synthesis of recombinant laminin-5 molecules retaining the biological properties of the normal counterpart. The typical basal polarized expression of laminin-5 was also observed in epithelia reconstructed in vitro using the laminin γ_2-transfected cells (Gagnoux-Palacios et al. 1996). These observations and the incorporation of the recombinant laminin-5 in the basement membrane were confirmed in cysts of immortalized cells formed in vivo after subcutaneous injection into nude mice (Gagnoux-Palacios et al. 1996). A similar approach, for keratinocytes deficient in the expression of integrin $a_6\beta_4$ or collagen XVII demonstrated that phenotypic reversion of these cells with the synthesis of hemidesmosomal structures in vitro was achieved using retroviruses expressing the appropriate wild-type transgene (Gagnoux-Palacios et al. 1997, Borradori et al. 1998). More recently, retroviral constructs expressing a human β_3 cDNA were used to transduce primary β_3-null keratinocytes with 100% efficiency. β_3-transduced keratinocytes synthesized and secreted mature heterotrimeric laminin-5. Gene correction fully restored the keratinocyte adhesion machinery including the capacity to assemble hemidesmosomes and prevented the loss of clonogenic potential (Vailly et al. 1998). Clonal analysis demonstrated that primary keratinocytes expressed the transgene permanently suggesting stable correction of epidermal stem cells (Dellambra et al. 1998).

Altered expression of collagen XVII causes mild clinical phenotypes because this transmembrane protein, which is not found in simple epithelia, displays a restricted tissue distribution and is not essential to hemidesmosome assembly. Seitz and co-workers have demonstrated that patients' primary keratinocytes genetically engineered with a retroviral vector to express a collagen XVII transgene display enhanced adhesion capacity in vitro (Seitz et al. 1999). These keratinocytes grafted to immune deficient mice regenerate firmly adhering epithelia that produce a basement membrane zone reactive to antibodies specific to collagen XVII (Seitz et al. 1999). These findings confirm the feasibility of phenotypic reversion of adhesion-defective epithelial cells expressing a recombinant basement membrane protein.

Efforts aimed at genetic correction of the dystrophic forms of epidermolysis bullosa are at an earlier stage. At present, all the mutations identified in patients with dystrophic epidermolysis bullosa have exclusively been performed in collagen VII. The type of mutation, its localization on defined regions of the gene, and the consequences with regard to the stability of the collagen VII RNA transcripts or the functionality of the corresponding polypeptide determine the clinical variability of the disorder. Genetic correction of the recessive and most severe form of the disease, which is generally characterized by absent expression of collagen VII, is hampered by the size (9 kb) of the collagen VII cDNA that cannot be easily accommodated in size-restricted retroviral vectors. Transfer of full-length collagen VII cDNAs has recently been achieved in vitro and in vivo in mouse and rat keratinocytes producing recombinant polypeptides immunoreactive with anti-collagen VII antibodies (Sawamura et al. 1999). However, evidence of homotrimerization of the recombinant polypeptides and formation of functional collagen VII molecules complementing the defect of keratinocytes from patients with dystrophic epidermolysis bullosa was not provided. Efficient delivery of a collagen VII "minigene" cDNA (2 kb) to collagen VII-defective keratinocytes has recently been reported to lead to the expression of a "minicollagen" molecule lacking the central collagenic domains (Chen et al. 1999). The gene-corrected cells acquired enhanced adhesion and increased proliferative potential in vitro. Grafting of these "cured" keratinocytes to immunodeficient mice and the generation of spatially intact epidermis will determine the use of shortened collagen VII molecule to reconstruct functional anchoring fibrils.

The full phenotypic reversion of primary human epidermal stem cells defective for proteins of the hemidesmosome-anchoring fibril complex and the reconstruction of transplantable epithelia from genetically engineered cell, has led to proposals for gene transfer strategies as possible therapeutic approaches to treat the main symptom (skin fragility) of inherited epidermolysis bullosa. Genomic gene therapy approaches using the type VII collagen locus (COL7A1) are being used for ex vivo gene therapy for recessive dystrophic EB. These experiments use a modified phage 1-based artificial chromosome containing the entire COL7A1 locus with its endogenous regulatory elements for transfection of cultured keratinocytes. Preliminary results show that the COL7A1 locus is functional and can be stably delivered to keratinocytes without breakage, thus demonstrating that this genomic approach could be of benefit for gene therapy of recessive dystrophic EB (A. Hovnanian, personal communication).

Disorders of Epithelial Cornification

Defective expression of enzymes and structural proteins involved in epithelial terminal differentiation and cutaneous barrier function has been associated with a variety of inherited skin diseases characterized by altered cornification of the epidermis (ichthyosis) (Rand and Bade 1983, Balc et al. 1996). Lamellar ichthyosis and X-linked ichthyosis, two recessive forms of these heterogeneous conditions, have been recently used to develop models of corrective gene therapy of disorders affecting the suprabasal layers of human skin.

The X-linked form of ichthyosis is characterized by a hypertrophic epidermis presenting with abnormal scaling (William and Elias 1987, Bale et al. 1996). The condition is caused by a deficiency in steroid sulfatase leading to the accumulation of cholesterol sulfate and abnormal desquamation (Yen et al. 1987). In vitro transfection with the cDNA encoding steroid sulfatase was shown to increase cell maturation and partially correct the phenotype of keratinocytes of patients with this disorder (Jensen et al. 1993). More recently, Freiberg and co-workers constructed a retroviral expression vector to transfer the steroid sulfatase cDNA into primary X-linked ichthyosis keratinocytes (Freiberg et al. 1997). Transduction resulted in the expression of full-length steroid sulfatase protein and restoration of sulfatase activity proportionally to the number of proviral integrations. The engineered keratinocytes grafted onto immunodeficient mice regenerated a full-thickness epidermis histologically indistinguishable from that formed by keratinocytes from healthy donors. Expression of steroid sulfatase was demonstrated *in vivo* by immunostaining at 5 weeks post-grafting as well as a normalization of barrier function parameters, while unmodified primary X-linked ichthyosis keratinocytes regenerated a hyperkeratotic epidermis lacking steroid sulfatase expression and presenting a defective skin barrier function.

Phenotypic reversion of the diseased phenotype was also achieved in keratinocytes from patients with lamellar ichthyosis, a condition much severer than X-linked ichthyosis. The infants with this disorder may die of complications (sepsis, protein and electrolyte loss). In most patients, lamellar ichthyosis results from defects in transglutaminase-1, a membrane-associated enzyme present in many epithelial as well as some non-epithelial tissue. In differentiating keratinocytes, transglutaminase-1 forms isopeptide bonds by transfer of an amine onto glutaminyl residues of cornified envelope precursor molecules (Kim et al. 1995). This enzyme can also form ester bonds between specific glutaminyl residues of human involucrin and a synthetic analog of epidermis-specific omega-hydroxy-ceramides, which indicates a dual role for transglutaminase-1 in barrier formation in the outer epidermis (Nemes et al. 1999). Restoration of functional transglutaminase-1 enzyme activity in the skin of transglutaminase-1 negative patients constitutes an attractive way of correcting the disease. In this perspective, Choate et al. have shown that in vitro retroviral transduction of primary keratinocytes taken from affected lamellar ichthyosis patients restores the expression of transglutaminase-1 and recovers the defective involucrin cross-linking (Choate et al. 1996a). When the genetically modified keratinocytes were grafted to immunodeficient mice to regenerate human epidermis in vivo, the neo-organ displayed expression of active transglutaminase-1 at levels comparable to those measured in epithelia formed by keratinocytes from healthy donors. The function of the cutaneous barrier was also restored, the corrective effect, however, failed to last beyond a few weeks (Choate et al. 1996b).

These studies on X-linked and lamellar ichthyosis indicate that while the transduced keratinocytes survive and differentiate in vivo in an epithelial tissue presenting the histological, clinical and functional features of human epidermis, virally-encoded genes are gradually inactivated by silencing of vector promoter elements (Choate and Khavari 1997). In these experiments, the decline of the transgene expression in transplanted keratinocytes constitutes an additional example of the instability of foreign gene expression in reconstituted tissues.

Ultraviolet Sensitive Skin Disorders

A multiprotein complex of about thirty gene products is involved in nucleotide excision repair following exposure to ultraviolet (UV) light. Mutations in one of these genes result in rare UV-sensitive disorders with a striking clinical heterogeneity: xeroderma pigmentosum, trichothiodystrophy, Cockayne's syndrome and xeroderma pigmentosum associated with Cockayne's syndrome (Cleaver et al. 1999). From the point of view of skin gene therapy, these diseases represent an example of disorders affecting all compartments of epidermis including melanocytes. Xeroderma pigmentosum is an autosomal recessive disease characterized by elevated photosensitivity resulting in a blistering rash on exposure to sunlight accompanied by atrophic lesions, scarring and keratoses. At the median age of eight years, the patients develop multiple tumors on exposed areas of the body. They include squamous cell carcinomas, basal cell carcinomas and melanomas. Progressive neurological degeneration is observed in some cases. Patients with trichothiodystrophy display brittle hair, ichthyosis, physical and mental retardation, photosensitivity in 50% of cases, but are not predisposed to cancer. Xeroderma pigmentosum associated with Cockayne's syndrome manifests as a combination of the cutaneous abnormalities of xeroderma pigmentosum with the severe neurological and developmental anomalies characteristic of Cockayne's syndrome (Cleaver et al. 1999).

These recessive diseases are genetically related, and each variant is subdivided into multiple complementation groups. Identification of the genetic groups to which a patient belongs is important for the understanding of the clinical symptoms and their evolution. The complementation of DNA repair defects by cell fusion assays has led to the identification of seven genetic groups (XP-A to XP-G) associated with 'classical' xeroderma pigmentosum and a variant group XP-V (Cleaver and Kraemer 1989). This observation confirmed the relationship between the genetic heterogeneity of these diseases and the heterogeneity of symptoms in affected patients. The tendency to develop skin tumors in the absence of neurological degeneration is prominent in patients belonging to XP-C, XP-E, XP-F and XP-V groups. Development of skin tumors associated with the metabolic dysfunction typical of the Cockayne's syndrome, which results in neurological degeneration, is observed in XP-B, XP-D and XP-G patients (Zeng et al. 1997, Cleaver et al. 1999).

The *XP-A* gene encodes a zinc metalloprotein that in connection with the XP-E protein binds to UV- or chemical carcinogen-induced damaged DNA. Synergistically with proteins belonging to the DNA repair/transcription factor TFIIH, which is required for transcription initiation by RNA polymerase II, the product of *XP-A* gene drives other proteins of the TFIIH complex towards the lesions and allows the excision of the damaged DNA strands (Schaeffer et al. 1993 and 1994). XP-B and XP-D proteins are two DNA helicases, both subunits of factor TFIIH, involved in the release of the damaged strand DNA after excision (Roy et al. 1994, Coin et al. 1998). XP-C protein is supposed to drive repair proteins to damaged DNA in non-transcribed strands. XPE is a DNA-binding protein recognizing UV-induced DNA damages and may function as a transcriptional partner of the E2F1 factor having a role in removing DNA lesions in chromatin (Rapic

Otrin et al. 1998, Shiyanov et al. 1999). XPF and XPG proteins are two endonucleases acting at the 5′ and 3′ sites of the DNA lesion, respectively (Sijbers et al.
1996, Constantinou et al. 1999). Recently, mutations in the gene encoding DNA
polymerase eta have been associated with the xeroderma pigmentosum variant
XP-V, which is characterized by an increased incidence of sunlight-induced skin
cancers with late onset (Masutani et al. 1999). This enzyme belongs to the
family of damage-bypass replication proteins. This indicates that a distinct DNA
repair pathway is affected in this group of XP patients.

In vitro studies have demonstrated that the defective DNA repair function of
primary skin fibroblasts derived from XP-A, XP-B, XP-C and XP-D patients can
be fully corrected after transfection of retroviral vectors introducing cDNAs expressing the appropriate DNA repair protein (Zeng et al. 1997). Expression of
the foreign transgene is stable in all types of fibroblast cell cultures and results
in full recovery of cell survival and repair activity after ultraviolet injury. The recovery of the cellular DNA repair properties is measured by evaluating the active
uptake of ^{3}H-labeled thymidine or uridine during unscheduled DNA synthesis or
restoration of RNA synthesis to normal levels. Expression of wild type DNA repair genes in these cells reverses a variety of cellular abnormalities observed in
xeroderma pigmentosum following UV-irradiation. These include reduced levels
of catalase activity (Quilliet et al. 1997), downregulation of ICAM-1 (Ahrens et
al. 1997) or abnormal stabilization of p53 (Dumaz et al. 1998). Correction of defective DNA repair is sufficient to counteract the metabolic alterations that may
accelerate tumor progression of skin cancer in patients with xeroderma pigmentosum. This finding implies that the cellular malfunctions associated with pre-
disposition to cancer in xeroderma pigmentosum are a consequence of the primary genetic defect.

This condition is rare, but in the Mediterranean area the number of potential
patients for clinical trials appears to be higher than expected from earlier eva-
luations (Kraemer et al. 1987). Most of these patients exclusively suffer from cutaneous cancers and do not present the complex pathological manifestations that
reduce the likelihood of enrollment in clinical trials.

From Gene Transfer to Therapy

Independent from the difficulties found in bypassing the biological and physical
barriers that hamper the introduction of foreign genetic information into a cell,
additional efforts are required to make gene therapy credible. The accessibility
of the integument facilitates the return of engineered cells to the patient. In addition, most of the inherited genodermatoses involve the keratinocytes and
fibroblasts, which are the major cellular components of epidermis and dermis,
respectively, and are, thus, easily manipulated in vitro. Indeed, the results obtained up to date clearly prove that gene transfer can achieve successful correction of recessive human skin diseases. We have learned in recent years that a
number of theoretical challenges may not represent insurmountable obstacles.

Regulated Expression of the Transgene

Ideally, treatment of inherited conditions by implantation of engineered cells supposes that complex regulatory pathways can be reconstituted when the curative transgene is delivered to the target cells. Indeed, the processes of adhesion, growth and terminal differentiation of keratinocytes are tightly regulated by the sequential expression of several genes from the basal layer to the different epidermal upper layers (Roop 1995). Mutations in the same gene may be responsible for different types of genodermatoses. It is therefore obvious that the proper correction of a cutaneous genetic defect may require the targeting of the exogenous wild type cDNA to a specific epidermal layer. This prerequisite may be particularly important, because little is known about the effect that a deregulated expression of a protein may have on keratinocyte function. Transgenic mouse models have nevertheless shown that aberrant expression of gene products in epidermal layers can cause alterations of epidermal proliferation and differentiation (Vassar and Fuchs 1991, Carroll et al. 1995). Controlled regulation of transfected genetic material, however, requires the surmounting of tremendous pitfalls before this goal can be achieved.

An interesting observation for cutaneous gene therapy is that targeted expression of the transgene is apparently not systematically required in keratinocytes from patients presenting with several forms of ichthyosis or epidermolysis bullosa. Indeed, the restored transcription of recombinant genes for steroid sulfatase and transglutaminase-1 in all the layers of the epithelium reconstructed with patients' keratinocytes that were initially devoid of these enzymes did not interfere with that proliferation and differentiation program (Choate et al. 1996b, Freiberg et al. 1997). Clearly, the availability of the respective substrates modulates the enzymatic activity of recombinant steroid sulfatase and transglutaminase-1, which is expected to be low in basal cells and enhanced in the suprabasal layer of the engineered epidermis.

The reconstitution of functional laminin-5 or collagen XVII trimers has also been achieved in a temporally appropriate and cell-type specific fashion. Transfer of recombinant laminin-5 and collagen XVII cDNAs using retroviral vectors sustained the ubiquitous expression throughout the epidermis. The manipulated cells preserved the epithelial polarity and differentiated into stratified tissues that correctly incorporated the recombinant molecules into the basement membrane (Vailly et al. 1998, Seitz et al. 1999). In the case of keratinocytes with defective expression of laminin β_3 or γ_2 chains, the regulated expression of the endogenous chains apparently governed the focal assembly of functional laminin-5 heterotrimers. The free recombinant polypeptides inappropriately produced by suprabasal cells or synthesized in excess by basal keratinocytes with respect to the 'partner' endogenous polypeptides are presumably degraded as observed in analogous pathologic situations (Aberdam et al. 1994, Vidal et al. 1995). In the case of collagen XVII, specific cell factors may be provided by the basal keratinocytes for post-transcriptional modifications mediating stable homotrimerization of the transgene protein. This may account for the focal expression and secretion of the corrected molecules by the patients' keratinocytes grafted to immunodeficient mice.

Such 'indirect' regulation of the curative molecule is not expected to apply to gene transfer in disorders affecting both basal and suprabasal compartments and the dermis. So far, the introduction of marker genes does not seem to induce detectable phenotypic changes in growth potential and differentiation of keratinocytes. A possibility, however, exists that lack of the precise control of the synthesized amount of therapeutic molecules may jeopardize the favorable effect of biological molecules that are optimally active at specific concentrations. Delivery of an unregulated gene may even lead to deleterious results as observed in the transgenic mouse models mentioned above (Vassar and Fuchs 1991, Carroll et al. 1995). In this respect, genetic correction of xeroderma pigmentosum in spatially reconstructed epidermis will provide useful information on potential problems of cell regulation induced by an unrestricted expression of recombinant polypeptides involved in cell functions as critical as RNA transcription and DNA repair in different skin compartments.

Permanent Expression of Curative Transgenes

Viral promoters are currently used to yield constitutive high levels of gene expression in keratinocytes. Expression of transduced genes in cultured keratinocytes is relatively stable, but loss of expression is obvious after transplantation of the cells back to the hosts. The mechanism underlying this loss of expression has not been clearly explored, but it was suggested that in vivo methylation of specific bases in the promoter region selectively inactivates viral regulatory elements in grafted cells (Fenjves et al. 1996). For instance, it was commonly observed that keratinocytes do not stably sustain appreciable levels of LTR-driven transgene expression in vivo. This idea has been recently challenged by the observation that persistent in vivo expression of retrovirally-mediated expression of a transgene is dependent on successful transduction of stem cells in culture (Kolodka et al. 1998). No sign of promoter inactivation was detected during a period of 20-weeks after transplantation of the transduced cells onto immunodeficient mice. Therefore, these studies indicate that failure to achieve stable gene transfer in vivo is mainly due to insufficient targeting of the transgene to long-lived stem cells that can assure transmission of the integrated gene to descendant keratinocytes.

During recent years, ex vivo gene therapy has been hampered by difficulties in harvesting, culturing and reimplanting human autologous cells. In the case of epidermis and other self-renewing tissues, the identification, sorting and stable transduction of stem cells has been an arduous task. In the absence of definite markers for epithelial stem cells, persistent transmission of an activated transgene by a cell to all daughter clones represents a criterion to measure stem cell behavior. We have recently shown by clonal analysis that the epidermal stem cells isolated from a patient with junctional epidermolysis bullosa can be stably corrected by transfer of a curative transgene restoring expression of laminin-5 (Dellambra et al. 1998). The transduced cells generated daughter colonies that constantly expressed laminin-5 in all their progeny for more than 140 generations. Gene correction fully restored the keratinocyte adhesion machinery including the capacity of proper hemidesmosomal assembly and prevented the loss of clonogenic potential, suggesting a direct link between adhesion to laminin-5 and preservation of keratinocyte proliferative capacity.

Despite recent achievements, the characterization of epidermal stem cells remains problematic and controversial (Cotsarelis et al. 1999). However, autologous cultured keratinocytes displaying the high clonogenic potential of stem cells are available for the permanent and self-renewing coverage in massive full-thickness burns. Permanent transgene expression in homogeneous primary cultures of highly clonogenic keratinocytes will open promising perspectives in the regeneration of corrected epithelia suitable for permanent coverage of lesional areas in patients with inherited skin diseases.

Direct in vivo introduction of genes into animals has also been extensively explored, because this approach is less complicated than procedures involving grafting of genetically modified cells. However, the different techniques currently used fail to efficiently target epithelial stem cells. The in vivo approach of genetic modification of keratinocytes has therefore suffered from short-lived expression of the transferred gene in a limited number of cells. For this reason, attempts to correct human lamellar ichthyosis by direct injection of naked plasmid into the skin from transglutaminase 1-deficient patients regenerated on immunodeficient mice was unsuccessful (Choate and Khavari 1997). A recent improvement of the classical in vivo gene transfer into the epidermis using viral vectors has been developed, in which transduction of follicular and interfollicular keratinocytes with high titer retroviruses sustained long-term transgene expression (Ghazizadeh et al. 1999). Considering that surgical grafting of ex vivo modified keratinocytes may require full thickness excision with the inherent risk of scarring and contracture, direct stable transduction of epidermis and hair follicles may represent a substantial progress in cutaneous gene therapy.

Lack of uniform expression of the transgene resulting from the inability of targeting 100% of the stem cells represents an additional difficulty. This may not be overwhelming in junctional epidermolysis bullosa, because it has been reported that recombinant laminin-5 secreted by patients' keratinocytes after gene correction exerts a paracrine effect on uncorrected neighbor cells (Vailly et al. 1998). This observation implies that efficient adhesion of self-renewing epidermis reconstituted with engineered keratinocytes re-expressing extracellular matrix components does not necessarily require a homogeneous population of transduced stem cells.

Immunogenicity of the Therapeutic Gene Product

In vivo gene delivery to the epidermis has been successful in stimulating the immune system of the skin even by low expression of exogenous gene products gaining access to Langerhans cells and dermal dendritic cells. Therefore, an important aspect of stable gene expression is the immune response that the de novo expressed polypeptide may elicit. In line with this possibility, it has recently been demonstrated that in vivo transduction of mouse epidermis with recombinant retroviral vectors sustains long-term expression of a LacZ reporter gene in immunocompetent transgenic animals constitutively expressing β-galactosidase. On the contrary, the transgene expression in immunocompetent mice intolerant to β-galactosidase is concurrently lost with the onset of the host immune response to the exogenous gene product (Ghazizadeh et al. 1999).

A strong immune response can also be elicited by antigens generated by secretion or processing of recombinant polypeptides synthesized by ex vivo transduced keratinocytes. Immunization against a protein may not be deleterious for the functionality and persistence of a corrected cell. Activation of the MHC class I pathway is, however, expected to lead to the destruction of the genetically transformed cells synthesizing the antigen(s). Because any protein containing novel epitopes is a potential target for host immune responses, genetic correction of inherited skin diseases with null mutations or caused by the synthesis of an aberrant protein is prone to danger of immunological clearance of the therapeutic factor. Such complications exists in junctional epidermolysis bullosa associated with defects in laminin-5 and collagen XVII, because these adhesion molecules, that are secreted in the extracellular matrix undergo active proteolytic cleavage, are also known to cause autoimmune disorders. Clearly, further investigation is necessary to evaluate the host tolerance to the delivered gene products and appraise the setbacks that undesired immune reactions may represent on the transfer from pre-clinical models to human clinical trials.

Animal Models

The actual therapeutic efficacy of a curative transgene and persistence of the corrected cells over very long periods of time in humans can only be determined by a clinical trial. Ideally, the clinical protocol requires prior evaluation in animal models. Animal models for human gene therapy have been developed using human skin reconstituted in vitro to form a spatially and histologically normal tissue grafted onto severe immunodeficient mice. This approach has permitted the regeneration of human skin presenting the clinical characteristic of the integument of patients suffering from inherited skin diseases and the successful correction of the genetic defect following gene transfer (Kim et al. 1992, Choate et al. 1996a and b, Choate and Khavari 1997, Seitz et al. 1999). The absence of an intact immune system is the major flaw of such models which, nevertheless, have substantially strengthened the idea that genetic correction of inherited skin disorders is a realistic goal. Models preserving the immune competence of the manipulated animals have been developed by disruption of the mouse genes homologous to the human counterparts. In several instances the mouse model recapitulates most of the clinical features of human disease and allows essential insights in the underlying pathomechanism, but their usefulness for testing therapeutic approaches and particularly gene replacement therapies is generally limited. This has been the case in strains of mice with null mutations in the genes for laminin-5, integrin $\alpha_6\beta_4$, and collagen VII. Targeted gene disruption reproduced the severe manifestations of the junctional and dystrophic forms of epidermolysis bullosa, but also resulted in the early death of the diseased animals (see also Chapter 3).

A variety of human inherited skin diseases amenable to genetic treatment have their corresponding manifestations in animals. However, most of the potential animal models either present poor genetic homology with the human disease, as observed in mice with X-linked ichthyosis (Salido et al. 1996) or are unsuitable for genetic manipulations.

The recent identification of breeds of dogs with inherited forms of epidermolysis bullosa provides the opportunity of verifying in a naturally occurring animal model the fulfillment of the basic requirements for successful gene therapy of these diseases. In short-haired dogs presenting a mild form of junctional epidermolysis bullosa with all the clinical manifestations characteristic of the human condition, the genetic defect underlying the disease has been identified and successfully corrected in vitro by retroviral transduction of the curative transgene (Spirito et al. 1999). Direct transgene delivery of retroviral vectors expressing the curative transgene successfully reverted the phenotype of the targeted canine keratinocytes. Subsequent autologous implantation of epithelial sheets obtained in vitro using these cells or grafts generated by populations of the engineered keratinocytes are expected to provide information on the host immune response to the corrected laminin-5 molecule and long-term persistence of the regenerated tissue. This approach provides the opportunity to better evaluate the therapeutic effects of gene transfer prior to clinical trials in humans. Similarly, dogs presenting with a mild form of recessive epidermolysis bullosa associated with aberrant expression of collagen VII can serve as a model to study the pathomechanism of the disease in visceral tissues (esophagus and gut) (Palazzi et al. 2000). Despite the differences between the human and canine integument, these dogs also provide a well defined system to test gene replacement therapies.

Future Developments

The final objective of gene therapy of inherited skin diseases is the improvement of the patients' condition. Recent progress in gene identification and pathogenesis of genodermatoses has been remarkable. At present, ex vivo gene transfer is efficient and effective, in vivo gene transfer has been remarkably improved, long-term expression of the transferred genes has been obtained, stem cell properties of primary keratinocytes appear preserved during manipulations, the grafting techniques are well established, and adequate animal models have been identified. Because of these achievements, are treatment protocols around the corner? Feasibility of keratinocyte-mediated autologous gene therapy still needs to be substantiated in animal models and awaits clinical trials. Junctional epidermolysis bullosa appears to best fulfill the conditions required for future realization: the variety of the well-defined mild forms of the disease provide the opportunity to ameliorate epithelial adhesion of very small areas of the skin for prevention and treatment.

The major objectives of future investigations obviously should include the establishment of methods for the correct evaluation of the biological effect associated with curative gene transfer. Tests must allow to assess the efficacy and dose response in vivo by measuring the correction of the epithelial defect and analyze insufficient rescue of the phenotype due to low expression of the curative polypeptide and toxicity of the constructs (van der Neut et al. 1999).

In the near future, the development of new viral vectors derived from the adenovirus-associated viruses (AAV) and/or lentiviruses will hopefully overcome the critical hurdles represented by efficient and safe gene transfer. Progress in vector refinement is expected to allow gene therapy to evolve from the stage of purely investigative studies to that of established clinical tools complementing conventional therapies. It is evident that a close collaboration between basic researchers and clinicians is required to overcome the impediments and problems related to gene therapy of skin diseases (Hengge et al. 1999) and make this idea work.

Acknowledgements. The authors would like to thank M. Mezzina for helpful discussions, M. S. Campo for critical reading of the manuscript, and V. Alison for editing. Part of the work reviewed in this manuscript was supported by grants from: EEC BIOMED 2 (BMH4–97–2062), the Programme Hospitalier de Recherche Clinique (France), and the DEBRA Foundation (U.K.).

References

Aberdam D, Galliano MF, Vailly J, Pulkkinen L, Bonifas J, Christiano K, Tryggvason K, Uitto J, Epstein EH Jr, Ortonne JP (1994) Herlitz's junctional epidermolysis bullosa is genetically linked to mutations in the nicein/kalinin (laminin-5) LAMC2 gene. Nat Genet 6:299–304

Ahrens C, Grewe M, Berneburg M, Grether-Beck S, Quilliet X, Mezzina M, Sarasin A, Lehmann AR, Arlett CF, Krutmann J (1997) Photocarcinogenesis and inhibition of intercellular adhesion molecule-1 expression in cells of DNA-repair-defective individuals. Proc Natl Acad Sci USA 94:6837–68341

Bale S, Compton J, Russell L, DiGiovanna J (1996) Genetic heterogeneity in lamellar ichthyosis. J Invest Dermatol 107:140–141

Borradori L, Sonnenberg A (1999) Structure and function of hemidesmosomes: more than simple adhesion complexes. J Invest Dermatol 112:411–418

Borradori L, Chavanas S, Schaapveld R, Gagnoux-Palacios L, Calafat J, Meneguzzi G, Sonnenberg A (1998) Role of the bullous pemphigoid antigen 180 (BP180) in the assembly of the hemidesmosomes and cell adhesion. Reexpression of the BP180 in generalized atrophic benign epidermolysis bullosa keratinocytes. Exp Cell Res 239:463–476

Carroll J, Romero M, Watt F (1995) Suprabasal integrin expression in the epidermis of transgenic mice results in developmental defects and a phenotype resembling psoriasis. Cell 83:957–968

Chen M, O'Toole EA, Liu Y-Y, Kasahara N (1999) Corrective gene transfer in dystrophic epidermolysis bullosa. J Invest Dermatol 112:552

Cheng J, Syder AJ, Yu QC, Letai A, Paller AS, Fuchs E (1992) The genetic basis of epidermolytic hyperkeratosis: a disorder of differentiation-specific epidermal keratin genes. Cell 70:811–819

Choate K, Khavari P (1997) Direct cutaneous gene delivery in a human genetic skin disease. Hum Gene Ther 8:1659–1665

Choate K, Kinsella T, Williams M, Nolan G, Khavary P (1996 a) Transglutaminase-1 delivery to lamellar ichtyosis keratinocytes. Hum Gene Ther 7:2247–2253

Choate K, Medalie D, Morgan J, Khavari P (1996b) Corrective gene transfer in the human skin disorder lamellar ichthyosis. Nat Med 2:263–67

Cleaver J, Kraemer K (1989) Xeroderma pigmentosum. Scriver C, Beaudet A, Sly W, Valle D (Eds). The metabolic and molecular bases of inherited disease. McGraw-Hill, New York, pp 2949–2971

Cleaver J, Thompson L, Richardson A, States J (1999) A summary of mutations in the UV-sensitive disorders: xeroderma pigmentosum, Cockayne syndrome, and trichothiodystrophy. Hum Mutat 14:9–22

Coin F, Marinoni J, Rodolfo C, Fribourg S, Pedrini A, Egly J (1998) Mutations in the XPD helicase gene result in XP and TTD phenotypes, preventing interaction between XPD and the p44 subunit of TFIIH. Nat Genet 20:184–188

Constantinou A, Gunz D, Evans E, Lalle P, Bates P, Wood R, Clarkson SG (1999) Conserved residues of human XPG protein important for nuclease activity and function in nucleotide excision repair. J Biol Chem 274:5637–5648

Cotsarelis G, Kaur P, Dhouailly D, Hengge U, Bickenbach J (1999) Epithelial stem cells in the skin: definition, markers, localization and functions. Exp Dermatol 8:80–88

Coulombe PA, Hutton ME, Letai A, Hebert A, Paller AS, Fuchs E (1991) Point mutations in human keratin 14 genes of epidermolysis bullosa simplex patients: genetic and functional analyses. Cell 66:1301–1311

Dellambra E, Vailly J, Pellegrini G, Bondanza S, Golisano O, Macchia C, Zambruno G, Meneguzzi G, De Luca M (1998) Corrective transduction of human epidermal stem cells in laminin-5 dependent junctional epidermolysis bullosa. Hum Gene Ther 9:1359–1370

Dumaz N, Drougard C, Quilliet X, Mezzina M, Sarasin A, Daya-Grosjean L (1998) Recovery of the normal p53 response after UV treatment in DNA repair-deficient fibroblasts by retroviral-mediated correction with the XPD gene. Carcinogenesis 19:1701–1704

Fenjves E, Yao S, Kurachi K, Taichman L (1996) Loss of expression of a retrovirus-transduced gene in human keratinocytes. J Invest Dermatol 106:576–578

Fine J, Eady R, Bauer E, Briggaman RA, Bruckner-Tuderman L, Christiano A, Heagerty A, Hintner H, Jonkman MF, McGrath J, Moshell A, Shimizu H, Tadini G, Uitto J (2000) Revised classification system for inherited epidermolysis bullosa: report of the second international consensus meeting on diagnosis and classification of epidermolysis bullosa. J Am Acad Dermatol 42:1051–1066

Freiberg R, Choate K, Deng H, Alperin E, Shapiro L, Khavari P (1997) A model of corrective gene transfer in X-linked ichthyosis. Hum Mol Genet 6:927–933

Gagnoux-Palacios L, Vailly J, Durand-Clement M, Wagner E, Ortonne J-P, Meneguzzi G (1996) Functional re-expression of laminin-5 in laminin-γ2 deficient human keratinocytes modifies cell morphology, motility, and adhesion. J Biol Chem 271:18437–18444

Gagnoux-Palacios L, Gache Y, Ortonne J, Meneguzzi G (1997) Hemidesmosome assembly assessed by expression of a wild type integrin β_4cDNA in junctional epidermolysis bullosa keratinocytes. Lab Invest 77:1–10

Ghazizadeh S, Harrington R, Taichman L (1999) In vivo transduction of mouse epidermis with recombinant retroviral vectors: implication for cutaneous gene therapy. Gene Ther 6: 1267–1275

Hahn H, Wicking C, Zaphiropoulous PG, Gailani MR, Shanley S, Chidambaram A, Vorechovsky I, Holmberg E, Unden AB, Gillies S, Negus K, Smyth I, Pressman C, Leffell DJ, Gerrard B, Goldstein AM, Dean M, Toftgard R, Chenevix-Trench G, Wainwright B, Bale AE (1996) Mutations of the human homolog of Drosophila patched in the nevoid basal cell carcinoma syndrome. Cell 85:841–851

Hengge U, Taichman L, Kaur P, Rogers G, Jensen T, Goldsmith L, Rees JL, Christiano AM (1999) How realistic is cutaneous gene therapy? Exp Dermatol 8:419–431

Jensen T, Jensen U, Jensen P, Ibsen H, Brandrup F, Ballabio A, Bolund L (1993) Correction of steroid sulfatase deficiency by gene transfer into basal cells of tissue-cultured epidermis from patients with recessive X-linked ichthyosis. Exp Cell Res 209:392–397

Kim S, Chung S, Steinert P (1995) Highly active soluble processed forms of the transglutaminase 1 enzyme in epidermal keratinocytes. J Biol Chem 270:18026–18035

Kim Y, Woodley D, Wynn K, Giomi W, Bauer E (1992) Recessive dystrophic epidermolysis bullosa phenotype is preserved in xenografts using SCID mice: development of an experimental in vivo model. J Invest Dermatol 98:191–197

Kolodka T, Garlick J, Taichman L (1998) Evidence for keratinocyte stem cells in vitro: long term engraftment and persistence of transgene expression from retrovirus-transduced keratinocytes. Proc Natl Acad Sci USA 95:4356–4361

Kraemer K, Lee M, Scotto J (1987) Xeroderma pigmentosum. Cutaneous, ocular, and neurologic abnormalities in 830 published cases. Arch Dermatol 123:241–250

Li L, Elledge SJ, Peterson CA, Bales ES, Legerski RJ (1994) Specific association between the human DNA repair proteins XPA and ERCC1. Proc Natl Acad Sci USA 91:5012–5016

Maestrini E, Monaco AP, McGrath JA, Ishida-Yamamoto A, Camisa C, Hovnanian A, Weeks DE, Lathrop M, Uitto J, Christiano AM (1996) A molecular defect in loricrin, the major component of the cornified cell envelope, underlies Vohwinkel's syndrome. Nat Genet 13:70–77

Maestrini E, Korge BP, Ocana-Sierra J, Calzolari E, Cambiaghi S, Scudder PM, Hovnanian A, Monaco AP, Munro CS (1999) A missense mutation in connexin26, D66H, causes mutilating keratoderma with sensorineural deafness (Vohwinkel's syndrome) in three unrelated families. Hum Mol Genet 8:1237–1243

Masutani C, Kusumoto R, Yamada A, Dohmae N, Yokoi M, Yuasa M, Araki M, Iwai S, Takio K, Hanaoka F (1999) The XPV (xeroderma pigmentosum variant) gene encodes human DNA polymerase eta. Nature 399:700–704

McGrath J, Gatalica B, Christiano A, Li K, Owaribe K, McMillan JR, Eady RA, Uitto J (1995) Mutations in the 180-kD bullous pemphigoid antigen (BPAG2), a hemidesmosomal transmembrane collagen (COL17A1), in generalized atrophic benign epidermolysis bullosa. Nat Genet 11:83–86

McLean WH, Rugg EL, Lunny DP, Morley SM, Lane EB, Swensson O, Dopping-Hepenstal PJ, Griffiths WA, Eady RA, Higgins C (1995) Keratin 16 and keratin 17 mutations cause pachyonychia congenita. Nat Genet 9:273–278

Milich L, Sullenger B (1997) Ribozymes as tools for the gene therapist. In: Strauss M and Barranger J (eds) Concepts in gene therapy. de Gruyter, New York, 197–232

Mulligan R (1993) The basic science of gene therapy. Science 260:926–931

Nemes Z, Marekov L, Fesus L, Steinert P (1999) A novel function for transglutaminase 1: attachment of long-chain omega-hydroxyceramides to involucrin by ester bond formation. Proc Natl Acad Sci USA 96:8402–8407

Palazzi X, Marchal T, Chabanne L, Spadafora A, Magnol JP, Meneguzzi G (2000) Canine dystrophic epidermolysis bullosa: a spontaneous model for gene therapy of the disease. J Invest Dermatol, in press

Pulkkinen L, Uitto J (1999) Mutation analysis and molecular genetics of epidermolysis bullosa. Matrix Biol 18:29–42

Quilliet X, Chevallier-Lagente O, Zeng L, Calvayrac R, Mezzina M, Sarasin A, Vuillaume M (1997) Retroviral-mediated correction of DNA repair defect in xeroderma pigmentosum cells is associated with recovery of catalase activity. Mutat Res 385:235–242

Rand R and Bade H (1983) The ichthyoses: a review. J Am Acad Dermatol 8:285–305

Rapic Otrin V, Kuraoka I, Nardo T, McLenigan M, Eker AP, Stefanini M, Levine AS, Wood RD (1998) Relationship of the xeroderma pigmentosum group E DNA repair defect to the chromatin and DNA binding proteins UV-DDB and replication protein A. Mol Cell Biol 18:182–190

Rickman L, Simrak D, Stevens HP, Hunt DM, King IA, Bryant SP, Eady RA, Leigh IM, Arnemann J, Magee AI, Kelsell DP, Buxton RS (1999) N-terminal deletion in a desmosomal cadherin causes the autosomal dominant skin disease striate palmoplantar keratoderma. Hum Mol Genet 8:971–976

Roop D (1995) Defects in the barrier. Science 267:474–475

Rothnagel JA, Traupe H, Wojcik S, Huber M, Hohl D, Pittelkow MR, Saeki H, Ishibashi Y, Roop DR (1994) Mutations in the rod domain of keratin 2e in patients with ichthyosis bullosa of Siemens. Nat Genet 7:485–490

Roy R, Schaeffer L, Humbert S, Vermeulen W, Weeda G, Egly J (1994) The DNA-dependent ATPase activity associated with the class II basic transcription factor BTF2/TFIIH. J Biol Chem 269:9826–9832

Ruzzi L, Gagnoux-Palacios L, Pinola M, Belli S, Meneguzzi G, D'Alessio M, Zambruno G (1997) A homozygous mutation in the integrin alpha6 gene in junctional epidermolysis bullosa with pyloric atresia. J Clin Invest 99:2826–8231

Sakuntabhai A, Ruiz-Perez V, Carter S, Jacobsen N, Burge S, Monk S, Smith M, Munro CS, O'Donovan M, Craddock N, Kucherlapati R, Rees JL (1999) Mutations in ATP2A2, encoding a Ca^{2+} pump, cause Darier disease. Nat Genet 21:271–277

Salido E, Li X, Yen P, Martin N, Mohandas T, Shapiro L (1996) Cloning and expression of the mouse pseudoautosomal steroid sulphatase gene. Nat Genet 13:83–86

Sawamura D, Meng X, Itai K, Kon S, Tamai K, Hanada H, Tanaka T, Hashimoto I (1999) In vitro and in vivo expression of full-length cDNA of type VII collagen: possibility of gene therapy for dystrophic epidermolysis bullosa (DEB). J Invest Dermatol 112:551

Schaeffer L, Roy R, Humbert S, Moncollin V, Vermeulen W, Hoeijmakers JH, Chambon P, Egly JM (1993) DNA repair helicase: a component of BTF2 (TFIIH) basic transcription factor. Science 260:58–63

Schaeffer L, Moncollin V, Roy R, Staub A, Mezzina M, Sarasin A, Weeda G, Hoeijmakers JH, Egly JM (1994) The ERCC2/DNA repair protein is associated with the class II BTF2/TFIIH transcription factor. EMBO J 15:2388–2392

Seitz C, Giudice G, Balding S, Marinkovich M, Khavari P (1999) BP180 gene delivery in junctional epidermolysis bullosa. Gene Ther 6:42–47

Shamsher MK, Navsaria HA, Stevens HP, Ratnavel RC, Purkis PE, Kelsell DP, McLean WH, Cook LJ, Griffiths WA, Gschmeissner S (1995) Novel mutations in keratin 16 gene underly focal non-epidermolytic palmoplantar keratoderma (NEPPK) in two families. Hum Mol Genet 4:1875–1881

Shiyanov P, Hayes S, Donepudi M, Nichols A, Linn S, Slagle BL, Raychaudhuri P (1999) The naturally occurring mutants of DDB are impaired in stimulating nuclear import of the p125 subunit and E2F1-activated transcription. Mol Cell Biol 19:4935–4943

Sijbers A, de Laat W, Ariza R, Biggerstaff M, Wei Y, Moggs JG, Carter KC, Shell BK, Evans E, de Jong MC, Rademakers S, de Rooij J, Jaspers NG, Hoeijmakers JH, Wood RD (1996) Xeroderma pigmentosum group F caused by a defect in a structure-specific DNA repair endonuclease. Cell 86:811–822

Smith FJ, Eady RA, Leigh IM, McMillan JR, Rugg EL, Kelsell DP, Bryant SP, Spurr NK, Geddes JF, Kirtschig G, Milana G, de Bono AG, Owaribe K, Wiche G, Pulkkinen L, Uitto J, McLean WH, Lane EB (1996) Plectin deficiency results in muscular dystrophy with epidermolysis bullosa. Nat Genet 13:450–457

Spirito F, Capt A, Ortonne J, Guaguere E, Meneguzzi G (1999) Mild junctional epidermolysis dullosa in dogs. A natural model for experimental gene therapy of the condition. J Invest Dermatol 113:445

Strauss M and Barranger J (eds) (1997) Concepts in gene therapy. De Gruyter, New York

Torchard D, Blanchet-Bardon C, Serova O, Langbein L, Narod S, Janin N, Goguel AF, Bernheim A, Franke WW, Lenoir GM (1994) Epidermolytic palmoplantar keratoderma cosegregates with a keratin 9 mutation in a pedigree with breast and ovarian cancer. Nat Genet 6:106–110

Vailly J, Gagnoux-Palacios L, Dell'Ambra E, Romero C, Pinola M, Zambruno G, De Luca M, Ortonne JP, Meneguzzi G (1998) Corrective gene transfer of keratinocytes from patients with junctional epidermolysis bullosa restores assembly of hemidesmosomes in reconstructed epithelia. Gene Ther 5:1322–1332

van der Neut R, Cachaco AS, Thorsteinsdottir S, Janssen H, Prins D, Bulthuis J, van der Valk M, Calafat J, Sonnenberg A (1999) Partial rescue of epithelial phenotype in integrin (beta)4 null mice by a keratin-5 promoter driven human integrin (beta)4 transgene. J Cell Sci 112:3911–3922

Vassar R, Fuchs E (1991) Transgenic mice provide new insights into the role of TGF-alpha during epidermal development and differentiation. Genes Dev 5:714–727

Vidal F, Aberdam D, Miquel C, Christiano AM, Pulkkinen L, Uitto J, Ortonne JP, Mene-
   guzzi G (1995) Integrin beta 4 mutations associated with junctional epidermolysis bul-
   losa with pyloric atresia. Nat Genet 10:229–234
William M, Elias P (1987) Genetically transmitted, generalized disorders of cornification.
   Ichth Dermatol Clin 5:155–178
Yanez R, Porter A (1998) Therapeutic gene targeting. Gene Ther 5:149–159
Yen P, Allen E, Marsh B, Mohandas T, Wang N, Taggart RT, Shapiro LJ (1987) Cloning
   and expression of steroid sulfatase cDNA and the frequent occurrence of deletions in
   STS deficiency: implications for X-Y interchange. J Cell Biol 49:443–454
Zeng L, Quilliet X, Chevallier-Lagente O, Eveno E, Sarasin A, Mezzina M (1997) Retro-
   virus-mediated gene transfer corrects DNA repair defect of xeroderma pigmentosum
   cells of complementation groups A, B and C. Gene Ther 4:1077–1084

8   Gene Transfer Strategies in Tissue Repair

S. A. EMING, J. M. DAVIDSON, T. KRIEG

Introduction

Recent technological advances in gene transfer in addition to a precise understanding of the molecular basis of many diseases have provided the tools necessary for a new approach to the treatment of both inherited and acquired diseases. This approach, called gene therapy, has the potential of providing long-term and cost effective treatment for some inherited diseases which have few other therapeutic options as well as enabling novel methods for the delivery of therapeutic proteins for the treatment of many acquired diseases. We and others are exploring the potential application of this technology in tissue repair. One primary focus has been to transfer genes encoding wound healing growth factors, a broad class of proteins which control local events in tissue repair such as cell proliferation, migration and the formation of extracellular matrix. Using several different strategies for gene transfer, wound healing growth factor genes have been successfully introduced and expressed in cells and tissues *in vitro* as well as *in vivo*. Various experimental models of wound healing and tissue repair have been used to evaluate the efficacy of this new and exciting approach to tissue repair and regeneration.

Molecular and Cellular Aspects of Wound Healing

The Physiological Wound Healing Process

The process of healing is an organized response to tissue injury that involves the interaction of diverse cells, extracellular matrix molecules and soluble mediators. To better understand this complex network of interacting mediators, the healing response has been divided into four broad categories that coincide with the temporal sequence of normal healing: hemostasis, inflammation, proliferation, and remodeling (reviewed in Martin 1997, Singer and Clark 1999).

The primary goal of biological repair is the termination of blood loss. Platelets adhere to freshly exposed tissue components such as collagen. Platelets and damaged cells release various mediators activating a cascade of factors finally transforming fibrinogen into fibrin. During the final stage of blood coagulation factor XIIIa is produced. By transforming soluble fibrin into its insoluble form, factor XIIIa stabilizes fibrin and stimulates monomeric fibrin to form net-like structures. This process provides the provisional matrix for fibroblast migration. In addition, factor XIIIa promotes the binding of fibroblasts to fibronectin and is therefore considered a connecting element between coagulation and cellular processes in wound healing. To keep blood coagulation and platelet aggregation within a physiological range, the endothelium produces regulatory factors such as prostacyclins, which inhibit platelet aggregation and protein C, which inactivates coagulation factors V and VIII, and t-plasminogen activator, which activates fibrinolysis.

Following thrombus formation, the inflammatory phase ensues as neutrophils and macrophages enter the wound site. As early as 1 hour following wounding there is increased expression of endothelial and granulocyte adhesion molecules (CD11/CD18) resulting in the enhanced adherence and migration of granulocytes and macrophages into the wound site. A variety of chemotactic factors attract both cell types to the site of injury including fibrinopeptides, fibrin degradation products, complement factors C3a and C5a, leukotriene B4, bacterial outer membrane proteins, platelet-activating-factor (PAF), platelet-derived growth factor (PDGF) and platelet factor 4 (PF-4). Neutrophils are primarily involved in debridement and bacterial defense. They carry granules loaded with a variety of proteolytic enzymes including elastase, acidic hydrolase, and lysozyme. Granulocytes destroy contaminating bacteria via phagocytosis and subsequent enzymatic and oxygen radical mechanisms. If substantial wound contamination has not occurred, neutrophil infiltration usually ceases within a few days.

In parallel to the invasion of neutrophils, macrophages accumulate at the wound site. As granulocytes, they synthesize tissue degrading agents including proteolytic enzymes such as elastase, collagenase, cathepsin B and plasmin activator. Besides promoting phagocytosis and debridement, macrophages play a central role in the initiation and propagation of the repair process by releasing proinflammatory cytokines (IL-1, TNF-α, IFN) and numerous growth factors (TGF-β, TGF-α, PDGF, IGF-1, VEGF, bFGF) (Bennett and Schultz 1993). A synopsis of growth factors and their activities are listed in Table 8.1. Thus, macrophages appear to play a pivotal role in the transition between inflammation and repair. Altering their number and function may influence a whole cascade of regulatory activities.

The formation of granulation tissue begins approximately 4 days following injury and is characterized by numerous new capillaries which endow the provisional extracellular matrix with its granular appearance. Besides new blood vessels, granulation tissue consists of macrophages, fibroblasts, and loose connective tissue. Fibroblasts, macrophages, and blood vessels move into the wound space as a unit, which correlates well with the proposed biological interdependence of these cells during tissue repair. In particular, macrophages provide a continuing source of cytokines necessary to stimulate fibroplasia and angiogenesis, fibroblasts construct new extracellular matrix necessary to support ingrowth of cells and blood vessels that carry oxygen and nutrients. The provisional extracellular matrix also promotes granulation tissue formation by providing scaffolding for contact guidance (fibronectin and collagen), low impedance for cell mobility (hyaluronic acid), a reservoir for cytokines, and direct signals to the cells through integrin receptors.

Reepithelialization of a wound begins within hours of injury. This process involves multiple processes including the formation of a provisional wound bed matrix, the migration and proliferation of epidermal keratinocytes from the wound edges, and finally the stratification and differentiation of the neoepithelium. Skin appendages such as hair follicles and wound margins are sources of cells for the wound epithelium. Epidermal cells undergo marked phenotypic alterations that include the dissolution of intercellular desmosomes and hemidesmosomal links between the epidermis and the basement membrane, which allow epidermal cell migration. The expression of a new spectrum of integrin receptors on epidermal cells allows the cells to interact with a variety of extracellular matrix proteins that are interspersed with stromal type I collagen at the margin of the wound and interwoven with the fibrin clot in the wound space. In addition, epidermal cell migration depends on the degradation of extracellular matrix, so that cells at the leading edge synthesize specific enzymes including collagenase I and stromelysins. Following migration, epidermal cells proliferate. The release of epidermal and dermal growth factors is believed to play a major role in the stimulation of epidermal cell migration and proliferation, such as TGF-a, KGF and EGF (Table 8.1). As reepithelialization ensues, basement membrane proteins reappear in a very ordered sequence from the margin of the wound inward. Epidermal cells revert to their normal phenotype, once again firmly attaching to the reestablished basement membrane and underlying dermis.

Remodeling is the last and longest phase of healing. During this period the exuberant vascularization of early granulation tissue recedes as repair continues. The principal processes occurring during this phase are the dynamic remodeling of collagen and the formation of the mature scar. During remodeling the tensile strength of the wound continues to increase despite a reduction in the rate of collagen synthesis. This gain in strength is a result of structural modification of the newly deposited collagen and crosslinking of collagen fibrils. However, the wound collagen never achieves the bundled, organized pattern of normal collagen and reflects the fact that the biomechanical properties of healed tissue never equal that of uninjured skin.

Clinical Aspects of Impaired Wound Healing

One consequence of the complexity of tissue repair is the variety of conditions that can impair it, including systemic factors such as malnutrition, underlying systemic disease, and therapeutic interventions (corticosteroids, immunosuppressants) or local factors such as bacterial infection, growth factor deficiency or increased proteolytic activity (Falanga 1993). Although, in recent years advances in cellular and molecular biology have greatly expanded the range of potential therapeutic treatments, impaired wound healing still remains a major health care problem. Therefore, more effective clinical strategies need to be developed.

Table 8.1. Growth factors that affect wound healing

Growth factor	Major source	Primary target cells/action
EGF	Platelets	Mitogen for most epithelial cells, fibroblasts, endothelial cells
HB-EGF	Macrophages	Mitogen for keratinocytes/fibroblasts
TGF-α	Macrophages, keratinocytes	Similar to EGF, but more angiogenic
KGF	Fibroblasts	Mitogen/motogen for keratinocytes
IGF-1	Fibroblasts, macrophages, platelets	Mitogen for keratinocytes, fibroblasts, endothelial cells
PDGF	Platelets, fibroblasts, macrophages	Chemotactic for fibroblasts, macrophages; mitogen for fibroblasts, matrix synthesis
TGF-β1, -2	Macrophages, fibroblasts, platelets	Keratinocyte migration, chemotactic for macrophages and fibroblasts
CTGF	Fibroblasts	Mitogen for fibroblasts
FGF-1, -2	Macrophages, endothelial cells	Angiogenic and mitogen for fibroblasts
VEGF	Keratinocytes, macrophages, mast cells	Mitogen and chemotactic for endothelial cells; chemotactic for macrophages
CSF-1	Multiple cells	Activation of macrophages, granulation tissue formation
Scatter factor	Fibroblasts	Mitogen for keratinocytes and endothelial cells
Activin	Fibroblasts, keratinocytes	Mitogen for keratinocytes
IL-1α, -β	Neutrophils	Activator of growth factor expression in macrophages, keratinocytes, fibroblasts
TNF-α	Neutrophils	Similar to IL-1

Chronic leg ulcers are the most common form of chronic wounds, with venous insufficiency being the predominant underlying cause (Phillips and Dover 1991). In such pathogenic situations, the obstruction of the deep veins leads to venous insufficiency and hypertension. This elevation in intravenous pressure then increases the vessel permeability towards large molecules such as albumin and fibrinogen, and leads to osmotically induced loss of fluid. Within the extracellular space, fibrin complexes can embed capillaries in a cuff-like manner, thereby blocking the diffusion of oxygen (Herrick et al. 1992). The resulting local hypoxia gives rise to the clinical feature of dermatosclerosis and is responsible for the subsequent cell death and necrosis, and ultimately leads to ulceration.

The most common cause of nonvenous leg ulcers is peripheral artery occlusive disease. Results from recent studies indicate that tissue damage may be a result of toxic mediators released by leukocytes, that are activated by ischemia and increased adherence to capillary endothelium.

Diabetes mellitus is another common clinical problem associated with multiple physiologic and biochemical defects that lead to impaired healing (Laing 1988, Apelquvist et al. 1993). Usually, neuropathy leads to the breakdown of skin after prolonged pressure or minor trauma. Ischemia, secondary to vascular disease, impedes the healing process by reducing the supply of oxygen and nutrients. Furthermore, diabetic ulcers are prone to infection due to impaired granulocyte function and chemotaxis.

Pressure or decubital ulcers are characterized by deep tissue necrosis. The application of an external force may cause the interstitial pressure to rise and consequently leads to reduced capillary filtration, edema, and cell autolysis.

Although the systemic mechanisms underlying each of these conditions are different, chronic wounds share the development of an inhibitory microenvironment. However, little is known about the epidermal/dermal mechanisms that cause and/or perpetuate the inability to heal successfully (reviewed in Falanga 1993). Therefore, the development of novel experimental approaches to address these issues is an essential step in understanding the pathogenesis of chronic wounds, that will likely lead to new therapeutic strategies.

Gene Transfer: A New Approach in Tissue Repair

Gene transfer refers to the genetic modification of mammalian cells for the purpose of gene therapy. Initial work in this field focused on the correction of inherited diseases for which no therapeutic approaches were available. However, it is now clear that the technique of gene therapy can potentially be applied to the treatment of acquired diseases, including impaired wound healing and tissue repair. Such approaches are often innovative and provide solutions to the problems inherent in cell-based, drug delivery methods.

Many of the therapeutic strategies currently available for the treatment of impaired wound repair are based on the delivery of a drug or protein that promotes healing of the injured tissue (Falanga 1992, Bennett and Schultz 1993, Scharffetter-Kochanek et al. 1999). Growth factors that stimulate wound healing processes such as cell proliferation and synthesis of extracellular matrix proteins, are obvious candidate genes for gene therapy-based approaches (Table 8.1). Other potential target genes include those that inhibit the catabolic factors found in the hostile wound environment, including protease inhibitors or receptor antagonists. Current drug delivery strategies, however, suffer from the inherent loss of drug activity due to the combined effects of physical inhibition and biological degradation.

Gene transfer techniques may aid in the sustained expression and release of proteins into the surrounding tissue. By inserting a gene into those cells involved in the healing process, it would be possible to engineer the synthesis and delivery of a specific therapeutic protein into the wound site using a permanent or transient gene expression system. This process could enhance the therapeutic benefit of the wound-healing agent and might create an environment that promotes tissue repair, rather than destruction.

Different delivery technologies for gene transfer have been investigated and have been successfully applied to ex vivo and in vivo gene therapy (Table 8.2). The ex vivo approach permits the introduction of genetic material directly into a particular cell type upon isolation of the involved cells from the patient, genetically manipulating these cells in culture, and then transplanting them back into the donor. Although ex vivo gene therapy is limited to those tissues for which culture conditions and transplantation techniques are well defined, this strategy allows for better control over the genetic modification of the target cell and modified cells can be combined with biomaterials prior to transplantation. In vivo gene therapy obviates the need for proper cell culture and transplantation, since the genes are delivered directly into the target tissue. This method simply requires that the DNA vector harboring the encoding sequence is inserted into host cells in vivo. This straightforward approach, besides being simple, is especially relevant to tissues where cells are difficult or impossible to culture and/or transplant, such as in the nervous system. Although there are clear advantages, it is sometimes difficult to target genes to specific cells of a particular tissue in vivo.

Gene Transfer Systems Applied to Tissue Repair

Viral Methods

Gene delivery systems can be classified as either viral or non-viral. Viruses are natural vehicles for gene delivery and were the first obvious choice (Friedmann 1992). Recombinant viruses had the sequences required for their self-replication removed and replaced with the foreign therapeutic DNA. The viral proteins necessary for efficient cell entry and gene delivery are supplied by packaging cell lines. Viruses, in general, efficiently transduce cells and in some cases permanently integrate the transgene into the host cell's genome. Retroviruses, adenoviruses and adeno-associated viruses are the most commonly used viral gene delivery systems.

Recombinant Retrovirus

Retroviruses are single-stranded RNA viruses with a genome of approximately 8 kilobases in size. Retroviruses used for gene transfer are derived from wild-type murine retroviruses. The recombinant viral particles are structurally identical to the wild type virus but carry a genetically engineered genome (retroviral vector) which encodes the therapeutic gene of interest. These viruses are incapable of self-replication but can infect and insert their genomes into the target cell's genome (Morgan et al. 1993).

  Recombinant retroviruses, like all other recombinant viruses, are produced by a two part system composed of a packaging cell line and a recombinant vector (Anderson 1992, Levine and Friedmann 1993). The packaging cell line expresses all the structural viral genes (*gag, pol and env*) necessary for the formation of an infectious virion. The retroviral vector is essentially the wild-type genome with all the viral genes removed. This vector encodes the transgene(s) and the

Table 8.2. Genetic strategies for tissue repair

Target cell	Transferred gene	Vector system	Clinical relevance	Reference
Keratinocyte	Growth hormone	Retrovirus (*in vitro*)	Skin	Morgan 1987
	LacZ	Retrovirus (*in vitro*)	Skin	Garlick 1991 Vogt 1994
	PDGF-A	Retrovirus (*in vitro*)	Wound healing, skin replacement	Eming 1995
	IGF-1	Retrovirus (*in vitro*)	Wound healing, skin replacement	Eming 1996
	EGF	Particle bombardment (*in vivo*)	Wound healing	Andree 1994
	TGF-β1	Particle bombardment (*in vivo*)	Wound healing	Benn 1996
	PDGF	Particle bombardment (*in vivo*)	Wound healing	Eming 1999
	LacZ, IL-8	Plasmid injection (*in vivo*)	Skin	Hengge 1995
	LacZ	Liposome (*in vivo*)	Skin appendages	Li 1995
Fibroblast	LacZ	Retrovirus (*in vitro*)	Skin replacement	Krueger 1994
	bFGF	Liposome (*in vivo*)	Wound healing	Sun 1997
Macrophages	LacZ	Liposome (*in vivo*)	Ligament healing	Nakamura 1998
	PDGF	Gene-activated matrix (*in vivo*)	Wound healing	Shea 1999
Chondrocytes	LacZ, IL-1ra	Adenovirus (*in vitro*)	Cartilage replacement	Baragi 1995
	PTH	Gene-activated matrix (*in vivo*)	Cartilage replacement	Bonadio 1999
Synovial cells	IL-1ra	Retrovirus (*in vitro*)	Rheumatoid arthritis	Bandara 1993
Endothelial cells	LacZ, tPA	Retrovirus (*in vitro*)	Local thrombolysis	Wilson 1989 Zweibel 1989 Dichek 1996
	VEGF	Plasmid injection (*in vivo*)	Restenosis prevention	Tio 1998
	bFGF	Adenovirus (*in vivo*)	Angiogenesis	Muhlhauser 1995 Sun 1997

regulatory sequences necessary for their expression as well as a special packaging sequence (ψ) which is required for encapsidation of the genome into an infectious viral particle (Morgan et al. 1993). The retroviral vector is transfected into the packaging cell line. The structural proteins expressed by the packaging cell line recognize the packaging sequence on RNAs transcribed from the transfected vector and encapsidate them into an infectious virion which is subsequently exocytosed by the cell and released into the culture medium. This medium containing infectious retroviral particles is harvested and used to transduce target cells. To achieve gene transfer the virus adsorbs on the target cell to a specific receptor and is internalized. The packaged RNA is uncoated, converted into DNA and the recombinant vector is stably integrated into the host genome.

Recombinant retroviruses have been one of the most successful methods for gene transfer and clinical application (Roemer and Friedmann 1992, Mulligan 1993). The molecular biology of these viruses is well understood, thus the manipulation of the viral genomes is straightforward and controllable. The major advantages of retroviral gene transfer are that recombinant retroviruses are capable of transferring genes into a wide range of different cell types including normal diploid cells, and at high efficiency, the genes are stably integrated into the chromosomal DNA. Disadvantages of retroviral gene transfer are that only genes of limited size (<6 kb) can be packaged and transferred, the producer cell lines produce virus in relatively low titers (10^5-10^7/ml) and methods to concentrate viral particles without loss of infectivity are difficult. Another significant disadvantage of recombinant retroviruses is that integration of the transferred gene occurs only in dividing cells, which limits the types of cells and tissues that can be modified. Recently, Naldini et al. described the construction of a retroviral vector based on a lentivirus which was able to integrate into the genome of non-proliferating cells and thereby overcame one of the major constraints in retroviral gene transfer (Naldini et al. 1996). Another area in need of development is the stability of gene expression of retrovirally transduced cells. Although long term gene expression has been reported in some systems, including fibroblasts and muscle cells, transient expression in retrovirally modified cells has also been described (Palmer et al. 1991). This in vivo instability of gene expression is unclear, however methylation or deletion of the proviral DNA are discussed (Challita and Kohn 1994).

The use of recombinant retroviruses has raised some safety concerns. These concerns have centered on two areas (Temin 1990, Cornetta et al. 1991, Roemer and Friedmann 1992). The early retroviral packaging cell lines occasionally produced replication competent virus by homologous recombination between the retroviral vector and the packaging cell line's retroviral sequences. Recent advances in the construction of these cell lines have made the emergence of replication competent viruses essentially impossible (Danos and Mulligan 1988). The other main safety concern was the possibility that the retrovirus, due to its integration into the host cell's genome, would activate a protooncogene and cause a neoplastic cell to become cancerous. However, the probability of insertion adjacent to a protooncogene is very low, and several mutations are required for a cell to become cancerous. Consequently, the risk of cellular transformation by retroviral vectors is extremely low and is typically outweighed by the potential therapeutic benefits for the patients (Temin 1990, Cornetta et al. 1991).

Recombinant Adenovirus

Adenoviruses are large (36 kb double stranded DNA genome) non-enveloped viruses. Most recombinant adenoviral vectors are based on a mutant of adenovirus type 5 (Ad5). The viral genome is organized into several early (E1-E4) and late (L1–L5) transcriptional regions depending on whether they are expressed before or after viral replication (Horwitz 1990). In general, early transcriptional units encode regulatory proteins that activate the transcription of other viral genes, whereas late transcriptional regions predominantly encode structural proteins that comprise the viral capsid. Most adenovirus vectors carry a deletion in the early region (E1), which renders the virus unable to replicate in many cell types and which creates space for the insertion of the gene of interest. Early genes in the E3 region may also be deleted to create further space for the insertion of additional genes. The recombinant adenoviral vector is generated by homologous recombination between the gene of interest (which is inserted into a plasmid vector so that it is flanked by adenovirus sequences) and the genome of an adenovirus with an E1 deletion. The recombinant vector is transfected into a packaging cell line (293 cells) which expresses the E1 gene products for virus production. This virus stock is screened for the rare event of correct homologous recombination in which the gene of interest has correctly recombined with the E1 minus mutant. The recombinant virus with the correct structure is isolated and grown on packaging cells to high titers.

Adenoviruses provide a useful alternative to retroviral gene transfer vectors. Their primary advantage is their ability to infect non-dividing cells (Mulligan 1993). This makes the in vivo transduction of tissues composed of fully differentiated or slowly dividing cells such as the liver and lung possible. Adenoviruses can be grown to high titers (10^{10}–10^{12} particles/ml) and can be concentrated another 100-fold without significant loss of infectivity (Roemer and Friedmann 1992). On the other hand significant technical issues limit the usefulness of adenoviral based vectors. Adenoviruses can only support the packaging of therapeutic genes that are smaller than 7 kb (Miller 1992). In addition, the genome of adenoviruses does not integrate into its host cells' genetic material but instead remains episomal (Miller 1992). Thus, gene expression is transient due to the loss of the vector DNA from the transduced cells over time. It is likely that repeated treatments of the patient will be required for continuous relief of chronic disorders. Unfortunately, repeated treatments may provoke an immune response to the viral proteins that could significantly reduce their effectiveness. Recombinant adenoviruses also tend to induce a mild, transient and dose-dependent inflammatory response that may also limit their usefulness for gene therapy. In addition, the current generation of adenoviral vectors expresses low levels of viral proteins that may be cytotoxic or may stimulate an immune response which may destroy the genetically modified cells (Roemer and Friedmann 1992, Levine and Friedmann 1993). However, strategies are being developed to limit the immune response to adenovirus particles (Schiedner et al. 1998).

Nonviral Methods

Effective nonviral gene transfer systems have been developed that deliver genes to target cells without the inherent disadvantages of viral-based systems such as antigenicity, potential for recombination with wild type viruses and possible cellular damage due to persistent or repeated exposure to the viral vectors (Felgner and Rhodes 1991). These synthetic systems are also easier to manufacture on a large scale because they typically use plasmid constructs that can be grown with existing fermentation technology. In addition, tedious measurements of viral titers and tests for replication competent virus are avoided. Direct plasmid application, lipofection and receptor-mediated delivery vectors are the most promising nonviral systems. There are many other nonviral transfection techniques which are too inefficient for clinical use (i.e. coprecipitation of DNA with calcium phosphate (Chen and Okayama 1987), DNA complexed with DEAE-dextran (Pagano et al. 1967), electroporation (Neumann et al. 1982) or laborious microinjection of DNA (Capecchi 1980).

Direct Plasmid Gene Delivery

The most straightforward application of DNA to the skin or into the tissue is the direct injection of "naked" plasmid DNA (Hengge et al. 1995, Fan et al. 1999). The mechanism by which keratinocytes take up naked DNA is not understood, although it may be related to uptake by semi-permanent membrane vesicles as suggested for monocytes (Dowty et al. 1995). There is evidence that plasmid DNA is not integrated into the cellular genome, remaining instead in a non-replicating episomal form (Wolff et al. 1992, Hengge et al. 1995).

Alternatively, plasmid DNA has been introduced into the skin by high-frequency puncturing of the skin with fine short needles (Ciernik et al. 1996, Eriksson et al. 1998), called puncture-mediated gene transfer or microseeding. Comparable studies demonstrated that the DNA delivery by this technique yields much higher levels of transgene expression than that mediated by single dermis injection.

Liposomes

Cationic liposomes coated with DNA have also been used for gene transfer. This technique relies upon the anionic properties of DNA, the cationic lipids and the negatively charged cell surface. Cationic liposomes are prepared by sonicating an aqueous suspension of cationic and neutral lipids. The unilamellar liposomes are mixed with the plasmid DNA, whose negatively charged backbone forms a noncovalent complex with the positively charged cationic lipids (Felgner and

Ringold 1989). For gene transfer or lipofection, the liposome-DNA complex is added to the target cells, adsorbs to the cell membrane and delivers the DNA into the cytoplasm. Stable integration of the DNA into the genome is low and comparable to calcium phosphate transfection (10^{-4}–10^{-5}).

Lipofection has been used with a variety of cell types in vitro and tissues in vivo, as well as in clinical trials (Nabel et al. 1990, Stribling et al. 1992, Nabel et al. 1993, Takeshita et al. 1994, Li and Hoffman 1995, Sun et al. 1997). The main advantages of liposomes are: 1) they can deliver DNA to virtually any cell type, 2) there are no constraints as to the size of the gene, 3) they are relatively non-toxic and 4) they can be applied repeatedly. Drawbacks of lipofection are the low frequency of stable transfection and the expense of the reagents.

Particle Mediated Gene Transfer

Another approach for gene transfer is a physical means of gene delivery by the bombardment of cells/tissues with DNA-coated particles or microprojectiles (Klein et al. 1987, Yang and Sun 1995, Yang et al. 1997). Microparticles (e.g. gold, tungsten) coated with the gene of interest are accelerated by a force (e.g. helium pressure) to penetrate the cells and to deliver the DNA. Using different mammalian cell culture lines, it was demonstrated that 3–15% of bombarded cells in monolayer culture expressed high levels of the transgene. However, similar to the other transfection methods, the transferred genes are expressed transiently and stable gene transfer occurred at a frequency of only 10^{-3}–10^{-4} (Yang et al. 1990, Cheng et al. 1993).

Advantages of this technology are the applicability to different cell types and tissues, the possibility to deliver large DNA molecules and the high loading capacity of the microprojectiles offering the ability to deliver multiple genes. This could facilitate the evaluation of the coordinate expression of multiple genes in the same tissue. Another significant advantage is the applicability of this technology for in vivo gene transfer. Bombardment of many tissues including the skin, liver pancreas, kidney and muscle resulted in readily detectable transgene activities (Williams et al. 1991, Lu et al. 1995, Sun et al. 1995, Benn et al. 1996, Mahvi et al. 1996, Eming et al. 1999). In skin and liver, transgene expression peaked between 1 and 3 days after bombardment and was minimal after 1 and 2 weeks, respectively. Current limitations of this technique are comparable to those of other transfection methods in that gene expression is transient and the frequency of stable gene integration is low.

Model Systems for Gene Transfer in Soft Tissue Repair

In Vitro Gene Transfer Techniques

As a surface tissue, the skin has several features that make it amenable to ex vivo and in vivo gene transfer (Khavari 1997, Khavari and Krueger 1997, Hengge et al. 1999). Epidermal keratinocytes are an attractive target for ex vivo gene therapy because they are easy to obtain, grow rapidly under appropriate culture conditions, and can be transplanted. The successful use of cultured epidermal sheet grafts as long-term wound coverage indicates that the epidermal stem cell survives in culture and can reconstitute a differentiated and renewable epidermis.

An alternative approach to the treatment of chronic wounds is the use of sheets of cultured autologous or allogeneic epidermal cells as a biological dressing (reviewed in Terskikh and Vasiliev 1999). Although the cells are eventually lost from the graft site, it is believed that the cells accelerate the healing process by providing an occlusive covering that sustains the synthesis and secretion of growth factors.

Several recombinant proteins have been evaluated in animals and humans for the acceleration of wound healing (Lawrence and Diegelman 1994, Scharffetter-Kochanek et al. 1999). Although the results in animal studies have been encouraging, human studies were less so. Several issues could contribute to the current limitations of the use of purified growth factor proteins. An important feature to the efficacy of these proteins appears to be the need for sustained delivery to achieve optimal wound repair.

One technology that could combine the epidermal cell-based biological dressing with the sustained delivery of high levels of a specific growth factor is retroviral gene transfer. Multiple studies have shown that keratinocytes can be effectively gene modified using retrovirus (Ghazizadeh et al. 1999), and different genes have been expressed including human growth hormone (Morgan et al. 1987), clotting factor IX (Gerrard et al. 1993), chloramphenicol acetyltransferase (Lee and Taichman 1989), apolipoprotein E (Fenjves et al. 1994) and laminin IV (Hoeffler et al. 1995). Recently, we used retroviral gene transfer to overexpress wound healing growth factors in keratinocytes, namely different PDGF isoforms or IGF-1 (Eming et al. 1995, Eming et al. 1996). PDGF is mitogenic and chemotactic for fibroblasts and mononuclear cells and is considered one of the master growth factors stimulating wound healing. IGF-1 besides stimulating keratinocyte proliferation and migration, induces angiogenesis and fibroblast proliferation. Genetically modified keratinocytes were shown to synthesize and secrete high levels of PDGF or IGF-1 in vitro. When modified cells were transplanted as an epithelial sheet to athymic mice, PDGF-expressing cells formed a differentiated epidermal structure, comparable to unmodified cells. The newly synthesized connective tissue layer subjacent to the PDGF-A-modified grafts was significantly thicker and showed an increase in cellularity, vascularity and fibronectin deposition, when compared to control grafts of unmodified cells or grafts expressing IGF-1. IGF-1-expressing keratinocytes also formed a stratified epidermis but showed an increase in the proliferation of modified cells, demonstrating that genetic modification can be used to modify the autocrine control of keratinocyte proliferation. These data demonstrate the feasibility of genetically modifying the cells of a skin substitute to secrete high levels of wound healing growth factors and the ability of this genetically modified skin substitute to affect the tissue formation process in vitro. Such modified skin substitutes may be useful in the future for the local and sustained delivery of wound healing growth factors (e.g. in chronic ulcers).

In addition to transplanting keratinocytes as epidermal sheets, more recent efforts have concentrated on developing a composite graft of cultured keratinocytes seeded onto a dermal analog so that both epidermal and dermal components are supplied. Composite grafts have been produced with keratinocytes seeded onto various dermal analogs, including collagen-GAG matrices (Hansbrough et al. 1989), fibroblast-contracted collagen lattices (Bell et al. 1981, Parenteau et al. 1991, Eaglstein and Falanga 1998), or acellular dermis (Medalie et al. 1996). Although the long-term outcome of these composite grafts is comparable to native skin autografts for the treatment of full-thickness burns, the composite grafts are more fragile, revascularize slower, and show a decreased percentage of initial engraftment resulting in an increased incidence of regrafting (Boyce et al. 1995). The molecular and cellular events that control the take of a graft are complex and unclear, but certainly involve the action of cells from the wound bed as well as from the graft. Genetically modified cells overexpressing potent growth factors could enhance the performance of composite skin grafts. To test this hypothesis we seeded gene-modified keratinocytes, which expressed the marker gene lacZ or PDGF, on acellular human dermis and transplanted these gene modified composite grafts to athymic mice (Eming et al. 1998). As indicated by lacZ expression numerous gene modified cells were present 1 week following transplantation (Fig. 8.1 a,b). Grafts overexpressing PDGF showed an increase in fibrovascular ingrowth in the dermal template and graft contraction was reduced (Fig. 8.1 c, d). These data indicate that genetic modification of cells combined with biomaterials can expand the potency of biomaterials.

Dermal fibroblasts have also been genetically modified to express various genes, including human growth hormone (Krueger et al. 1994), adenosine deaminase (Palmer et al. 1991), β-galactosidase (Krueger et al. 1994), β-glucuronidase (Moullier et al. 1993), and PDGF-AA (Machens et al. 1998). The primary gene transfer strategy chosen in these studies was the genetic modification of fibroblasts by retroviral vectors in vitro and autologous transplantation to the recipient either by injection or by seeding the cells onto a dermal matrix. Both transplantation approaches resulted in active transgene expression in vivo, and serum levels of the corresponding proteins could be temporarily detected. These studies demonstrate the potential of autologous implants of genetically modified fibroblasts as an approach to gene replacement therapy.

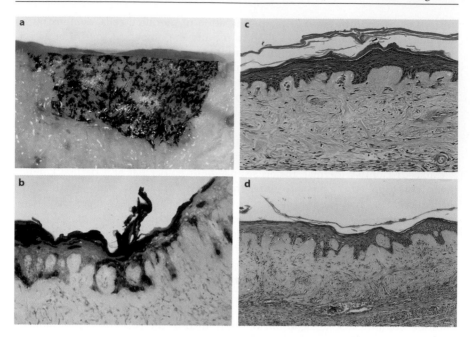

Fig. 8.1 a–d. Genetically modified keratinocytes persist on the acellular dermis after transplantation. Keratinocytes modified with the a-SGC-LacZ (**a,b**) or PDGF-A (**d**). Retroviruses were seeded onto acellular dermis and transplanted to athymic mice. At day 7 grafts were harvested and LacZ gene expression was visualized by X-Gal staining of whole tissue (**a**) or cryosection (**b**). In comparison to grafts of unmodified keratinocytes (**c**) grafts expressing PDGF-A (**d**) are characterized by enhanced cellularity and vascularity

In Vivo Gene Transfer Techniques

Alternative to the in vitro gene transfer strategy several in vivo gene transfer approaches have been investigated (Andree et al. 1994, Hengge et al. 1995, Eriksson et al. 1998, Eming et al. 1999, Ghazizadeh et al. 1999). All these strategies aimed to alter the inhibitory local wound environment.

One of the most practical methods to deliver DNA to the skin is the direct injection. This approach was first described by Hengge and co-workers, who demonstrated that the direct injection of naked DNA encoding the lacZ gene subepidermally, resulted in the transient expression by epidermal keratinocytes (Hengge et al. 1995). Injection of the gene encoding interleukin-8, a potent chemoattractant for neutrophils, resulted in significant dermal neutrophil recruitment. This study demonstrates that DNA directly injected into the skin can be taken up by keratinocytes and its transient expression can induce a biological response.

A more sophisticated technique for the delivery of naked DNA has recently described by Ciernik et al. and Eriksson et al. and was termed puncturemediated gene transfer or microseeding, respectively (Ciernik et al. 1996, Eriksson et al. 1998). These techniques deliver DNA directly to the target cells by multiple perforations using oscillating solid microneedles. Using this technique in a pig model, partial thickness wounds were gene modified with an EGF expression construct. Two days following transfection significant levels of EGF protein could be detected in tissue and wound fluids collected from transfected wound sites. The authors state that transgene expression by microseeding is more efficient than delivering DNA by a single dermal injection.

Another physical method for introducing DNA into cells is the so-called particle bombardment. This technology is based on the acceleration of DNA-coated microprojectiles using high-pressure helium as propellant (Yang et al. 1997). By varying the propellant pressure, the DNA-loaded particles can be targeted to individual epidermal cell layers and optimal gene expression is achieved when most of the gold particles are present in the basal epidermal layer. Increasing the pressure to target deeper connective tissue cells results in many particles lodging in the extracellular matrix rather than in the cytoplasm.

Recently, we used this technique to evaluate the expression of different PDGF isoforms on wound healing in a rat incisional wound healing model (Eming et al. 1999). Using RT-PCR analysis transgene expression was readily detected up to day 3 after transfection, but expression of the transgene fell below detection limits by day 5. To examine the biological effect of transient local PDGF expression we determined the wound breaking strength 7 and 14 days after a single administration of recombinant DNA to the skin. On average we obtained 75–100% increase in mechanical strength of incisions for up to 2 weeks after transfection. These findings indicate that particle-mediated gene transfer is a promising tool for the delivery of growth factor DNA to the skin and can significantly augment the wound healing response. These findings are supported by studies of other groups using this technique. Benn et al. demonstrated that overexpression of TGF-β also resulted in the significant increase of tensile strength of healing rat tissue (Benn et al. 1996). Another group demonstrated that the in vivo transfection of porcine partial-thickness wounds with a vector expressing EGF increased the rate of reepithelialization and shortened the time of wound closure (Andree et al. 1994). Overall these studies demonstrate that particle-mediated transfection using appropriate expression vectors, might be a simple and effective means of enhancing the rate of wound repair in an animal model.

Recently, several groups reported DNA delivery in vivo from polymer coatings, microspheres and synthetic matrices (Bonadio et al. 1999, Shea et al. 1999). In the study of Shea and co-workers plasmid DNA was entrapped within porous polymer matrices of polylactide-co-glycolide (Shea et al. 1999). After immersion in water, DNA was slowly released from the matrix for as long as 30 days and plasmid was shown to be biological active. When transplanted into the subcutaneous tissue of rats a large number of transfected cells were observed in the implant periphery. Matrices carrying the gene for PDGF resulted in a significant increase in the thickness of granulation tissue and the number of blood vessels two and four weeks after transplantation. Alternatively, Bonadio and co-workers investigated the induction of bone in a canine bone defect model following the implantation of a polymer matrix loaded with plasmid encoding the gene for parathyroid hormone (Bonadio et al. 1999). The study demonstrated that normal new bone could be effectively generated through local plasmid gene transfer of parathyroid hormone. In summary, both studies demonstrated that gene activated matrices can lead to sustained gene delivery and are sufficient to cause tissue formation.

Further, adenoviral vectors have been investigated for gene transfer in animal wound healing models. Yamasaki and co-workers demonstrated the reversal of impaired wound repair in inducible nitric oxide synthase-deficient mice (iNOS) by the topical adenoviral-mediated iNOS gene transfer (Yamasaki et al. 1998). Most evidence suggests that adequate rates of nitric oxide (NO) production are essential for normal wound healing. iNOS synthesizes NO in a sustained manner and iNOS knockout mice show a significant delay in repair. The study demonstrated that a single short-term topical application of an adenoviral vector expressing the iNOS gene improved wound healing in the knockout mice. Expression of the mRNA transgene was present up to 10 days after transfection. These data suggest that adenoviral-mediated gene transfer is applicable to deliver potent mediators with wound healing properties.

Liechty et al. investigated the topical application of an adenoviral vector expressing PDGF-B in an ischemic impaired rabbit wound healing model (Liechty et al. 1999). In these studies control animals received an adenoviral vector expressing the marker gene lacZ. In support of the studies from Yamasaki, these studies also demonstrated that adenoviral vectors could efficiently deliver genes to a wound. However, Liechty reported that wounds treated with the adenoviral vector showed a significant defect in reepithelialization. This phenomenon might be the result of an inflammatory response to the adenovirus or a direct cytotoxic effect of the adenovirus.

In addition to cutaneous wound repair, gene transfer has been investigated in other target cells involved in soft tissue repair, as well as cartilage and bone. Although a detailed discussion of the many applications investigated is beyond the scope of this review, several examples will illustrate the promising application of this technique. Ligaments are specialized connective tissues that link bone to bone, consisting of parallel bundles of collagen fibers, dermatan sulfate and interspersed fibroblasts. Ligaments may be subject to a variety of injuries and rapid restoration of the function is wanted. Therefore, methods aimed to stimulate cell proliferation and synthesis of extracellular matrix could provide more rapid and stronger ligament healing. Recently, the introduction of growth factor genes into the healing patellar ligament has been investigated in this regard (Nakamura et al. 1998). Although the efficiency of transfection in these studies was modest, they demonstrated the feasibility to augment the healing response by gene transfer.

Similarly, endothelial cells have been the target for gene transfer of factors stimulating angiogenesis to treat ischemic disease and also cutaneous tissue repair (Muhlhauser et al. 1995, Sun et al. 1997, Tio et al. 1998). Further, chondrocytes have been genetically modified by adenovirus. Thereby, interleukin-1 receptor antagonist (IL-1ra)-expressing chondrocytes were seeded onto the surface of osteoarthritic cartilage in organ culture and were able to protect the osteoarthritic cartilage from IL-1-induced matrix degradation (Baragi et al. 1995). Additionally, it might be possible to augment cartilage formation by gene modifying chondrocytes with growth factor genes, including bFGF, TGF-β, IGF-1 and

PDGF, which are important regulators of chondrocyte proliferation, differentiation and matrix synthesis (Fujisate et al. 1996, Shida et al. 1996).

Future Developments

Molecular medicine holds considerable therapeutic promise and the potential range and versatility of gene therapy in tissue repair has been outlined in this article. Numerous experimental investigations have demonstrated the feasibility of gene transfer to various cell types involved in soft tissue repair. Viral based methods, including retroviral and adenoviral methods have been shown to transduce cells with high efficiency. Also nonviral methods, which use a variety of physical/chemical techniques for gene transfer have been successfully used to augment the wound healing response.

A key challenge which remains to be addressed to advance cutaneous gene transfer in general and gene transfer in wound healing is the development of vehicles that can provide safe, efficient, selective, and targeted gene delivery in a nontoxic, noninflammatory and nonimmunogenic manner. Recently, several groups reported the exciting approach to deliver plasmid DNA by combining functional genes with biocompatible materials, which have been used for tissue engineering (Bonadio et al. 1999, Shea et al. 1999). Thereby, a gene-activated matrix was generated, which is characterized by controlled and sustained gene delivery into the periphery. Interestingly, gene transfer using this technique appeared to be more effective than direct dermal injection of the plasmid. It might be speculated that slow gene delivery may enhance the efficiency of gene transfer beyond the enhancement obtained by gene replacement itself. This work could stimulate new approaches that integrate physical and genetic signals in tissue regeneration.

To date, genetic strategies in tissue repair have been predominantly developed in various animal models. However, factors which are essential for efficient gene transfer and gene expression are different in animal models than in the human system including the gene-regulating milieu, interacting proteins, tissue architecture, and finally, the disease phenotype. Therefore, one major advance in the development of genetic strategies in tissue repair is the evaluation of the efficacy of local gene therapy in the human system. Grafting human gene modified cells or human skin to immunodeficient animals offers one model system to answer these questions. However, only evaluating the efficiency of gene transfer in the human system will give proof whether gene transfer offers an alternative approach to tissue repair.

References

Anderson WF (1992) Human gene therapy. Science 256:808–813

Andree C, Swain WF, Page CP, Macklin MD, Slama J, Hatzis D, Eriksson E (1994) In vivo transfer and expression of a human epidermal growth factor gene accelerates wound repair. Proc Natl Acad Sci USA 91:12 188–12 192

Apelquvist J, Larsson J, Agardt CD (1993) Longterm prognosis for diabetic patients with food ulcers. J Internal Med 233:485–491

Bandara G, Mueller GM, Galea-Lauri J, Tindal MH, Georgescu HI, Suchanek MK, Hung GL, Glorioso JC, Robbins PD, Evans CH (1993) Intraarticular expression of biologically active IL-1 receptor antagonist protein by ex vivo gene transfer. Proc Natl Acad Sci USA 90:10 764–10 768

Baragi VM, Renkiewicz RR, Jordan H, Bonadio J, Hartman JW (1995) Transplantation of transduced chondrocytes protects articular cartilage from IL-1 induced extracellular matrix degradation. J Clin Invest 96:2454–2460

Bell E, Ehrlich HP, Buttle DJ, Nakatsuji T (1981) Living tissue formed in vitro and accepted as skin-equivalent tissue of full thickness. Science 211:1052–1054

Benn SI, Whitsitt JS, Broadley KN, Nanney LB, Perkins D, He L, Patel M, Morgan JR, Swain WF, Davidson JM (1996) Enhancement of wound healing in rat skin following particle bombardment with cDNAs encoding TGF-β1. J Clin Invest 98:2894–2902

Bennett NT, Schultz GS (1993) Growth factors and wound healing: biochemical properties of growth factors and their receptors. Am J Surg 165:728–737

Bonadio J, Smily E, Patil P, Goldstein S (1999) Localized, direct plasmid gene delivery in vivo: prolonged therapy results in reproducible tissue regeneration. Nat Med 5:753–759

Boyce ST, Goretsky MJ, Greenhalgh DG, Kagan RJ, Rieman MT, Warden GD (1995) Comparative assessment of cultured skin substitutes and native skin autografts for treatment of full-thickness burns. Ann Surg 222:743–752

Capecchi M (1980) High efficiency transformation by direct microinjection of DNA into cultured mammalian cells. Cell 22:479–488

Challita PM, Kohn DB (1994) Lack of expression from a retroviral vector after transduction of murine hematopoietic stem cells is associated with methylation in vivo. Proc Natl Acad Sci USA 91:2567–2571

Chen C, Okayama H (1987) High efficiency transformation of mammalian cells by plasmid DNA. Mol Cell Biol 7:2745–2752

Cheng L, Ziegelhoffer PR, Yang NS (1993) In vivo promoter activity and transgene expression in mammalian somatic tissues evaluated by using particle bombardment. Proc Natl Acad Sci USA 90:4455–4459

Ciernik IF, Krayenbühl BH, Carbone DP (1996) Puncture-mediated gene transfer to the skin. Hum Gen Ther 7:893–899

Cornetta K, Morgan RA, Anderson WF (1991) Safety issues related to retroviral-mediated gene transfer in humans. Hum Gen Ther 2:5–14

Danos O, Mulligan R (1988) Safe and efficient generation of recombinant retroviruses with amphotropic and ecotropic host ranges. Proc Natl Acad Sci USA 85:6460–6464

Dichek DA, Neville RF, Zweibel JA, Freeman SM, Leon MB, Anderson WF (1996) Seeding of intravascular stents with genetically engineered endothelial cells. Circulation 80: 1347–1353

Dowty ME, Williams P, Zhang G, Hagstrom JE, Wolff JA (1995) Plasmid entry into postmitotic nuclei of primary rat myoblasts. Proc Natl Acad Sci USA 92:4572–4576

Eaglstein WH, Falanga V (1998) Tissue engineering and the development of Apligraf, a human skin equivalent. Adv Wound Care 11:1–8

Eming SA, Lee J, Snow RG, Tompkins RG, Yarmush ML, Morgan JR (1995) Genetically modified human epidermis overexpressing PDGF-A directs the development of a cellular and vascular connective tissue stroma when transplanted to athymic mice. J Invest Dermatol 105:756–763

Eming SA, Snow RG, Yarmush ML, Morgan JR (1996) Targeted expression of IGF-1 to human keratinocytes: modification of the autocrine control of keratinocyte proliferation. J Invest Dermatol 106:113–120

Eming SA, Medalie DA, Tompkins RG, Yarmush ML, Morgan JR (1998) Genetically modified human keratinocytes overexpressing PDGF-A enhance the performance of a composite skin graft. Hum Gen Ther 9:529–539

Eming SA, Whitsitt JS, He L, Krieg T, Morgan JR, Davidson JM (1999) Particle-mediated gene transfer of PDGF isoforms promotes wound repair. J Invest Dermatol 112:297–302

Eriksson E, Yao F, Svensjö T, Winkler T, Slama J, Macklin MD, Andree C, McGregor M, Hinshaw V, Swain WF (1998) In vivo gene transfer to skin and wound by microseeding. J Surg Res 78:85–91

Falanga V (1992) Growth factors and chronic wounds: the need to understand the microenvironment. J Dermatol 19:667–672

Falanga V (1993) Chronic wounds: pathophysiologic and experimental considerations. J Invest Dermatol 100:721–725

Fan H, Lin Q, Morrissey GR, Khavari PA (1999) Immunization via hair follicles by topical application of naked DNA to normal skin. Nat Biotechnol 17:870–872

Felgner PL, Ringold GM (1989) Cationic liposome-mediated transfection. Nature 337:387–388

Felgner PL, Rhodes G (1991) Gene therapeutics. Nature 349:351–352

Fenjves ES, Smith J, Zaradic S, Taichman LB (1994) Systemic delivery of secreted protein by grafts of epidermal keratinocytes: Prospects for keratinocyte gene therapy. Hum Gene Ther 5:1241–1248

Friedmann T (1992) A brief history of gene therapy. Nat Genet 2:93–98

Fujisate T, Sajiki T, Liu O, Ikada Y (1996) Effects of bFGF on cartilage regeneration in chondrocyte-seeded collagen sponge scaffold. Biomaterials 17:155–162

Garlick JA, Katz AB Fenjves ES, Taichman LB (1991) Retrovirus mediated transduction of cultured epidermal keratinocytes. J Invest Dermatol 97:824–829

Gerrard AJ, Hudson DL, Brownlee GG, Watt FM (1993) Towards gene therapy for haemophilia B using primary human keratinocytes. Nat Genet 3:180–183

Ghazizadeh S, Harrington R, Taichman L (1999) In vivo transduction of mouse epidermis with recombinant retroviral vectors: implications for cutaneous gene therapy. Gene Ther 6:1267–1275

Hansbrough JF, Boyce ST, Cooper ML, Foreman TJ (1989) Burn wound closure with cultured autologous keratinocytes and fibroblasts attached to a collagen-glycosaminoglycan substrate. J Am Med Assn 262:2125–2130

Hengge UR, Chan EF, Foster RA, Walker PS, Vogel JC (1995) Cytokine gene expression in epidermis with biological effects following injection of naked DNA. Nat Genet 10:161–166

Hengge UR, Taichman LB, Kaur P, Rogers G, Jensen TG, Goldsmith LA, Rees JL, Christiano AM (1999) How realistic is cutaneous gene therapy? Exp Dermatol 8:419–431

Herrick SE, Sloan P, McGurk M, Freak L, McCollum CN, Ferguson MWJ (1992) Sequential changes in histologic pattern and extracellular matrix deposition during the healing of chronic venous ulcers. Am J Path 141:1085–1095

Hoeffler WK, Wang CK, Matsui C (1995) Phenotypic reversion of junctional epidermolysis bullosa keratinocytes by introduction of a therapeutic laminin 5 chain gene. J Invest Dermatol 104:597

Horwitz MS (1990) Adenoviruses. In: Fields BN, Knipe DM (eds) Virology, Raven Press, New York, pp 1723–1741

Khavari PA (1997) Therapeutic gene delivery to the skin. Mol Med Today 3:533–538

Khavari PA, Krueger GG (1997) Cutaneous gene delivery. Adv Clin Res 5:27–35

Klein TM, Wolf ED, Wu R, Sanford JC (1987) High-velocity microprojectiles for delivering nucleic acids into cells. Nature 327:70–73

Krueger GG, Morgan JR, Jorgensen CM, Schmidt L, Li HL, Kwan MK, Boyce ST, Wiley HS, Kaplan J, Petersen MJ (1994) Genetically modified skin to treat disease: potential and limitations. J Invest Dermatol 103:76S–84 S

Laing P (1988) The development and complications of diabetic foot ulcers. Am J Surg 176:5S-10S

Lawrence T, Diegelman RF (1994) Growth factors in wound healing. Clinics Dermatol 12:157-169

Lee JI, Taichman LB (1989) Transient expression of a transfected gene in cultured epidermal keratinocytes: implications for future studies. J Invest Dermatol 92:267-271

Levine F, Friedmann T (1993) Gene therapy. Am J Dis Child 147:1167-1174

Li L, Hoffman RM (1995) The feasibility of targeted selective gene therapy of the hair follicle. Nat Genet 1:705-706

Liechty KW, Nesbit M, Herlyn M, Radu A, Adzick NS, Crombleholme TM (1999) Adenoviral-mediated overexpression of PDGF-B corrects ischemic impaired wound healing. J Invest Dermatol 113:375-383

Lu B, Scott G, Goldsmith LA (1995) A model for keratinocyte gene therapy: Preclinical and therapeutic considerations. Proc Ass Am Phys 108:165-172

Machens HG, Morgan JR, Berthiaume F, Stefanovich P, Reimer R, Berger AC (1998) Genetically modified fibroblasts induce angiogenesis in the rat epigastric island flap. Langenbecks Arch Surg 383:345-350

Mahvi DM, Burkholder JK, Turner J, Culp J, Malter JS, Sondel PM, Yang NS (1996) Particle-mediated gene transfer of GMCSF cDNA to tumor cells: implications for a clinically relevant tumor vaccine. Hum Gene Ther 7:1535-1543

Martin P (1997) Wound healing - Aiming for perfect skin regeneration. Science 276:75-81

Medalie DA, Eming SA, Tompkins RG, Yarmush ML, Krueger GG, Morgan JR (1996) Evaluation of human skin reconstituted from composite grafts of cultured keratinocytes and human acellular dermis transplanted to athymic mice. J Invest Dermatol 107:121-127

Miller AD (1992) Human gene therapy comes of age. Nature 357:455-460

Morgan JR, Barrandon Y, Green H, Mulligan RC (1987) Expression of an exogenous growth hormone gene by transplantable human epidermal cells. Science 237:1476-1479

Morgan JR, Tompkins RG, Yarmush ML (1993) Advances in recombinant retroviruses for gene delivery. Advanced Drug Delivery Reviews 12:143-158

Moullier P, Bohl D, Heard JM, Danos O (1993) Correction of lysosomal storage in the liver and spleen of MPS VII mice by implantation of genetically modified skin fibroblasts. Nat Genet 4:154-159

Muhlhauser J, Pili R, Merrill MJ, Maeda H, Passaniti A, Crystal RG, Capogrossi MC (1995) In vivo angiogenesis induced by recombinant adenovirus vectors coding either for secreted or nonsecreted forms of aFGF. Hum Gene Ther 6:1457-1465

Mulligan RC (1993) The basic science of gene therapy. Science 260:926-932

Nabel EG, Plautz G, Nabel GJ (1990) Site-specific gene expression in vivo by direct gene transfer into arterial wall. Science 249:1285-1288

Nabel GJ, Nabel EG, Yang ZY, Fox BA, Plautz GE, Gao X, Huang L, Shu S, Gordon D, Chang AE (1993) Direct gene transfer with DNA-liposome complexes in melanoma: expression, biologic activity, and lack of toxicity in humans. Proc Natl Acad Sci USA 90:11307-11311

Naldini L, Blömer U, Gallay P, Ory D, Mulligan R, Gage FH, Verma IM, Trono D (1996) In vivo delivery and stable transduction of nondividing cells by a lentiviral vector. Science 272:263-267

Nakamura N, Shino K, Natsuume T, Horibe S, Matsumoto N, Kaneda Y, Ochi T (1998) Early biological effect of in vivo gene transfer of PDGF-B into healing patellar ligament. Gene Ther 5:1165-1170

Neumann E, Schaefer-Ridder M, Wang Y, Hofschneider PH (1982) Gene transfer into mouse lyoma cells by electroporation in high electric fields. EMBO J 1:841-845

Pagano J, McCutchan JH, Vaheri A (1967) Factors influencing the enhancement of the infectivity of poliovirus ribonucleic acid by diethylaminoethyl-dextran. J Virol 1:891-897

Palmer TD, Rosman GJ, Osborne WRA, Miller AD (1991) Genetically modified skin fibroblasts persist long after transplantation but gradually inactivate introduced genes. Proc Natl Acad Sci USA 88:1330-1334

Parenteau NC, Nolte CM, Belbo PR, Rosenberg M, Wilkins LM, Johnson EW, Watson S, Mason VS, Bell E (1991) Epidermis generated in vitro: Practical considerations and applications. J Cell Biochem 45:245-251

Phillips TJ, Dover JS (1991) Leg ulcers. J Am Acad Dermatol 25:965–987

Roemer K, Friedmann T (1992) Concepts and strategies for human gene therapy. Eur J Biochem 208:211–225

Scharffetter-Kochanek K, Meewes C, Eming SA, Dissemond J, Hani N, Wenk J, Wlaschek M, Brenneisen P (1999) Chronische Wunden und Wachstumsfaktoren. Z Hautkrankheiten 74:664–672

Schiedner G, Moral N, Parks RJ, Wu Y, Koopamans SC, Langston C, Graham FL, Beaudet AL, Kochanek S (1998) Genomic DNA transfer with high-capacity adenovirus vector results in improved in vivo gene expression and decreased toxicity. Nat Genet 18:180–183

Shea LD, Smiley E, Bonadio J, Mooney DJ (1999) DNA delivery from polymer matrices for tissue engineering. Nat Biotechnol 17:551–554

Shida J, Jingushi S, Izumi T, Iwaki A, Sugioka Y (1996) bFGF stimulates articular cartilage enlargement in young rats in vivo. J Orthop Res 14:265–272

Singer AJ, Clark RAF (1999) Cutaneous wound healing. Lancet 341:738–746

Stribling R, Brunette E, Liggitt D, Gaensler K, Debs R (1992) Aerosol gene delivery in vivo. Proc Natl Acad Sci USA 89:11 277–11 281

Sun WH, Burkholder JK, Sun J, Culp J, Turner J, Lu XG, Pugh TD, Ershler WB, Yang NS (1995) In vivo cytokine gene transfer by gene gun reduces tumor growth in mice. Proc Natl Acad Sci USA 92:2889–2893

Sun L, Xu L, Chang H, Henry FA, Miller RM, Harmon JM, Nielsen TB (1997) Transfection with a FGF cDNA improves wound healing. J Invest Dermatol 108:313–318

Takeshita S, Gal D, Leclere GJ (1994) Increased gene expression after liposome-mediated arterial gene transfer associated with intimal smooth muscle cell proliferation. In vitro and in vivo findings in a rabbit model of vascular injury. J Clin Invest 93:652–661

Terskikh VV, Vasiliev AV (1999) Cultivation and transplantation of epidermal keratinocytes. Int Rev Cytol 188:41–72

Temin HM (1990) Safety considerations in somatic gene therapy of human disease with retrovirus vectors. Hum Gene Ther 1:111–123

Tio RA, Isner JM, Walsh K (1998) Gene therapy to prevent restenosis, the Boston experience. Semin Interv Cardiol 3:205–210

Vogt PM, Thompson S, Andree C, Liu P, Breuing K, Hatzis D, Brown H, Mulligan RC, Eriksson E (1994) Genetically modified keratinocytes transplanted to wounds reconstitute the epidermis. Proc Natl Acad Sci USA 91:9307–9311

Williams RS, Johnston SA, Riedy M, DeVit MJ, McElligott SG, Sanford JC (1991) Introduction of foreign genes into tissues of living mice by DNA-coated microprojectiles. Proc Natl Acad Sci USA 88:2726–2730

Wilson JM, Birinyi JK, Salomon RN, Libby P, Callow AD, Mulligan RC (1989) Implementation of vascular grafts lined with genetically modified endothelial cells. Science 244:1344–1348

Wolff JA, Ludtke JJ, Acsadi G, Williams P, Jani A (1992) Long-term persistence of plasmid DNA and foreign gene expression in mouse muscle. Hum Mol Genet 1:363–369

Yang NS, Sun WH (1995) Gene gun and other non-viral approaches for cancer gene therapy. Nat Med 1:481–483

Yang NS, Burkholder J, Roberts B, Martinell B, McCabe D (1990) In vivo and in vitro gene transfer to mammalian somatic cells by particle bombardment. Proc Natl Acad Sci USA 87:9568–9572

Yang NS, McCabe DE, Swain WF (1997) Methods for particle-mediated gene transfer into skin. In: Robbinson PD (ed) Gene Therapy Protocols. Humana Press, Totowa, New Jersey, pp 281–296

Yamasaki K, Edlington HDJ, McClosky C, Tzeng E, Lizonova A, Kovesdi I, Steed DL, Billiar TR (1998) Reversal of impaired wound repair in iNOS-deficient mice by topical adenoviral-mediated iNOS gene transfer. J Clin Invest 101:967–971

Zweibel JA, Freeman SM, Xantoff PW, Cornett K, Ryan U, Anderson WF (1989) High-level recombinant gene expression in rabbit endothelial cells transduced by retroviral vectors. Science 243:220–224

Systemic Effects of Skin Gene Therapy

9 The Use of Skin-Directed Gene Therapy in the Treatment of Systemic Diseases

T. G. JENSEN, K. G. CSAKY

Introduction

Easy access for gene transfer and the existence of sophisticated cultivation and transplantation methods makes the skin an attractive target for somatic gene therapy. An additional advantage includes the theoretical possibility of topical regulation of gene expression. The use of the skin to deliver or remove proteins from the circulation is theoretically possible in that the blood supply to the skin is considerable (5–10% of the cardiac output), can be regulated, and exceeds the demand at least 10-fold (Odland 1983). For safety reasons, the skin is also an attractive organ since genetically modified cells can be easily monitored and, if necessary, be removed.

Genetically modified skin cells, both keratinocytes and fibroblasts, have the capacity of over-producing medically relevant proteins which can then be transported into the circulation (skin as a "neo-organ") (Fenjves et al. 1989). Alternatively, skin cells can be engineered to produce enzymes that are capable of degrading toxic substances accumulating in certain disorders (skin as a "metabolic sink") (Fenjves et al. 1997) (Table 9.1).

Sustained epidermal gene therapy, which is a prerequisite for both cutaneous and systemic epidermal gene therapy, requires gene transfer into stem cells. Although several studies have suggested that this might be possible (Mathor et al. 1996, Deng et al. 1997, Levy et al. 1998, White et al. 1998, Ghazizadeh et al. 1999), the advance in characterization of these cells and defining their location in the skin will probably further enhance the possibilities of specific stem cell targeting (Jensen et al. 1999). Recently, Kolodka et al. were able to successfully transduce stem cells ex vivo and showed persistence of transgene expression for up to 40 weeks when these cells were subsequently transplanted (Kolodka et al. 1998).

Epidermal gene therapy with the purpose of achieving sustained gene expression has mostly focused on the use of retroviral vectors. Delivery of retroviral vectors directly to the skin (in vivo gene therapy) with resulting tissue expression has been difficult to achieve and therefore retrovirally-mediated gene transfer into the skin has been performed mostly ex vivo followed by grafting. It is important to note that most of the work done with ex vivo retroviral transduction utilizes transgenes driven by a viral LTR promoter. This promoter has pre-

Table 9.1. Transfected neo-organs

Neo-organ		Reference
Transgenic keratinocytes	FIX	Alexander and Akhurst 1995
	hGH	Wang et al. 1997
	IGF-II	Da Costa et al. 1994
	TNF-alpha	Cheng et al. 1992
Grafted keratinocytes	ApoE	Fenjves et al. 1989
	hGH	Morgan et al. 1987
	IL-6	Mathor et al. 1996
	Alpha1AT	Setoguchi et al. 1994
	FIX	Gerrard et al. 1993
Keratinocytes in vivo	IL-6	Sun et al. 1995
	IL-8	Hengge et al. 1995
	IL-10	Meng et al. 1998
	α1-antitrypsin	Setoguchi et al. 1994
Fibroblasts in vitro	FVIII	Hoeben et al. 1993
	Alpha-galactosidase	Medin et al. 1996
Fibroblasts in vivo	FIX	Chen et al. 1998
	Beta-glucuronidase	Moullier et al. 1993
	Erythropoietin	Naffakh et al. 1995
	Transferrin	Petersen et al. 1995
Metabolic sink		
Keratinocytes in vitro	Adenosine deaminase	Fenjves et al. 1997
	Ornithine aminotransferase	Sullivan et al. 1997

viously been shown to be downregulated when transduced human keratinocytes are grafted to immunodeficient mice (Fenjves et al. 1996). Due to the complexity and surgical trauma of skin transplantation, methods allowing direct in vivo delivery with long-term expression would be of great value. Chimeric viral vector systems that incorporate the favorable attributes of two different viral vectors such as the efficient in vivo transduction properties of adenoviral vectors and the stable integration of retroviral vectors, might be a solution to these problems (Ramsey et al. 1998). Combination of viral and nonviral gene transfer methods, such as the use of plasmovirus (Noguiez-Hellin et al. 1996), might also be feasible.

Skin as Secretory Organ

Genetically manipulated keratinocytes may be advantageous to use as a neo-organ for the production of secretory proteins. Genetic modification of skin fibroblasts has also been achieved and resulted in overexpression and secretion of numerous potentially therapeutic proteins.

Several rate-limiting steps may inhibit the delivery of a protein from the epidermis to the circulation. The efficiency of synthesis and secretion varies substantially among different proteins. The transport across the basement membrane may be limited by size and hydrophobicity of the protein and many proteins are rapidly degraded in the circulation.

Apolipoprotein E (ApoE)

Human keratinocytes transfected with the human ApoE gene have been shown to increase the secretion of ApoE. When these cells were transplanted onto mice, human ApoE could be detected in the circulation (Fenjves et al. 1989 and 1994). The amount detected in vivo was higher than expected from in vitro measurements, probably due to the fact that the ApoE was mainly produced in suprabasal cells which are the predominant epidermal cell type in vivo. The maximal concentrations obtained from a graft of 7 mm^2 in size was 77 ng/ml. Thus, a graft size of 340 cm^2 (corresponding to 2% of the total body surface in an adult) would be expected to result in a serum ApoE concentration of 374 µg/ml, an amount which greatly exceeds the normal concentration (40 µg/ml).

Human Growth Hormone (hGH)

Because of its therapeutic use and ease of quantification even at low levels, human growth hormone (hGH) has been used as a model protein to study the secretion into the circulation by genetically engineered cells (Morgan et al. 1987, Teumer et al. 1990, Jensen et al. 1994, Wang et al. 1997).

Morgan et al. described the first attempt to engineer keratinocytes secreting hGH into the circulation (Morgan et al. 1987). Retrovirally-transduced primary human keratinocytes did secrete hGH in vitro, but after grafting no hGH could be detected in the circulation. Secretion of hGH into the circulation was later shown by grafting sheets of a human keratinocyte cell line (SCC13) stably transfected with an hGH construct onto mice (Teumer et al. 1990). The secretion rate in vitro was 0.8–5.3 µg/day/10^6 cells. A graft occupying approximately 2% of the surface area was transplanted which resulted in therapeutic serum hGH concentrations of 0.6–1.5 ng/ml for more than 4 weeks.

Primary human keratinocytes transfected with an EBV-based expression vector containing the hGH gene resulted in high expression and secretion into the media (Jensen et al. 1994). A daily secretion of more than 1 µg of biologically active hGH from a 25 cm^2 culture could be obtained. Four days after transplantation of these hGH transfected cultures to mice, hGH could still be detected in mouse serum. This is significant considering that the half-life of hGH in mouse serum is less than four minutes (highest concentration obtained: 2.6 ng/ml). Ten days after transplantation no hGH could be measured.

In contrast, hGH expression driven by a keratin promoter (K14) in transgenic mice resulted in stable expression of the hormone leading to physiological levels in the circulation (Wang et al. 1997). The levels in the circulation ranged from 25 to 50 ng/ml hGH in adult mice, higher than the endogenous mouse GH and resulted in an increase in the size of the mice. Skin from these transgenic mice were subsequently grafted to SCID mice. Transgenic skin grafts from these adults continued to produce and secrete hGH stably (range: 0.15 to 0.40 ng/ml) corresponding to approximately 1/10 of physiological levels in the bloodstream of nontransgenic recipient mice.

Hemophilia

Somatic gene therapy is being explored as a treatment for hemophilia B. Various tissues have been investigated as potential sources for genetically manipulated secretion of Factor IX including liver, skin, muscle, gut, and hematopoietic cells. Long-term expression and correction of animal models following in vivo gene delivery to liver and muscle tissue has recently been reported (Herzog et al. 1999, Snyder et al. 1999).

Two groups described that human coagulation Factor IX secreted from retro-virally-transduced human keratinocytes transplanted onto nude mice could be detected in the circulation (Gerrard et al. 1993, Fenjves et al. 1996). However, the protein could only be measured in the circulation for a limited period. The transport of this protein from the graft to the circulation was found to be ineffi-cient with only 1–5% of the total protein produced entering the circulation (Gerrard et al. 1993).

Recently, White et al. showed that sustained expression of Factor IX from pri-mary human keratinocytes could be achieved using the retroviral vector MFG (White et al. 1998). Transduced keratinocytes, which secreted on average 830 ng of Factor IX/10^6 cells/24 hr in tissue culture, were used to form a bilayered (composite) skin equivalent and grafted onto nude mice under a silicone trans-plantation chamber. Concentrations ranging from 0.1 and 2.75 ng/ml of human Factor IX were found in mouse plasma for more than 1 year.

Alexander and Akhurst developed transgenic mice with targeted expression of human Factor IX from the epidermis (Alexander and Akhurst 1995). The most effective Factor IX expression (46 ng/ml steady-state levels of circulating human Factor IX) was obtained utilizing the human homologue of the keratin 10 pro-moter, which is exclusively active in differentiated keratinocytes. Thus, it was demonstrated that human Factor IX can be efficiently synthesized and secreted from keratinocytes in situ and can cross the epidermal basement membrane to reach the systemic circulation.

Skin fibroblasts have also been the target for Factor IX synthesis. Chen et al. reported that low level (20 ng/ml) expression could be achieved long-term (>600 days) after subcutaneous implantation of primary skin fibroblasts genetically en-gineered to secrete Factor IX into rabbits (Chen et al. 1998). Factor VIII has also been expressed in skin fibroblasts (Hoeben et al. 1993), although its large size may limit its secretion into the circulation.

Lysosomal Storage Diseases

Genetically engineered skin fibroblasts producing and secreting lysosomal proteins may be used to treat inherited metabolic diseases caused by genetic defects of lysosomal enzymes. Mice lacking the enzyme β-glucuronidase develop a disease homologous to human mucopolysaccharidosis type VII (Sly syndrome), and autologous implants of genetically modified skin fibroblasts produced and secreted the enzyme (Moullier et al. 1993). β-glucuronidase accumulated in various tissues and disappearance of the lysosomal storage lesions was observed in both liver and spleen. Fabry's disease, a lysosomal storage disease due to a deficiency of a-galactosidase, has also been attempted as target for skin-directed gene therapy. Skin fibroblasts from Fabry patients were corrected for the metabolic defect by transduction with a retroviral vector containing the a-galactosidase A gene, and secreted enzyme could be detected (Medin et al. 1996). Interestingly, the secreted enzyme was also found to be taken up by uncorrected cells.

Interleukins

Tissue specific expression of interleukins in the skin results in the secretion of biologically active proteins into the blood. Da Costa et al. developed transgenic mice containing extra copies of the mouse insulin-like growth factor-II (IGF-II) gene driven by the bovine keratin 10 promoter (Da Costa et al. 1994). In one line of animals, adult plasma IGF-II levels were elevated at least three times above normal resulting in a lowered lipid content of both brown and white adipose depots at 2–4 months of age.

Cheng et al explored the role of TNF alpha synthesis in keratinocytes (Cheng et al. 1992). The authors used a keratin 14 (K14) promoter to target human TNF alpha expression to the epidermis and other stratified squamous epithelia of transgenic mice. Most mice expressing the K14-TNF alpha transgene stopped gaining weight within 1 week after birth and exhibited retarded hair growth. Over time, the epidermis exhibited an increased stratum corneum and signs of necrosis of the skin.

Interleukins can also be secreted into the blood using the ex vivo delivery approach. Mathor et al. transduced normal human keratinocytes with retroviral constructs expressing a bacterial beta-galactosidase gene or a human interleukin-6 (hIL-6) cDNA. When epidermal sheets prepared from basal cells transduced with hIL-6 were grafted onto athymic animals, the serum levels (range 16–70 pg/ml) of hIL-6 were found to be proportional to the rate of secretion in vitro and to the number of proviral integration events (Mathor et al. 1996).

Genes encoding interleukins have also been directly transferred into the skin and have resulted in secretion into the blood (in vivo gene delivery). Following direct injection of naked plasmid DNA into the skin, transient expression could be measured in epidermal keratinocytes (Hengge et al. 1995). Injection of an interleukin-8 plasmid into the skin resulted in a biological response consisting of neutrophil recruitment indicating secretion of a biologically active gene product. Using similar transfection techniques, Meng et al. examined the systemic effects

of a circulating gene product, human interleukin 10 (IL-10), released from transduced keratinocytes (Meng et al. 1998). An expression vector (phIL-10) was constructed for human IL-10 and was injected into the dorsal skin of hairless rats.
Analysis showed that the amount of IL-10 in local keratinocytes and in the circulation increased with the dose of phIL-10. To determine whether circulating
IL-10 could inhibit the effector phase of contact hypersensitization at a site distant from the site of injection, various doses of phIL-10 were injected into the
dorsal skin of sensitized rats prior to an ear-challenge injection. It was found
that the degree of ear swelling in phIL-10-treated rats was significantly lower
than in negative control animals. Thus, these results suggested that IL-10 released from transfected keratinocytes could enter the bloodstream and cause
biological effects at sites distant from the injection. Other studies utilizing gene
gun mediated gene transfer to the skin have shown successful secretion of various cytokines into the plasma (Sun et al. 1995). In vivo skin transfection with
the human interleukin 6 gene reduced the methylcholanthrene-induced fibrosarcoma growth. Additionally, direct skin transfection of a combination of murine
tumor necrosis factor alpha and interferon gamma genes inhibited the tumor
growth in a renal carcinoma tumor model. Significant serum levels of interleukin 6 or interferon gamma were detected in these experiments demonstrating effective secretion of transgenic proteins into the bloodstream.

Other Proteins

Naffakh et al. showed that secretion of erythropoietin (Epo) from genetically
modified cells could represent an alternative to repeated injections of the recombinant hormone for treating chronic anemia responsive to Epo (Naffakh et al.
1995). Primary mouse skin fibroblasts were transduced with a retroviral vector
in which the murine Epo cDNA was expressed under the control of the murine
phosphoglycerate kinase promoter. "Neo-organs" containing the genetically modified fibroblasts embedded in collagen lattices were implanted into the peritoneal
cavity of mice. Increased hematocrit (>80%) and elevated serum Epo concentrations (ranging from 60 to 408 milliunits/ml) were observed in recipient animals
over a 10-month observation period. Hematocrit values measured in recipient
mice correlated with the number of implanted Epo-secreting fibroblasts (ranging
from 2.5 to 20×10^6).

Setoguchi et al. used a replication-deficient recombinant adenoviral vector
coding for human α1-antitrypsin (human α1AT) in both ex vivo and in vivo approaches to alleviate α1AT deficiency (Setoguchi et al. 1994). Syngeneic keratinocytes were transduced ex vivo and subsequently transplanted. Serum measurements in mice receiving these transplants (10^5 cells/mouse) demonstrated human α1AT for at least 14 days with maximum levels of 41 ng/ml. Direct subcutaneous injection of the adenoviral vector into the mice also gave significant serum levels of human α1AT (53 ng/ml at day 4), with the protein being detectable
for at least 14 days.

Other attempts of dermal protein secretion were performed by Krueger et al.
who reported the secretion of human chorionic gonadotropin (hCG) in trans-

duced keratinocytes in vitro (Krueger et al. 1994) and Petersen et al. demonstrating the production of human transferrin by transduced fibroblasts implanted subcutaneously into athymic mice (Petersen et al. 1995).

In conclusion, a wide range of different proteins has been successfully expressed in the skin through various gene transfer strategies with subsequent detection in the circulation. Both, in vivo and ex vivo delivery strategies as well as transgenic animal models have been used. Not only has protein expression in keratinocytes revealed promising results, but also dermal fibroblasts have served as bioreactors. Although the technology has been applied for various purposes, potential limitations as caused by the size and charge of the protein product have not yet been resolved.

Epidermis as a Metabolic Sink

In another respect, skin can be used as a source of metabolizing enzymes for detoxification ("the metabolic sink"). The use of the epidermis for this purpose, was first suggested by Flowers et al. in 1990 (Flowers et al. 1990). Although this approach has several potential applications, the "metabolic sink" technology is complicated by biochemical limitations. As illustrated by attempts to clear ornithine from the skin (Jensen et al. 1997, Sullivan et al. 1997), the metabolic capacity of an epidermal graft not only depends on the amount of enzyme produced in the cells, but also on parameters such as co-factor supply, regional substrate concentrations and clearance of downstream metabolites. In fact, genetic manipulation at several points along the metabolic pathway will most likely be required to obtain a clinical benefit. Additionally, it is not clear if cutaneous expression of an enzyme that the host is lacking, might elicit an immune response.

In several inherited metabolic diseases toxic substances accumulate in the circulation due to the defect of an enzyme catalyzing a distinct biochemical process. Somatic gene therapy performed by direct injection into the affected organ (predominantly the liver) is not possible with currently available technology. An alternative way to treat these diseases could be to genetically modify keratinocytes in such a way that the cells provide the necessary enzymes for metabolization following uptake of the toxic metabolites from the circulation (Taichman 1994).

Keratinocytes normally not only secrete a variety of proteins which reach the systemic circulation, but it is also well known that these cells take up and metabolize substances, such as provitamin D (Holick 1981). As mentioned earlier, the secretion of proteins synthesized in genetically manipulated keratinocytes into the circulation can be problematic due to transport barriers. However, for smaller metabolites accumulating in metabolic diseases this limitation may not exist.

Adenosine Deaminase

In 1987 Palmer et al. constructed a retroviral vector containing a human adenosine deaminase (ADA) cDNA and used it to infect ADA-fibroblasts from a patient with ADA deficiency (Palmer at al. 1987). A 12-fold increase in ADA levels as compared to fibroblasts from normal individuals was obtained and the cells were able to rapidly metabolize exogenous deoxyadenosine and adenosine. This was important since these metabolites accumulate in the plasma of ADA-deficient patients and play a role in producing the phenotype of the severe combined immunodeficiency syndrome. These experiments indicated the potential of retrovirally-mediated gene transfer into human fibroblasts to increase therapeutically important catabolic enzymes. It was calculated that 4×10^8 cells would be sufficient to treat an ADA patient assuming unlimited access of the cells to the plasma. However, a serious problem with using a metabolic sink to treat this particular disease is the fact that the adenosine mainly accumulates intracellularly with a high concentration found in circulating cells but almost normal levels found in the serum. Thus, a low serum concentration makes the use of skin-directed removal of the toxic metabolites in ADA deficiency problematic.

Fenjves et al. measured the capacity of keratinocytes from ADA patients transduced with an ADA-containing retroviral vector to metabolize adenosine (Fenjves et al. 1997). Transduced patient keratinocytes deaminated adenosine 5.5-times more efficiently than normal controls. At a clinically relevant substrate concentration (10 µM), the rate of deamination did not demonstrate a saturation kinetics indicating that the metabolic capacity of these cells was well below the maximum. Furthermore, it was demonstrated that the increase in the deamination rate correlated with an increase in ADA mRNA, suggesting that the transport of adenosine did not limit the availability in the intercellular compartment. It was calculated that a graft occupying 2% of the total body area had the capacity to metabolize 337 µmol adenosine per day or 10% of the normal daily load. It was further suggested that increasing the blood flow to the graft, for instance by increasing the skin temperature, might improve the kinetics of substrate elimination.

Ornithine Aminotransferase

Another inborn error of metabolism that could be a candidate disease for the metabolic sink approach, is ornithine aminotransferase (OAT) deficiency or gyrate atrophy (GA). This condition results in high serum levels of ornithine and leads to the atrophy of the choroid and retina with a consecutive loss of vision. Evidence suggests that it is of therapeutic benefit to decrease the concentration of ornithine in the circulation. One advantage of selecting this disease for epidermal gene therapy is that compared to the adenosine in ADA deficiency, ornithine is readily transported across cell membranes and is thus, also present at high concentrations in the plasma.

Ornithine aminotransferase (OAT) is a mitochondrial enzyme catalyzing the conversion of ornithine to glutamate semialdehyde (Quastel and Witty 1951, Peraino 1972, Valle and Simell 1995). The deficiency of the enzyme results in plasma ornithine levels 10- to 15-fold higher than normal (Takki and Simell 1976). About 150 biochemically confirmed cases of this rare autosomal recessive disorder are known, and more than 50 different mutations have been identified (Brody et al. 1992, Valle and Simell 1995). The mechanisms of how OAT deficiency and hyperornithinemia leads to retinal degeneration is not fully understood (Hayakama et al. 1980). Retina pigment epithelial (RPE) damage could result from local OAT deficiency or from an increased sensitivity of the RPE to ornithine accumulation. High concentrations of ornithine have been found to be toxic towards isolated RPE cells (Kuwabara et al. 1981). Decreasing serum ornithine through dietary arginine restriction has been shown to slow the progression of the retinal degeneration in gyrate atrophy patients (Kaiser-Kupfer et al. 1981 and 1991). The hyperornithinemia or metabolic abnormalities appear to play a role in the development of the retina pathology (Rao and Cotler 1984, Ratzlaff and Batch 1987, Wang et al. 1995). This observation, although based on a small number of patients, suggests that ornithine accumulation plays an essential role in the disease process. Thus, reducing the systemic ornithine load by skin gene therapy is being explored as a treatment modality.

Adenoviral-mediated overexpression of OAT in keratinocytes demonstrated that GA keratinocytes have a significant capacity of OAT expression, and that ornithine uptake and metabolism can be increased to levels exceeding normal (Sullivan et al. 1996 and 1997). An approximately 16-fold overexpression of OAT resulted in a six-fold enhancement of ornithine metabolism. Interestingly, the kinetics of ornithine metabolism in these transduced keratinocytes demonstrated saturation at levels well below that expected for OAT. Further work revealed an accumulation of downstream metabolites that appeared to limit the ornithine metabolism. Thus, it appears that for keratinocytes to efficiently degrade ornithine, other downstream catabolic enzymes, such as pyrroline-5-carboxylate (P5 C) dehydrogenase or P5 C reductase, would also need to be overexpressed (Fig. 9.1).

In order to achieve stable OAT expression in keratinocytes, which would be required for gene therapy to be clinically useful, retrovirally-mediated transfer of the OAT gene was investigated. Retrovirally-mediated transfer of the OAT gene into CHO cells and mouse fibroblasts has been reported (Rivero et al. 1994, Lacorazza and Jendoubi 1995). However, the biochemical and clinical usefulness of retroviral vectors used in these studies was limited by the low level of OAT expression and the presence of a neomycin resistance gene, which might elicit an immune response in GA patients (Riddell et al. 1996). A method to identify retrovirus producing clones based on immunofluorescence of target patient cells was used to develop a highly efficient OAT retroviral vector (GCsamOAT) lacking a selectable marker. Transduced patient keratinocytes contained 25–75 times more OAT activity than normal keratinocytes (Jensen et al. 1997). The ability of patient keratinocytes transduced with the vector GCsamOAT to eliminate ornithine from media was also higher than those of normal keratinocytes. After 4 hours of incubation at 37 °C, less than 50% of the initial amount of ornithine was left in the media as opposed to 80% in control keratinocytes. No detectable change in ornithine catabolism was measured following air-liquid interphase culturing and differentiation of transduced keratinocytes. Additionally, clonal selec-

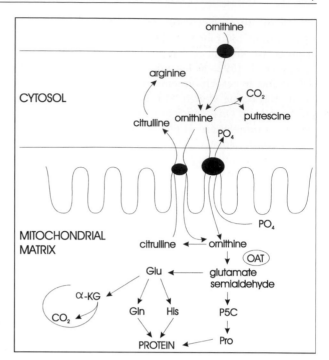

Fig. 9.1. Ornithine metabolism. *OAT*, ornithine-δ-aminotransferase; *P5 C*, pyrroline-5-carboxylate

tion of these retrovirally-transduced keratinocytes indicated that OAT overexpression was maintained over multiple passages (T. G. Jensen and K. G. Csaky, unpublished results).

As mentioned above, one problem with OAT expression in the skin of GA patients is the potential of the development of an immune response against OAT. To study potential interventions in such an immune response, the mechanism for immunologic rejection of normal C57BL/10 (B10) myoblasts in dystrophin-deficient mdx mice, an animal model of Duchenne muscular dystrophy, was investigated (Ohtsuka et al. 1998). Mdx mice developed an immune response to dystrophin. Immunologic tolerance against dystrophin was successfully induced by i.v. injection of dystrophin peptides before B10 myoblast transplantation. The induced tolerance resulted in sustained preservation of dystrophin-expressing myoblasts in mdx mice. These results demonstrated that dystrophin is antigenic in dystrophin-deficient mice and that an immunologic intervention would be necessary to achieve persistent expression of the introduced dystrophin in muscles of dystrophin-deficient individuals.

The initial study of correcting the genetic defect in GA has prompted the institution of a clinical gene therapy trial. Published work has laid the groundwork for this first clinical gene therapy trial for the treatment of an ocular disease using GMP grade retrovirus, GCsamOAT. Previous work with this vector has already established its ability to overexpress ornithine aminotransferase in keratinocytes obtained from patients with gyrate atrophy. Additionally, transduction is sufficiently high to allow these cells to clear ornithine at a markedly in-

Table 9.2. Potential future applications for the skin as a bioreactor or metabolic sink

Phenylalanine hydroxylase
Insulin
Ornithine transcarbamylase
Angiostatins
Lecithin-cholesterol acyltransferase
ApoA1
Lipoprotein receptors

creased rate compared with normal keratinocytes. The clinical trial will involve the transplantation of a five by five-centimeter patch of autologous keratinocytes transduced ex vivo with GCsamOAT. Endpoints of the study include the change in serum ornithine, the determination of duration of expression of epidermal OAT and the examination of possible immune responses against OAT.

Other diseases where a metabolic sink approach in the skin could be relevant are listed in Table 9.2. For several reasons, epidermis is an attractive target for gene therapy of certain metabolic disorders. Advanced methods to culture the cells are available, much is known about the cellular heterogeneity in this tissue, and efficient gene transfer is possible both in vivo and in vitro. However, many challenges still remain. Specific gene targeting of stem cells would be highly advantageous (Jensen et al. 1999). Methods allowing high and sustained gene expression in vivo, or even better, regulated expression, have to be developed. The transport of proteins from the epidermis to the circulation is not well understood, and the biochemical knowledge of the flux in complex metabolic pathways must be further investigated to allow therapeutic manipulation. In conclusion, in spite of the challenges associated with gene therapy of skin diseases, there are no indications so far that systemic metabolic diseases will be a straightforward target for epidermal gene therapy.

Conclusions

The easy access for gene transfer and clinical evaluation and the possibility of topical regulation of gene expression make the skin an attractive target for somatic gene therapy. There are still several problems to be overcome before cutaneous gene therapy may become a clinical reality. These include overcoming the difficulties in inducing sustained expression of the desired gene in vivo and the challenge of targeting genes to long-lived stem cells. They might be resolved in conjunction with an improved understanding of basic biological properties of the skin, strategies for stem cell isolation and manipulation, and advanced approaches to regulate gene delivery and expression. Altogether, these advances will increase the likelihood of moving cutaneous gene therapy into the clinic and, thus, improve the treatment of both cutaneous and systemic diseases.

References

Alexander MY, Akhurst RJ (1995) Liposome-mediated gene transfer and expression via the skin. Hum Mol Gen 4:2279–2285

Brody LC, Mitchell GA, Obie C, Michaud J, Steel G, Fontaine G, Robert MF, Sipila I, Kaiser-Kupfer M, Valle D (1992) Ornithine delta-aminotransferase mutations in gyrate atrophy. Allelic heterogeneity and functional consequences. J Biol Chem 267:3302–3307

Chen L, Nelson DM, Zheng Z, Morgan RA (1998) Ex vivo fibroblast transduction in rabbits results in long-term (>600 days) Factor IX expression in a small percentage of animals. Hum Gene Ther 9:2341–2351

Cheng J, Turksen K, Yu QC, Schreiber H, Teng M, Fuchs E (1992) Cachexia and graft-vs.-host-disease-type skin changes in keratin promoter-driven TNF alpha transgenic mice. Genes Dev 6:1444–1456

Da Costa TH, Williamson DH, Ward A, Bates P, Fisher R, Richardson L, Hill DJ, Robinson IC, Graham CF (1994) High plasma insulin-like growth factor-II and low lipid content in transgenic mice: measurements of lipid metabolism. J Endocrinol 143:433–439

Deng H, Lin Q, Khavari PA (1997) Sustainable cutaneous gene delivery. Nat Biotechnol 13:1388–1391

Fenjves ES, Gordon DA, Pershing LK, Williams DL, Taichman LB (1989) Systemic distribution of apolipoprotein E secreted by grafts of epidermal keratinocytes: implications for epidermal function and gene therapy. Proc Natl Acad Sci USA 86:8803–8807

Fenjves ES, Smith J, Zaradic S, Taichman LB (1994) Systemic delivery of secreted protein by grafts of epidermal keratinocytes: prospects for keratinocyte gene therapy. Hum Gene Ther 5:1241–1248

Fenjves ES, Yao SN, Kurachi K, Taichman LB (1996) Loss of expression of a retrovirus-transduced gene in human keratinocytes. J Invest Dermatol 106:576–578

Fenjves ES, Schwartz PM, Blaese RM, Taichman LB (1997) Keratinocyte gene therapy for adenosine deaminase deficiency: a model approach for inherited metabolic disorders. Hum Gene Ther 8:911–917

Flowers ME, Stockschlaeder MA, Schuening FG, Niederwieser D, Hackman R, Miller AD, Storb R (1990) Long-term transplantation of canine keratinocytes made resistant to G418 through retrovirus-mediated gene transfer. Proc Natl Acad Sci USA 87:2349–2353

Ghazizadeh S, Harrington R. Taichman L (1999) In vivo transduction of mouse epidermis with recombinant retroviral vectors: implications for cutaneous gene therapy. Gene Ther 6:1267–1275

Gerrard AJ, Hudson DL, Brownlee GG, Watt FM (1993) Towards gene therapy for haemophilia B using primary human keratinocytes. Nat Genet 3:180–183

Hayakama S, Shiono T, Takaku Y, Mizuno K (1980) Ornithine ketoacid aminotransferase in the bovine eye. Invest Ophthalmol 19:1457–1460

Hengge UR, Chan EF, Foster RA, Walker PS, Vogel JC (1995) Cytokine gene expression in epidermis with biological effects following injection of naked DNA. Nat Genet 10:161–166

Herzog RW, Yang EY, Couto LB, Hagstrom JN, Elwell D, Fields PA, Burton M, Bellinger DA, Read MS, Brinkhous KM, Podsakoff GM, Nichols TC, Kurtzman GJ, High KA (1999) Long-term correction of canine hemophilia B by gene transfer of blood coagulation Factor IX mediated by adeno-associated viral vector. Nat Med 5:56–63

Hoeben RC, Fallaux FJ, Van Tilburg NH, Cramer SJ, Van Ormondt H, Briet E, Van Der Eb AJ (1993) Toward gene therapy for hemophilia A: long-term persistence of factor VIII-secreting fibroblasts after transplantation into immunodeficient mice. Hum Gene Ther 4:179–186

Holick MF (1981) The cutaneous photosynthesis of previtamin D3: a unique photoendocrine system. J Invest Dermatol 77:51–58

Jensen TG, Sullivan DM, Morgan RA, Taichman LB, Nussenblatt RB, Blaese RM, Csaky KG (1997) Retrovirus-mediated gene transfer of ornithine-delta-aminotransferase into keratinocytes from gyrate atrophy patients. Hum Gene Ther 8:2125–2132

Jensen UB, Jensen TG, Jensen PK, Rygaard J, Hansen BS, Fogh J, Kolvraa S, Bolund L (1994) Gene transfer into cultured human epidermis and its transplantation onto immunodeficient mice: an experimental model for somatic gene therapy. J Invest Dermatol 103:391–394

Jensen UB, Lowell S, Watt FM (1999) The spatial relationship between stem cells and their progeny in the basal layer of human epidermis: a new view based on whole-mount labeling and lineage analysis. Development 126:2409–2418

Kaiser-Kupfer MI, de Monasterio F, Valle D, Walser M, Brusilow S (1981) Visual results of a long-term trial of a low-arginine diet in gyrate atrophy of choroid and retina. Ophthalmology 88:307–310

Kaiser-Kupfer MI, Caruso RC, Valle D (1991) Gyrate atrophy of the choroid and retina. Long-term reduction of ornithine slows retinal degeneration. Arch Ophthalmol 109:1539–1548

Kolodka TM, Garlick JA, Taichman LB (1998) Evidence for keratinocyte stem cells in vitro: long term engraftment and persistence of transgene expression from retrovirus-transduced keratinocytes. Proc Natl Acad Sci USA 95:4356–4361

Krueger GG, Morgan JR, Jorgensen CM, Schmidt L, Li HL, Kwan MK, Boyce ST, Wiley HS, Kaplan J, Petersen MJ (1994) Genetically modified skin to treat disease: potential and limitations. J Invest Dermatol 103:76 S–84 S

Kuwabara T, Ishikawa Y, Kaiser-Kupfer MI (1981) Experimental model of gyrate atrophy in animals. Ophthalmology 88:331–335

Lacorazza HD, Jendoubi M (1995) Correction of ornithine-delta-aminotransferase deficiency in a Chinese hamster ovary cell line mediated by retrovirus gene transfer. Gene Ther 2:22–28

Levy L, Broad S, Zhu AJ, Carroll JM, Khazaal I, Peault B, Watt FM (1998) Optimised retroviral infection of human epidermal keratinocytes: long-term expression of transduced integrin gene following grafting on to SCID mice. Gene Ther 5:913–922

Mathor MB, Ferrari G, Dellambra E, Cilli M, Mavilio F, Cancedda R, De Luca M (1996) Clonal analysis of stably transduced human epidermal stem cells in culture. Proc Natl Acad Sci USA 93:10371–10376

Medin JA, Tudor M, Simovitch R, Quirk JM, Jacobson S, Murray GJ, Brady RO (1996) Correction in trans for Fabry disease: expression, secretion and uptake of alpha-galactosidase A in patient-derived cells driven by a high-titer recombinant retroviral vector. Proc Natl Acad Sci USA 93:7917–7922

Meng X, Sawamura D, Tamai K, Hanada K, Ishida H, Hashimoto I (1998) Keratinocyte gene therapy for systemic diseases. Circulating interleukin 10 released from gene-transferred keratinocytes inhibits contact hypersensitivity at distant areas of the skin. J Clin Invest 101:1462–1467

Morgan JR, Barrandon Y, Green H, Mulligan RC (1987) Expression of an exogenous growth hormone gene by transplantable human epidermal cells. Science 237:1476–9

Moullier P, Bohl D, Heard JM, Danos O (1993) Correction of lysosomal storage in the liver and spleen of MPS VII mice by implantation of genetically modified skin fibroblasts. Nat Genet 4:154–159

Naffakh N, Henri A, Villeval JL, Rouyer-Fessard P, Moullier P, Blumenfeld N, Danos O, Vainchenker W, Heard JM, Beuzard Y (1995) Sustained delivery of erythropoietin in mice by genetically modified skin fibroblasts. Proc Natl Acad Sci USA 92:3194–3198

Noguiez-Hellin P, Meur MR, Salzmann JL, Klatzmann D (1996) Plasmoviruses: nonviral/viral vectors for gene therapy. Proc Natl Acad Sci USA 93:4175–4180

Odland GF (1983) Structure of the skin. In: Goldsmith LA (ed) Biochemistry and physiology of the skin. Vol I. Oxford University Press, New York, pp. 3–63

Ohtsuka Y, Udaka K, Yamashiro Y, Yagita H, Okumura K (1998) Dystrophin acts as a transplantation rejection antigen in dystrophin-deficient mice: implication for gene therapy. J Immunol 160:4635–4460

Palmer TD, Hock RA, Osborne WR, Miller AD (1987) Efficient retrovirus-mediated transfer and expression of a human adenosine deaminase gene in diploid skin fibroblasts from an adenosine deaminase-deficient human. Proc Natl Acad Sci USA 84:1055–1059

Peraino C (1972) Functional properties of ornithine-ketoacid aminotransferase from rat liver. Biochem Biophys Acta 289:117–127

Petersen MJ, Kaplan J, Jorgensen CM, Schmidt LA, Li L, Morgan JR, Kwan MK, Krueger GG (1995) Sustained production of human transferrin by transduced fibroblasts implanted into athymic mice: a model for somatic gene therapy. J Invest Dermatol 104:171–176

Quastel, J, Witty, R (1951) Ornithine transaminase. Nature 167:556

Ramsey WJ, Caplen NJ, Li Q, Higginbotham JN, Shah M, Blaese RM (1998) Adenovirus vectors as transcomplementing templates for the production of replication defective retroviral vectors. Biochem Biophys Res Commun 246:912–919

Rao G, Cotler E (1984) Ornithine delta-aminotransferase activity in retina and other tissues. Neurochem Res 9:555–562

Ratzlaff K, Batch A (1987) Comparison of ornithine activities in the pigment epithelium and retina of vertebrates. Comp Biochem Physiol 88:35–37

Riddell SR, Elliott M, Lewinsohn DA, Gilbert MJ, Wilson L, Manley SA, Lupton SD, Overell RW, Reynolds TC, Corey L, Greenberg PD (1996) T-cell mediated rejection of gene-modified HIV-specific cytotoxic T lymphocytes in HIV-infected patients. Nat Med 2:216–223

Rivero JL, Lacorazza HD, Kozhich A, Nussenblatt RB, Jendoubi M (1994) Retrovirus-mediated gene transfer and expression of human ornithine delta-aminotransferase into embryonic fibroblasts. Hum Gene Ther 5:701–707

Setoguchi Y, Jaffe HA, Danel C, Crystal RG (1994). Ex vivo and in vivo gene transfer to the skin using replication-deficient recombinant adenovirus vectors. J Invest Dermatol 102:415–421

Snyder RO, Miao C, Meuse L, Tubb J, Donahue BA, Lin HF, Stafford DW, Patel S, Thompson AR, Nichols T, Read MS, Bellinger DA, Brinkhous KM, Kay MA (1999) Correction of hemophilia B in canine and murine models using recombinant adeno-associated viral vectors. Nat Med 5:64–70

Sullivan DM, Chung DC, Anglade E, Nussenblatt RB, Csaky KG (1996) Adenovirus mediated gene transfer of ornithine aminotransferase in cultured human RPE. Invest Ophthalmol Vis Sci 37:766–774

Sullivan DM, Jensen TG, Taichman LB, Csaky KG (1997) Ornithine-d-aminotransferase expression and ornithine metabolism in cultured epidermal keratinocytes: toward metabolic sink therapy for gyrate atrophy. Gene Therapy 4:1036–1044

Sun WH, Burkholder JK, Sun J, Culp J, Turner J, Lu XG, Pugh TD, Ershler WB, Yang NS (1995) In vivo cytokine gene transfer by gene gun reduces tumor growth in mice. Proc Natl Acad Sci USA 92:2889–2893

Taichman LB (1994) Epithelial gene therapy. In: The Keratinocyte Handbook. Leigh IM, Lane EB (eds). Cambridge University Press, New York, pp. 543–551

Takki K, Simell O (1976) Gyrate atrophy of the choroid and retina with hyperornithinemia. Birth Defects Orig Artic Ser 12:373–384

Teumer J, Lindahl A, Green H (1990) Human growth hormone in the blood of athymic mice grafted with cultures of hormone-secreting human keratinocytes. FASEB J 4:3245–3250

Valle D, Simell O (1995) The Hyperornithinemias. In: The Metabolic Basis of Inherited Disease. Scriver CR, Beaudet AL, Sly WS, Valle D (eds), McGraw-Hill, New York. 1147–85

Wang T, Lawler AM, Steel G, Sipila I, Milam AH, Valle D (1995) Mice lacking ornithine-delta-aminotransferase have paradoxical neonatal hypoornithinaemia and retinal degeneration. Nat Genet 11:185–190

Wang X, Zinkel S, Polonsky K, Fuchs E (1997) Transgenic studies with a keratin promoter-driven growth hormone transgene: prospects for gene therapy. Proc Natl Acad Sci USA 94:219–226

White SJ, Page SM, Margaritis P, Brownlee GG (1998) Long-term expression of human clotting Factor IX from retrovirally transduced primary human keratinocytes in vivo. Hum Gene Ther 9:1187–1195

Keratinocyte Gene Therapy Using Cytokine Genes

D. SAWAMURA

Cytokines and Keratinocyte Gene Therapy

The epidermis is the outermost organ of the body and a terminally differentiated, stratified squamous epithelium. Its major cell type, approximately 95%, consists of keratinocytes. Several advantages of employing keratinocytes for gene therapy have been proposed (Vogel 1993, Fenjves 1994, Greenhalgh et al. 1994). The furthermost characteristic is their accessibility. Keratinocytes can be easily obtained and monitored. Secondly, keratinocytes have many important biological functions, such as crucial barrier and immunological functions. Furthermore, they produce cytokines and hormones (Chakraborty et al. 1995). These pluripotent cells can also synthesize mature proteins from a variety of introduced transgenes. Thirdly, keratinocytes are highly proliferative. If their proliferative capacity is preserved following gene transfer, keratinocytes should be appropriate target cells for repopulating wounds such as observed in burn patients or individuals with chronic venous insufficiency.

Cytokines are soluble proteins, which are effective at pico- or nanomolar concentrations. They build a complex network to regulate immunological and non-immunological, probably all responses of cells, and are also involved in the pathogenesis of many diseases. They affect the very cells that secreted them in an autocrine manner and act as well in a paracrine and endocrine manner. Since recombinant cytokines are now used in clinical practice for treating patients with various cancers and viral diseases, gene therapy using cytokine genes holds great promise. Since keratinocytes are known to synthesize many cytokines that are known to modulate keratinocyte function, transduced keratinocytes can not only be used as a bioreactor, but also to improve intractable skin diseases (Vogel 1993, Greenhalgh et al. 1994, Meng et al. 1998).

In Vivo Method for Introducing Cytokine Genes into Keratinocytes

Successful keratinocyte gene therapy requires the development of highly efficient methods of gene transfer. Several methods, including particle bombardment (Cheng et al. 1993), adenoviral transfer (Setoguchi et al. 1994), needle injection of naked DNA (Hengge et al. 1995), hemagglutinating virus of Japan (HVJ)-liposomes (Sawamura et al. 1997), and herpes viral transfer (Lu et al. 1997) have been reported for in vivo gene transfer to keratinocytes. Also, topical application of liposome-entrapped DNA could target genes to hair follicles (Li and Hoffman 1995). As each method has both advantages and disadvantages, a combination of several methods will be most likely used for clinical practice.

Of these methods, needle injection of naked DNA method is simple and relatively efficient (Hengge et al. 1995, Sawamura et al. 1997). Hengge et al. succeeded in transferring the interleukin-8 gene into pig and human keratinocytes in vivo (Hengge et al. 1995 and 1996). It is hypothesized that intradermally injected DNA moves to the epidermis and enters keratinocytes through mechanisms that have not been fully elucidated. Using the HVJ-liposome method (Kaneda et al. 1989), DNA associated with high mobility group (HMG)-1 proteins is encapsulated in HVJ-liposomes. HVJ enhances liposome fusion with cell membranes and facilitates the intracellular delivery of the complex. The liposome is thereby introduced into the cytoplasm about 100- to 1000-times more efficiently by HVJ-liposomes than by liposomes alone (Nakanishi et al. 1989). Furthermore, 3- to 10-times more DNA was transferred to the nucleus when bound to HMG-1 than when introduced alone. HMG-1 binds DNA, stabilizes its molecular structure, and improves its nuclear localization through the nuclear localization signal (Kato et al. 1991). In terms of transfer efficiency to keratinocytes, needle injection of naked DNA has been found advantageous compared to the HVJ-liposome method (Sawamura et al. 1997). We hypothesized that co-introduction of DNA with HMG-1 might further increase the transfer efficiency of naked DNA. Therefore, we performed gel mobility shift assays and confirmed DNA binding to HMG-1 in vitro. Then, we injected the DNA-HMG-1 complex, which contained a β-galactosidase (β-gal) expression vector, into the skin of rats and measured the β-gal activity in keratinocytes. The activity of samples containing HMG-1 was 3- to 4-times higher than that of specimens without HMG-1 (Ina et al. 2000). The localization pattern of transfected keratinocytes did not differ between the two samples. Semiquantitative analysis of the transferred-DNA amount and a time course of transgene expression in keratinocytes suggested that HMG-1 might increase the transfer of DNA from the cytoplasm to the nucleus (Ina et al. 2000).

Promoter/Enhancer Cassettes for Keratinocyte Gene Therapy

Successful keratinocyte gene therapy requires transcriptional cassettes that express the therapeutic gene properly in keratinocytes. Several expression cassettes may have to be used depending on the experimental model and purpose. We usually use cassettes that result in high transgene expression levels and ideally choose inducible cassettes that express transgenes for an appropriate period and at a desired level. In order to establish the basis for strong cassettes in keratinocytes in vivo, we transferred plasmids that were constructed by introducing various promoter/enhancers fused with the lacZ (reporter) gene into rat keratinocytes by needle injection of naked DNA (Hengge et al. 1995) and measured β-gal expression (Sawamura et al. 1999 a). The following promoters were used for the experiments: viral promoters such as the SV40 early promoter, Rous sarcoma (RS) virus promoter and cytomegalovirus (CMV) immediate early (IE) promoter and ubiquitous cellular promoters such as the chicken modified β-actin promoter and the mouse metallothionein promoter. They were compared with the keratinocyte-specific promoters i.e. the bullous pemphigoid antigen 1 (BPAG1) promoter, the keratin 5 (K5) promoter and the keratin 10 (K10) promoter. All constructs contained the lacZ indicator gene and the SV40 polyadenylation signal. Figure 10 a shows that the specific β-gal activity of these constructs varied considerably. Of the viral promoters, the CMV-IE promoter exhibited a much stronger activity than the SV40 promoter and the RS virus long terminal repeat. Of the promoters expressed almost specifically in keratinocytes, the K10 promoter resulted in relatively high-level β-gal expression, whereas the BPAG1 promoter had a weak effect. Since the CMV-IE promoter was the strongest among the simple promoters excised from original genes, we examined two other constructs, pCAGS-lacZ (Miyazaki et al. 1989) and pCAGGS-lacZ (Niwa et al. 1991) to determine the effects of the CMV-IE enhancer and the 3'-flanking sequence of the rabbit β-globin gene on the transcriptional activity of keratinocytes. The CMV-IE enhancer was introduced into the β-actin promoter, resulting in the construct pCAGS-lacZ (Miyazaki et al. 1989). Plasmid pCAGGS-lacZ was obtained by replacing the SV40 polyadenylation signal of pCAGS-lacZ with the 3'-flanking sequence of the rabbit β-globin gene (Niwa et al. 1991). The activity of pCAGS-lacZ was about 15-times greater than that of pAGS-lacZ, and that of pCAGGS-lacZ was about two- and six-times that of pCAGS-lacZ and pCMZ, respectively (Fig. 10.1b). These results demonstrated the contribution of the CMV-IE enhancer and the 3'-flanking sequence of the rabbit β-globin gene with regard to increased transgene expression in keratinocytes in vivo (Sawamura et al. 1999a). These experiments provide useful information for developing potential promoter/enhancer cassettes for keratinocyte gene therapy.

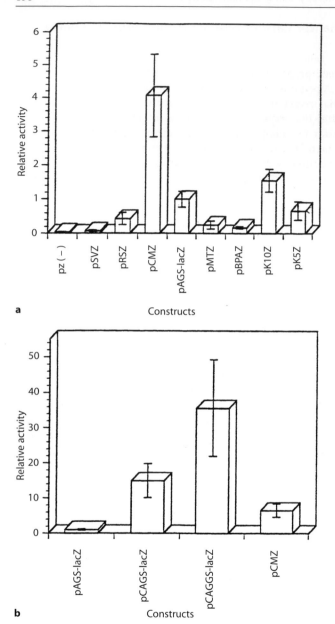

Fig. 10.1 a, b. Comparison of the β-gal activities in keratinocytes *in vivo* after transfer of various constructs. **A** The following promoters were used for this experiment: the SV40 early promoter in pSVZ, Rous sarcoma (RS) virus long terminal repeat in pRSZ, the CMV-IE promoter in pCMZ, the chicken modified β-actin promoter in pAGS-lacZ, the mouse metallothionein promoter in MTZ, the 1.1-kb mouse BPAG1 promoter in pBPAZ, the K10 promoter in pK10Z, the K5 promoter in pK5Z, no promoter in pz(–). **B** The chicken modified β-actin promoter with the CMV-IE enhancer in pCAGS-lacZ and the β-actin promoter with CMV-IE enhancer and the 3′-flanking sequence of the rabbit β-globin gene in pCAGGS-lacZ were also examined. β-Gal activity was assayed 24 h after transfer. Each value shown represents the mean±SD

Introduction of Several Cytokine Genes into Keratinocytes

Although many biological effects of cytokines on keratinocytes and other skin cells have been reported, these effects were predominantly studied on the basis of in vitro investigations. Considering keratinocyte gene therapy using cytokine genes for clinical applications, their effects should be evaluated in vivo. Therefore, we cloned cDNAs of several cytokines (Table 10.1), constructed expression vectors by subcloning them into the pCAGGS or pCY4B expression vector (Niwa et al. 1991) that contained the β-actin promoter with the CMV-IE enhancer and the 3'-flanking sequence of the rabbit β-globin gene, and expressed the inserted DNA strongly in rat keratinocytes in vivo as described above. We evaluated eventual skin changes by routine histological examination. Of 12 cytokine genes tested (Table 10.1), the introduction of the IL-6 and TNF-α genes by needle injection of naked DNA induced significant histological changes. We also introduced the TGF-α and -β genes bound to HMG-1 by DNA injection that led to significant histological changes (Ina et al. 2000).

Introduction of the IL-6 Gene into Keratinocytes Induces Skin Inflammation

IL-6 is a cytokine that possesses pleiotropic effects on a wide range of target cells: growth and differentiation of B lymphocytes, differentiation and activation of T lymphocytes, enhancement of multipotent hematopoietic colony formation, and induction of acute-phase proteins in the liver (Kishimoto 1989, Van Snick 1990, Akira et al. 1993). Grossman et al. have demonstrated that IL-6 stimulates the proliferation of cultured human keratinocytes (Grossman et al. 1989). The above-mentioned evidence suggested that overexpression of IL-6 in skin may induce leukocyte infiltration and keratinocyte proliferation. However, transgenic mice in which IL-6 was specifically overexpressed in keratinocytes did not show enhanced keratinocyte proliferation or leukocytic infiltration of the skin

Table 10.1. Cytokine genes introduced into keratinocytes

Interleukins
Interleukin 4 (IL-4), Interleukin 6 (IL-6), Interleukin 10 (IL-10)
Interferons
Interferon γ (IFN-γ)
Cytotoxic factors
Tumor necrosis factor α (TNF-α)
Growth factors
Transforming growth factor α (TGF-α), Transforming growth factors $\beta 1$, $\beta 2$ and $\beta 3$ (TGF-$\beta 1$, $\beta 2$ and $\beta 3$), Platelet derived growth factor (PDGF)
Chemokines
Monocyte chemotactic and activating factor (MCAF)
Hematopoietic factors
Granulocyte-macrophage colony stimulating factor (GM-CSF)

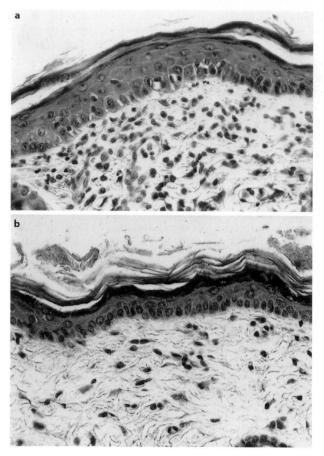

Fig. 10.2 a, b. Histological demonstration of skin changes after the transfer of an IL-6 expression plasmid. Biopsy specimens were obtained 48 h after introduction of the human IL-6 gene. **a** The specimen shows epidermal thickening and lymphocytic infiltration of the dermis. **b** Skin specimen treated with ph(–) as a control shows no changes

(Suematsu et al. 1992, Turksen et al. 1992). Furthermore, the intradermal injection of recombinant IL-6 did not induce these changes in treated skin (Turksen et al. 1992). On the other hand, increased IL-6 production by keratinocytes in patients with inflammatory skin diseases such as psoriasis (Grossman et al. 1989, Neuner et al. 1991) and lichen planus (Yamamoto and Osaka 1995) strongly suggests that IL-6 is involved in skin inflammation in vivo. Thus, the biological functions of IL-6 in vivo have not been fully elucidated under normal and abnormal skin conditions.

We next constructed a human IL-6 expression vector that strongly expressed human IL-6 in keratinocytes and introduced it into hairless rat keratinocytes in vivo by needle injection of naked DNA (Sawamura et al. 1998). We macroscopically observed an erythema in the treated area of the skin. The erythema started to develop in the treated area at 12 h after injection. The degree of erythema reached a maximum at 48 h after injection. Thereafter, the erythema gradually decreased and disappeared about 7 days after injection. Biopsy specimens obtained at 48 h after gene transfer showed thickening and hypergranulosis of the epidermis, a lymphocytic infiltration and telangiectasia in the upper dermis (Fig. 10.2). The introduction of a control vector ph(–) did not induce any particular changes in the treated skin. These histological changes showed some resemblance to those of psoriasis and lichen planus, in which IL-6 production by keratinocytes is also enhanced. Since previous studies using IL-6 transgenic mice have not shown skin inflammation, our results provide the first direct evidence that IL-6 is responsible for the development of these unique inflammatory skin diseases. High levels of IL-6 expression were achieved by the strong expression cassette and the rapid induction of IL-6 following needle injection of naked DNA was responsible for the observed expression pattern.

Suppression of IL-6-Induced Inflammation by Transfer of a Mutant IL-6 Gene

The IL-6 receptor a interacts specifically with IL-6 and keeps it in a conformation suitable for interaction with gp130, resulting in the activation of intracellular signaling. It has been proposed that IL-6 folds as a bundle of four a-helices (A, B, C and D) (Bazan 1991), and recently it has been predicted to possess three topologically distinct receptor binding sites: site 1 for binding to the subunit specific chain IL-6Ra and sites 2 and 3 for interaction with two subunits of the signaling chain gp130 (Savino et al. 1994a). Mutation of residues Y31, G35, S118 and V121 in site 2 gave rise to mutant IL-6 with no bioactivity but unimpaired binding to the IL-6Ra, mutations in residues K70 and S60 at site 1 increased the binding to the IL-6Ra (Savino et al. 1994b, Sporeno et al. 1996). We mutated these residues using in vitro mutagenesis as shown in Table 10.2, constructed the expression vectors, and introduced them into keratinocytes to assess the resulting skin reaction. The size of the erythema induced by each construct decreased with the injected dose, and was shown to be a good indicator of erythema-inducing activity (Fig. 10.3). The activities of the mutant forms of IL-6 were lower than that of

Table 10.2. Amino acid substitutions to produce mutant IL-6 molecules

No. of residue	31	35	118	121
Wild type	Y	G	S	V
Form A	D	E	–	–
Form B	D	F	H	D
Form C	D	F	R	D
Form D	D	E	H	D

For each mutant IL-6, the amino acid substitutions at the respective positions are indicated. Residues 31, 35, 118 and 121 interact with the two subunits of the signaling chain gp130

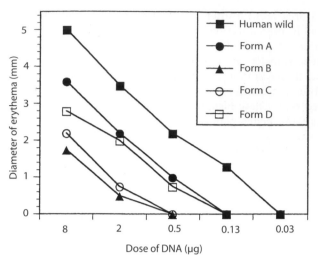

Fig. 10.3. Erythema size induced by mutated IL-6 genes at several doses. We introduced each vector expressing the wild-type IL-6 and the mutant IL-6 (Table 10.2) at doses of 8, 2, 0.5, 0.13 and 0.03 µg, and measured erythema size 48 h after gene transfer

the human wild-type form; the A and D forms showed slightly decreased activity, whereas the B and C forms showed a decrease of about 16-fold (Fig. 10.3).

On the basis of the results, we selected the B and C mutants because of their low erythema-inducing activities. Forms B and C, which were the maximum doses not causing erythema, were used at 0.5 µg for transfection 24 h before administration of 0.5 µg of the wild-type IL-6 gene, with the erythema size being measured 24 h after introduction of the mutant genes. We injected 8 µg of ph(–), of pCAGGS-lacZ (Niwa et al. 1991), and PBS as controls. The erythema size was expressed as the percentage relative to the PBS control. The obtained results 24 h after transfer showed that the erythema produced by the mutants B and C was significantly smaller than that in the controls (Fig. 10.4). Consequently, the mutant IL-6 genes exerted an inhibitory effect which was believed to block wild-type IL-6 binding to the IL-6Rα on keratinocytes. This result indicates that keratinocyte gene therapy may be possible in order to treat inflammatory skin diseases using IL-6 mutant genes (Sawamura et al. 1998).

Introduction of the TNF-α Gene into Keratinocytes Induces Apoptosis

Apoptosis is known as programmed cell death and recognized as an active regulator of cell proliferation and differentiation. Tumor necrosis factor (TNF)-α is an inflammatory cytokine that is generally thought to have an anti-tumor effect. TNF-α can also induce apoptosis in hepatocytes (Senaldi et al. 1998), keratinocytes (Reinartz et al. 1996) and cytotrophoblasts (Garcia-Lloret et al. 1996) in vitro. However, a contrary report recently demonstrated that TNF-α does not in-

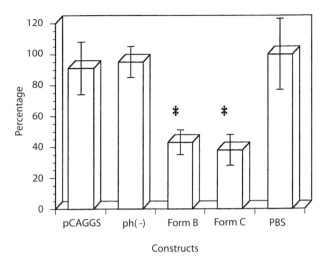

Fig. 10.4. Suppression of phIL6-induced erythema by pre-treatment with a mutated IL-6 gene. We introduced 0.5 μg of the C and D mutants of the human IL-6 gene 24 h before administration of 0.5 μg of the wild-type IL-6 gene, and measured the erythema size 24 h later. 8 μg of ph(–) and pCAGGS-lacZ, and PBS were injected as controls. The erythema size was expressed as the percentage relative to the PBS-treated site. Each value represents the mean ± SD. *Significant difference ($p < 0.01$)

duce apoptosis of cultured human keratinocytes (Bemasii et al. 1997). In addition, apoptosis of keratinocytes has never been observed in TNF-α transgenic mice. Therefore, we constructed an expression vector of human TNF-α and introduced it into hairless rat keratinocytes in vivo by needle injection of naked DNA. We confirmed TNF-α expression and protein in keratinocytes in the treated area by RT-PCR and ELISA, respectively. Histological examination revealed that some keratinocytes appeared eosinophilic and pyknotic (Meng et al. 1999). The terminal deoxynucleotidyl transferase-mediated dUTP-biotin nick end labeling (TUNEL) technique was used to confirm the development of apoptosis. It showed that eosinophilic and pyknotic keratinocytes were TUNEL-positive, indicating that TNF-α caused apoptosis of epidermal keratinocytes in vivo (Meng et al. 1999). Keratinocyte gene therapy using TNF-α gene might therefore be considered in the treatment of malignant epithelial tumors.

Introduction of the TGF-α Gene into Keratinocytes Induces Proliferation

An in vitro study revealed that TGF-α enhanced keratinocyte proliferation (Coffy et al. 1987), which was confirmed by a transgenic mouse study showing TGF-α-induced epidermal thickening in vivo (Vassar and Fuchs 1991). Furthermore, topical application of viral vectors expressing the TGF-α gene in keratinocytes caused epidermal thickening in the treated skin area (Lu et al. 1997). We expressed a TGF-α expression vector in rat keratinocytes using the HMG-1-DNA injection method (Ina et al. 2000). Although we showed that this method allowed high gene transfer efficiency, we did not detect a systemic effect of the transgenic protein. We performed histological examination confirming epidermal hypertrophy, indicating a biologically active protein (Ina et al. 2000). Since there are many intractable skin diseases displaying epidermal atrophy, keratinocyte gene therapy with the TGF-α gene may be useful for the treatment of these atrophic skin diseases. Moreover, it might be applicable to skin transplantation in surgery, with the TGF-α gene being inserted into the excised meshed skin graft and transplanted to the ulcer, where rapid epithelization between the gaps of the graft might occur.

Introduction of the TGF-β Gene into Keratinocytes Induces Proliferation

TGF-β is a growth factor that has pleiotropic effects on a wide range of target cells. The TGF-β family comprises TGF-β1, β2, and β3 and the biological activities of these molecules are very similar. In vitro studies demonstrated that TGF-β enhances the differentiation of keratinocytes (i.e. enhancement of keratinization and suppression of growth). Transgenic mice with K14 driving the TGF-β1 gene showed hyperkeratosis, hypogranulosis, and epidermal thinning (Sellheyer et al. 1993). When we transfected the TGF-β gene into keratinocytes again using the HMG-1-DNA injection method, we found parakeratosis and epidermal thickening besides hyperkeratosis. There was no clear difference in the histological changes among TGF-β1, β2, and β3 expressing constructs. It is well known that TGF-β also activates collagen synthesis in fibroblasts. Although dermal thickening was not observed in the TGF-β transgenic mice (Ina et al. 2000), we noted thickening of the skin where the TGF-β gene was introduced. Our previous results showed that the cassette used in this study increased gene expression about 25- to 50-times over the keratin promoter cassette which has been widely used in transgenic mouse experiments (Sawamura et al. 1999a). We postulated that the combination of this strong cassette and the HMG-1-DNA injection method provided high level expression of TGF-β in the epidermis, which affected fibroblasts and led to dermal thickening. However, dermal cells, including fibroblasts, endothelial cells, and leukocytes, are activated by transgenic TGF-β and may release factors that cause epidermal thickening via indirect effects. This suggests that further investigation is necessary to clarify the interactions between keratinocytes and dermal cells.

Keratinocytes as Bioreactor for Systemic Cytokine Delivery

Keratinocytes might be applied in the future for intractable skin diseases. More-over, keratinocytes can be employed as bioreactors releasing transgenic proteins into the circulation which have endocrine and systemic effects (Fig. 10.5). Using ex vivo gene transfer methods, apolipoprotein E (Fenjves et al. 1989), human growth hormone (Teumer et al. 1990), human factor IX (Gerrard et al. 1993) produced by transduced keratinocytes were reported to reach the bloodstream after keratinocyte grafting. In addition, α1-antitrypsin was detected in mouse serum after in vivo introduction of the gene into the skin using adenoviral transfer (Setoguchi et al. 1994). Although these reports showed the existence of transgenic products in serum, systemic and endocrine effects of the circulating gene products were generally not assessed when exogenous genes were trans-ferred into keratinocytes. Therefore, we performed several experiments using the IL-10 gene to investigate systemic effects.

IL-10 is known to play a major role in suppressing immune and inflammatory responses by inhibiting the production of proinflammatory cytokines. Although IL-10 was first isolated from T helper 2 cells, keratinocytes are also known to be capable of producing IL-10 (Li et al. 1994). Recent studies have shown that intra-cutaneous or intraperitoneal injection of recombinant IL-10 suppresses the effec-tor phase of contact hypersensitivity (CHS) in the skin (Kondo et al. 1994, Schwarz et al. 1994). When we introduced an IL-10 expression vector using needle injection of naked DNA, no histological changes in the treated skin occurred. Therefore, an animal model of CHS was selected to evaluate the bio-logical effects of circulating IL-10 released from transfected keratinocytes.

First, we measured the amount of human IL-10 in rat serum after the intro-duction of a human IL-10 expression plasmid into rat keratinocytes. Consider-able amounts of IL-10 were detected in the serum of treated rats after the injec-tion of 160 µg plasmid. A maximum concentration (about 10 pM) was obtained 18–24 h after transfer that was high enough to exert biological activities (Meng et al. 1998). To determine whether transgenic IL-10 had a suppressive effect on

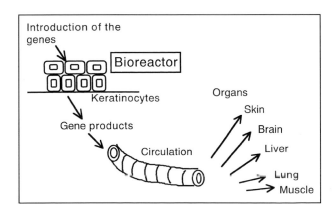

Fig. 10.5. Keratinocytes as bioreactors for pro-viding gene products into the circulation

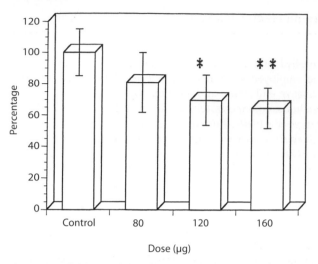

Fig. 10.6. Inhibition of the effector phase of contact hypersensitivity by transfer of the IL-10 gene to keratinocytes. An IL-10 expression plasmid at doses of 80, 120 and 160 µg was injected subepidermally into rats sensitized by dinitrochlorobenzene (DNCB) 12 h before DNCB challenge. Ear swelling was measured 24 h after challenge. The degree of ear swelling is expressed as the percentage relative to rats treated with control vector. Each value represents the mean±SEM. Significant difference (* $p<0.05$, ** $p<0.01$)

CHS at a distant site, we sensitized hairless rats by dinitrochlorobenzene (DNCB), injected the IL-10 plasmid into the back skin 12 h before DNCB challenge to the ear and measured the ear swelling 24 h thereafter. Gene transfer of 120 and 160 µg of the plasmid significantly inhibited the effector phase of CHS whereas 80 µg of the plasmid did not (Fig. 10.6). These results indicate a relationship between the serum level of IL-10 and its inhibitory effect of CHS. Recently, IL-10 was shown to prevent autoimmune diabetes (Moritani et al. 1996), suppress tumor metastasis (Zheng et al. 1996) and inhibit apoptosis (Kitabayashi et al. 1995). Moreover, psoriasis can be treated by systemic administration of recombinant IL-10 (Asadullah et al. 1999). Keratinocyte gene therapy using IL-10 gene will eventually be applied against these diseases in the future.

At this point, we wondered whether all transgenic cytokines released from transduced keratinocytes gained access to the circulation. We chose 7 additional cytokines including IL-4, IL-6, TGF-β1, MACF, GM-CSF, TNF-α, and IFN-γ. We analyzed local mRNA and protein expression in treated epidermis and assessed the circulating proteins systemically after subepidermal injection of the respective plasmids. Whereas considerable mRNA and protein amounts of all cytokine genes were detected in the local epidermis, only the serum concentrations of IL-4, IL-6, IL-10 and TGF-β1 reached detectable levels, whereas those of MACF, GM-CSF, TNF-α and INF-γ were very low or undetectable (Meng et al., submitted). The properties of cytokines released from keratinocytes obviously differed from injected recombinant proteins, although detailed mechanisms have not been fully elucidated.

Gene Transfer into Human Skin

To be able to perform keratinocyte gene therapy in the future, fundamental experiments have still to be performed using human skin. Hengge et al. transplanted human skin onto SCID mice and succeeded in transferring the bacterial β-gal gene into the human keratinocytes in vivo using hypodermic needle injection of naked DNA (Hengge et al. 1996). We transplanted human skin onto a nude rat, injected a β-gal expression vector into the transplanted human skin, and finally detected its activity within the grafted human keratinocytes. However, our experiments using the bacterial gene did not reveal biologically active

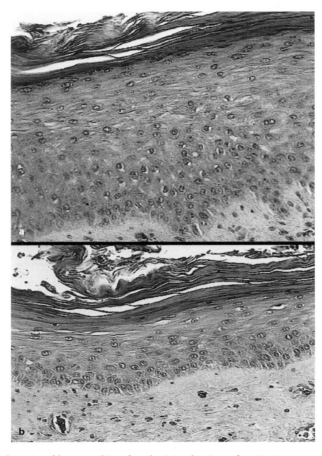

Fig. 10.7 a, b. Histological changes of human skin after the introduction of an IL-6 expression plasmid. 8 µg of IL-6 expression plasmid and control plasmid ph(–) were injected into the grafts and biopsies were taken 48 h later from the treated areas. Epidermal thickening was found in the skin treated with the expression plasmid (**a**), whereas no changes were observed in the ph(–)-treated skin (**b**)

protein. Since we previously showed epidermal proliferation and lymphocytic infiltration following IL-6 gene injection into rat skin (Sawamura et al. 1998), we examined whether these skin changes would also occur in human skin upon transfer of the human IL-6 gene.

By doing so, human skin grafts on nude rats demonstrated epidermal thickening, but no lymphocytic infiltration in the upper dermis (Fig. 10.7) (Sato et al. 1999). The absent lymphocyte infiltration might be due to rat lymphocytes that did not recognize the human skin components. Inter-species differences between adhesion molecules were suggested between rat lymphocytes and human skin cells. To prove keratinocyte proliferation, proliferating cell nuclear antigen (PCNA) staining was performed (Furukawa et al. 1992). PCNA is an acidic non-

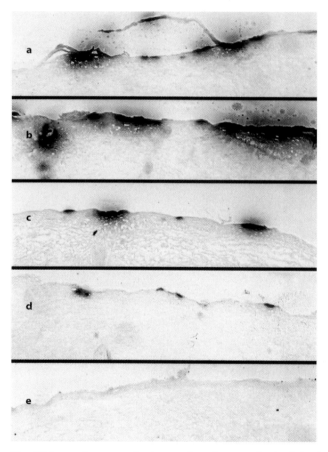

Fig. 10.8 a–e. Gene transfer into rat keratinocytes by jet injection of naked DNA. Plasmids pCAGGS-lacZ and pG(–) were diluted in PBS to 0.1 µg/µl. The injector was placed at various distances from the back skin of hairless rats and the DNA solution was fired into the skin. The injection volume was 100 µl per injection site. Skin specimens were taken from the injected sites 48 h after jet injection and sections were stained for β-gal. Distance: **a,** 20 cm; **b,** 10 cm; **c,** 5 cm; **d,** 0 cm; **e,** control plasmid pG(–)

histone nuclear protein that appears in proliferating cells. An immunohistochemical study using an anti-PCNA antibody showed that PCNA was strongly expressed in the area of epidermal thickening that was initially injected with the IL-6 gene (Sato et al. 1999).

Jet injection of naked DNA can alternatively be used to transfer genes to skin, muscle, fat, and mammary tissue (Furth et al. 1992). Brandsma et al. have induced papilloma lesions after jet injection of the cottontail rabbit papillomavirus genome into skin by an air-pressure propulsion system (Brandsma et al. 1991). We tried to introduce DNA into keratinocytes using this gene transfer method and investigated the efficiency of this method. Several jet injectors have been developed and are commonly used in dermatology to deliver corticosteroid and anesthetic solutions into human skin by air propulsion (Sparrow and Abell 1975). A MADAJET® injector (Mada Equipment, Carlstadt, NJ) was used for our experiments when we attempted to introduce the β-gal expression vector pCAGGS-lacZ into skin (Sawamura et al. 1999b). Since the force of the injection affected the gene transfer efficiency (Furth et al. 1995) but cannot be changed in MADAJET®, we fired the DNA into rat skin from several distances. The keratinocyte sample from 10 cm above the skin surface showed the highest activity among all samples. As the distance became shorter than 10 cm, the β-gal activity decreased (Fig. 10.8). When the time course of gene expression was analyzed, a rapid decrease was detected, indicating no chromosomal integration of the transgene. Next, we transplanted human skin onto nude rats and sucessfully introduced the β-gal expression plasmid into human keratinocytes by jet injection of naked DNA. In addition, we compared the jet with needle injection by subepidermal application of the same amount of DNA into human skin. A strong β-gal activity was found in the skin specimen at 48 h when DNA was fired from a distance of 10 cm, whereas little activity was found from the 0 cm firing distance (Fig. 10.9). Little or no expression was shown when control vector was introduced. Interestingly, jet injection exhibited higher activity than needle injection. It is conceivable that following needle injection, the plasmid moves to the epidermis and enters keratinocytes. On the other hand, some of the plasmid that is jet-injected towards the skin surface is thought to remain within the epidermis. Besides offering greater transfer efficiency, the jet injection method was quicker and easier to perform than needle injection. Jet injection of naked DNA will probably become a useful method for keratinocyte gene therapy in the future (Sawamura et al. 1999b).

Keratinocyte Gene Therapy Using Cytokine Genes in Clinical Practice

We have suggested to use cytokine genes to improve intractable skin disorders. Of the various in vivo methods, needle- and jet-injection of naked DNA are simple and relatively efficient (Hengge et al. 1995 and 1996, Sawamura et al. 1997 and 1999b). The needle and jet injection methods do not induce genetic or chromosomal changes in host keratinocytes, since integration of the transgene does not occur. They have not been found to induce antibodies to DNA

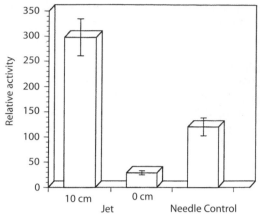

Fig. 10.9. Gene transfer into human keratinocytes by jet injection of naked DNA. Human skin was excised, dissected from the underlying soft tissue, and transplanted onto the back of nude rats. The jet injection was carried out 7 days later. The injector was placed between 0- and 10-cm distance from the human skin and 0.1 µg/µl pCAGGS-lacZ solution used; the injection volume was 100 µl per injection site. pG(−) was fired at 10 cm as a control. Also, 0.2 µg/µl pCAGGS-lacZ solution were injected into the human skin using a 29 G needle and an injection volume of 50 µl per site. Skin biopsies were taken 48 h after jet-injection and subjected to β-gal activity quantification. Each value shown represents the mean±SD

(Gilkeson et al. 1995). These results were confirmed in about 300 hairless rats without side effects (own unpublished results).

However, a thoughtful safety assessment of plasmid DNA is warranted before its widespread clinical use can be recommended.

Acknowledgement. I gratefully appreciate important contributions of the following collaborators in the Department of Dermatology, Hirosaki University School of Medicine, Drs. Meng Xianmin, Ina Shinsuke, Itai Koji, Sato Masanori, Nakano Hajime, Tamai Katsuto, Nomura Kazuo, Hanada Katsumi, Hashimoto Isao. I also thank Prof. Miyazaki Jun-ichi (Department of Nutrition and Physiological Chemistry, Graduate School of Medicine, Osaka University) and Prof. Yasui Akira, (Institute of Development, Aging and Cancer, Tohoku University) for the pAGS-lacZ, pCAGS-lacZ, pCAGGS-lacZ and pCY4B plasmids, respectively. I am also grateful to Ms Uno Youko and Ms Hanada Komaki for excellent technical assistance. This works was supported in part by a grant from the Japanese Ministry of Education.

References

Akira S, Taga T, Kishimoto T (1993) Interleukin-6 in biology and medicine. Adv Immunol 54:1–78
Asadullah K, Doecke WD, Ebeling M, Friedrich M, Belbe G, Audring H, Volk HD, Sterry W (1999) Interleukin 10 treatment of psoriasis: Clinical results of a phase 2 trial. Arch Dermatol 135:187–192
Bazan JF (1991) Neuropoietic cytokines in the hematopoietic field. Neuron 7:197–208

Bemasii L, Ottani D, Fantini F, Chiodino C, Giannetti A, Pincelli C (1997) 1,25-Dihydroxy-vitamin D3 transforming growth factor β1, calcium, and ultraviolet B radiation induce apoptosis in cultured human keratinocytes. J Invest Dermatol 109:276–282

Brandsma J, Yang ZH, Barthold SW, Johnson EA (1991) Use of a rapid, efficient inoculation method to induce papillomas by cottontail rabbit papillomavirus DNA shows that the E7 gene is required. Proc Natl Acad Sci USA 88:4816–4820

Chakraborty A, Slominski A, Ermak G, Hwang J, Pawelek J (1995) Ultraviolet B and melanocyte-stimulating hormone (MSH) stimulate mRNA production for alpha MSH receptors and proopiomelanocortin-derived peptides in mouse melanoma cells and transformed keratinocytes. J Invest Dermatol 105:655–659

Cheng L, Ziegelhoffer PR, Yang NS (1993) In vivo promoter activity and transgene expression in mammalian somatic tissues evaluated by particle bombardment. Proc Natl Acad Sci USA 90:4455–4459

Coffy RJ, Derynck R, Wilcox JN, Bringman TS, Coustin AS, Moses HL, Pittelkow MR (1987) Production and auto-induction of transforming growth factor-alpha in human keratinocytes. Nature 328:817–820

Fenjves ES (1994) Approaches to gene transfer in keratinocytes. J Invest Dermatol 103:70S–75S

Fenjves ES, Gordon DA, Pershing LK, Williams DL, Taichman LB (1989) Systemic distribution of apolipoprotein E secreted by grafts of epidermal keratinocytes: Implications for epidermal function and gene therapy. Proc Natl Acad Sci USA 86:8803–8807

Furth PA, Shamay A, Wall RJ, Hennighausen L (1992) Gene transfer into somatic tissues by jet injection. Anal Biochem 205:365–368

Furth PA, Shamay A, Hennighausen L (1995) Gene transfer into mammalian cells by jet injection. Hybridoma 14:149–152

Furukawa F, Imamura S, Fujita M, Kinoshita K, Yoshitake K, Brown WR, Norris DA (1992) Immunohistochemical localization of proliferating cell nuclear antigen/cyclin in human skin. Arch Dermatol Res 284:86–91

Garcia-Lloret MI, Yui J, Winkler-Lowen B, Guilbert LJ (1996) Epidermal growth factor inhibits cytokine-induced apoptosis of primary human trophoblasts. J Cell Physiol 167:324–332

Gerrard, AJ, Hudson DL, Brownlee GG, Watt FM (1993) Towards gene therapy for haemophilia B using primary human keratinocytes. Nat Genet 3:180–183

Gilkeson GS, Pippen AM, Pisetsky DS (1995) Induction of cross-reactive anti-dsDNA antibodies in preautoimmune NZB/NZW mice by immunization with bacterial DNA. J Clin Invest 95:1398–1402

Greenhalgh DA, Rothnagel JA, Roop DR (1994) Epidermis: an attractive target tissue for gene therapy. J Invest Dermatol 103:63S–69S

Grossman RM, Krueger J, Yourish D, Granelli-Piperno A, Murphy DP, May LT, Kupper TS, Sehgal PB, Gottlieb AB (1989) Interleukin 6 is expressed in high levels in psoriatic skin and stimulates proliferation of cultured human keratinocytes. Proc Natl Acad Sci USA 86:6367–6371

Hengge UR, Chan EF, Foster RA, Walker PS, Vogel JC (1995) Cytokine gene expression in epidermis with biological effects following injection of naked DNA. Nat Genet 10:161–166

Hengge UR, Walker PS, Vogel JC (1996) Expression of naked DNA in human, pig, and mouse skin. J Clin Invest 97:2911–2916

Ina S, Sawamura D, Meng X, Tamai K, Hanada H, Hashimoto I (2000) In vivo transfer of transforming growth factor (TGF)-α and -β-genes to keratinocytes by intradermal injection of naked DNA complexed with high mobility group-1 protein (HMG-1). Acta Derm Venerol 80:10–13

Kaneda Y, Iwai K, Uchida T (1989) Increased expression of DNA cointroduced with nuclear protein in adult rat liver. Science 243:375–378

Kato K, Nakanishi M, Kaneda Y, Uchida T, Okada Y (1991) Expression of hepatitis B virus surface antigen in adult rat liver. J Biol Chem 266:3361–3364

Kishimoto T (1989) The biology of interleukin-6. Blood 74:1–10

Kitabayashi A, Hirokawa M, Miura AB (1995) The role of interleukin-10 (IL-10) in chronic B lymphocytic leukemia: IL-10 prevents leukemic cells from apoptotic cell death. Int J Hematol 62:99–106

Kondo S, McKenzie RC, Sauder DN (1994) Interleukin-10 inhibits the elicitation phase of allergic contact hypersensitivity. J Invest Dermatol 103:811–814

Li L, Elliott JF, Mosmann TR (1994) IL-10 inhibits cytokine production, vascular leakage, and swelling during T helper 1 cell-induced delayed type hypersensitivity. J Immunol 153:3967–3977

Li L, Hoffman RM (1995) The feasibility of targeted selective gene therapy of the hair follicle. Nat Med 1:705–706

Lu B, Federoff HJ, Wang Y, Goldsmith LA, Scott G (1997) Topical application of viral vectors for epidermal gene transfer. J Invest Dermatol 108:803–808

Meng X, Sawamura D, Tamai K, Hanada K, Ishida H, Hashimoto I (1998) Keratinocyte gene therapy for systemic diseases: circulating interleukin-10 released from gene-transferred keratinocytes inhibited contact hypersensitivity at distant areas of the skin. J Clin Invest 101:1462–1467

Meng X, Sawamura D, Baba T, Ina S, Ita K, Tamai K, Hanada K, Hashimoto I (1999) Transgenic TNF-alpha causes apoptosis in epidermal keratinocytes after subcutaneous injection of TNF-alpha DNA plasmid. J Invest Dermatol 113:856–857

Miyazaki J, Takaki S, Araki K, Tashiro F, Tominaga A, Takatsu K, Yamanura K (1989) Expression vector system based on the chicken beta–actin promoter directs efficient production of interleukin–5. Gene 79:269–277

Moritani M, Yoshimoto K, Ii S, Kondo M, Iwahana H, Yamaoka T, Sano T, Nakano N, Kikutani H, Itakura M (1996) Prevention of adoptively transferred diabetes in non-obese diabetic mice with IL-10-transduced islet-specific Th1 lymphocytes. A gene therapy model for autoimmune diabetes. J Clin Invest 98:1851–1859

Nakanishi M, Uchida T, Sugawa H, Ishiura M, Okada Y (1989) Efficient introduction of content of liposomes into cells using HVJ (Sendai virus). Exp Cell Res 159:399–409

Neuner P, Urbanski A, Trautinger F, Moller A, Kirnbauer R, Kapp A, Schopf E, Schwarz T, Luger TA (1991) Increased IL-6 production by monocytes and keratinocytes in patients with psoriasis. J Invest Dermatol 97:27–33

Niwa H, Yamamura K, Miyazaki J (1991) Efficient selection for high-expression transfectants with a novel eukaryotic vector. Gene 108:193–200

Reinartz J, Bechtel MJ, Kramer MD (1996) Tumor necrosis factor-alpha-induced apoptosis in a human keratinocytes cell line (HaCaT) is counteracted by transforming growth factor-alpha. Exp Cell Res 228:334–340

Sato M, Sawamura D, Ina S, Yaguchi T, Hanada K, Hashimoto I (1999) In vivo introduction of the IL-6 gene into human keratinocytes: Induction of epidermal proliferation by the fully spliced form of IL-6 but not by the alternatively spliced form. Arch Dermatol Res, in press

Savino R, Lahm A, Salvati AL, Ciapponi L, Sporeno E, Altamura S, Paonessa G, Toniatti C, Ciliberto G (1994a) Generation of interleukin-6 receptor antagonists by molecular modeling-guided mutagenesis of residues important for gp130 activation. EMBO J 13:1357–1363

Savino R, Ciapponi L, Lahm A, Demartis A, Cabibbo A, Toniatti C, Delmastro P, Altamura S, Ciliberto C (1994b) Rational design of a receptor super-antagonist of human interleukin-6. EMBO J 13:5863–5870

Sawamura D, Meng X, Ina S, Ishikawa H, Tamai K, Nomura K, Hanada K, Hashimoto I, Kaneda Y (1997) In vivo transfer of a foreign gene to keratinocytes using the hemagglutinating virus of Japan-liposome method. J Invest Dermatol 108:195–199

Sawamura D, Meng X, Ina S, Sato M, Tamai K, Hanada K, Hashimoto I (1998) Induction of keratinocyte proliferation and lymphocyte infiltration by in vivo introduction of the IL-6 gene into keratinocytes and possibility of keratinocyte gene therapy for inflammatory skin diseases using IL-6 mutant genes. J Immunol 161:5633–5639

Sawamura D, Meng X, Ina S, Nakano H, Tamai K, Nomura K, Hanada K, Miyazaki J, Hashimoto I (1999a) Promoter/enhancer cassettes for keratinocyte gene therapy. J Invest Dermatol 112:829–830

Sawamura D, Ina S, Itai K, Meng X, Kon A, Tamai K, Hanada K, Hashimoto I (1999b) In vivo gene introduction into keratinocytes using jet injection. Gene Ther 6:1785–1787

Schwarz A, Grabbe S, Riemann H, Aragane Y, Simon M, Manon S, Andrade S, Luger TA, Zlotnik A, Schwarz T (1994) In vivo effects of interleukin-10 on contact hypersensitivity and delayed-type hypersensitivity reactions. J Invest Dermatol 103:211–216

Sellheyer K, Bickenbach JR, Rothnagel JA, Budman D, Longley MA, Krieg T, Roche NS, Roberts AB, Roop DR (1993) Inhibition of skin development by overexpression of transforming growth factor $\beta 1$ in the epidermis of transgenic mice. Proc Natl Acad Sci USA 90:5237–5241

Senaldi G, Shaklee CL, Simon B, Rowan CG, Lacey DL, Hartung T (1998) Keratinocyte growth factor protects murine hepatocytes from tumor necrosis factor-induced apoptosis in vivo and in vitro. Hepatology 27:1584–1591

Setoguchi Y, Jaffe HA, Dane C, Crystal RG (1994) Ex vivo and in vivo gene transfer to the skin using replication–deficient recombinant adenovirus vectors. J Invest Dermatol 102:415–421

Sparrow G, Abell E (1975) Granuloma anulare and necrobiosis lipoidica treated by jet injector. Br J Dermatol 93:85–89

Sporeno E, Savino R, Ciapponi L, Paonessa G, Cabibbo A, Lahm A, Pulkki K, Sun X-R, Toniatti C, Klein B, Ciliberto G (1996) Human interleukin-6 receptor super-antagonists with high potency and wide spectrum on multiple myeloma cells. Blood 87:4510–4519

Suematsu S, Matsusaka T, Matsuda T, Ohno S, Miyazaki J, Yamamura K, Hirano T, Kishimoto T (1992) Generation of plasmacytomas with the chromosomal translocation t(12;15) in interleukin 6 transgenic mouse. Proc Natl Acad Sci USA 89:232–235

Teumer T, Lindahl A, Green H (1990) Human growth hormone in the blood of athymic mice grafted with cultures of hormone-secreting human keratinocytes. FASEB J 4:3245–3250

Turksen K, Kupper T, Degenstein L, Williams I, Fuchs R (1992) Interleukin 6: Insights to its function in skin by overexpression in transgenic mice. Proc Natl Acad Sci USA 89:5068–5072

van Snick J (1990) Interleukin-6: an overview. Annu Rev Immunol 8:253–278

Vassar R, Fuchs E (1991) Transgenic mice provide new insights into the role of TGF-α during epidermal development and differentiation. Genes Dev 5:714–727

Vogel JC (1993) Keratinocyte gene therapy. Arch Dermatol 129:1478–1483

Yamamoto Y, Osaka T (1995) Characteristic cytokines generated by keratinocytes and mononuclear infiltrates in oral lichen planus. J Invest Dermatol 104:784–788

Zheng LM, Ojcius DM, Garaud F, Roth C, Maxwell E, Li Z, Rong H, Chen J, Wang XY, Catino JJ, King I (1996) Interleukin-10 inhibits tumor metastasis through an NK cell-dependent mechanism. J Exp Med 184:579–584

Genetic Vaccination Using the Skin

11   Principles of Genetic Immunization

D. J. Lee, K. Takabayashi, M. Corr, E. Raz

Summary

Using plasmids to express protein antigens in vivo has opened many opportunities in the areas of vaccination against infectious diseases, allergy, and cancer immunotherapy. While the initial experiments showing in vivo expression were performed in muscle, similar results have been obtained in the skin. Targeting the skin has allowed DNA vaccines (also known as gene vaccines, genetic vaccines, or DNA immunization) to take advantage of the abundance of antigen-presenting cells in the skin. Although there are several advantages to the use of plasmid DNA vaccination, some disadvantages will be described as well. Most importantly, DNA immunization results in very strong cell mediated immune responses. While immunostimulatory sequences (ISS) present in the plasmid are required, the mechanism by which DNA vaccines induce these potent immune responses are still not fully elucidated. This review will discuss these various aspects of genetic immunization in greater detail.

Introduction

The surprising finding that a gene encoded on plasmid DNA injected intramuscularly (i.m.) could be expressed in vivo (Wolff et al. 1990) opened an entirely new approach to vaccine development. Since that discovery, an explosion of studies have embarked upon a number of applications using direct plasmid injection including prevention of infectious disease, treatment of cancer, and treatment of allergic diseases. While most studies have used i.m. and intradermal (i.d.) routes of immunization, other routes of injection such as intravenous, intranasal, subcutaneous, and intraperitoneal methods have been tested (Fynan et al. 1993).

The Skin as an Immune Organ

Tissues that serve as barriers against the entry of pathogens such as the skin have associated lymphoid tissues that provide high levels of local immune surveillance. The skin-associated lymphoid tissue (SALT) (Fig. 11.1) has a variety of cells involved in immunity. A unique cell type not commonly associated with the immune system, the keratinocyte, produces an array of cytokines to help separate the microenvironment of the intraepidermal space (Nickoloff 1993). Therefore, they directly influence the functional properties of Langerhans cells, lymphocytes, macrophages, dendritic cells, endothelial cells, fibroblasts and other cells that reside in or migrate to this compartment. Furthermore, exogenous stimulation may cause keratinocytes to increase cell adhesion molecule expression that will subsequently attract lymphocytes and other migrating blood-borne cells. Immature dendritic cells or epidermal Langerhans cells are the primary antigen-presenting cells of the skin. These cells pick up antigen from the epidermis, carry it across the dermal/epidermal junction and present the anti-

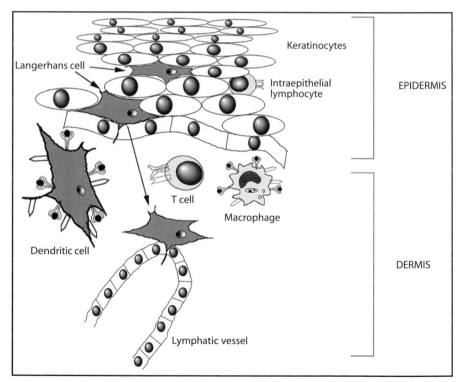

Fig. 11.1. Schematic drawing of the skin immune system. Within the epidermal layer antigen-presenting cells such as Langerhans cells reside along with T cells. Langerhans cells migrate from tissues to lymph nodes via the draining lymphatic vessels. The dermis also contains dendritic antigen-presenting cells

gen in the draining lymph node. In addition to the epidermis, MHC class II-expressing antigen-presenting cells can also be detected in the dermis (Tse and Cooper 1990). In fact, the total number of dermal macrophages significantly exceeds the number of epidermal Langerhans cells in any given section of skin (Weber-Matthiesen and Sterry 1990). By taking advantage of these elements in the skin, the expression of genetically introduced antigens in the microenvironment of the skin may advance the fields of vaccinology and immunotherapy.

Genetic Vaccination: An Overview

Genetic immunization in the skin is highly effective in inducing potent and long-lived immune responses (Raz et al. 1994). Genetic immunization refers to the use of DNA encoding a protein antigen as a vaccine. The plasmid DNA is circular, with several elements (Fig. 11.2). An origin of replication, along with an antibiotic resistance gene allows the plasmid to be replicated and produced in high quantities in *E. coli* under selective pressure. Expression of the gene encoding the antigen is usually under the control of a strong eukaryotic promoter, such as the human cytomegalovirus (CMV) E1 promoter. The appropriate termination and polyadenylation sequences follow the antigen gene sequence so that any mammalian cell that takes up the plasmid can express the protein. The DNA is purified from *E. coli* by a method resulting in very low or no associated endotoxin, and injected without any

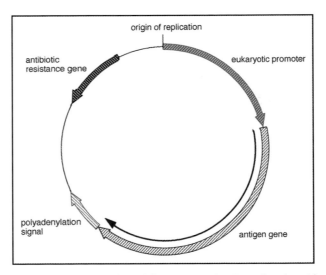

Fig. 11.2. Schematic drawing of a typical plasmid used for DNA vaccination. The plasmid contains an origin of replication, an antibiotic resistance gene, and a sequence that encodes the antigen of interest. The gene encoding the antigen is preceded by a strong eukaryotic promoter sequence and followed by termination and polyadenylation signal sequences

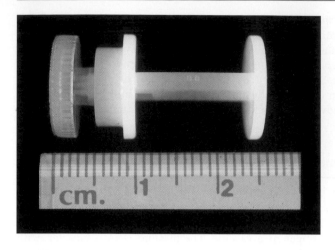

Fig. 11.3. The Tine device used for allergy testing can also be used to deliver DNA to the skin for genetic immunization

associated proteins or lipids to facilitate transfection of cells in vivo. Thus, it is termed "naked" DNA immunization.

Delivery of the DNA to the skin can be performed in a variety of ways. The plasmid may simply be dissolved in normal saline and injected i.d. (Raz et al. 1994, Hengge et al. 1995). Alternatively, a "gene gun" can be used to transfect the skin cells with gold microprojectiles coated with plasmid DNA encoding the antigen (also known as particle-mediated gene delivery technology) (Haynes et al. 1994, Hui et al. 1994, Johnston and Tang 1994, Pertmer et al. 1995). Lastly, the Tine device used in allergy immunotherapy for skin testing (Fig. 11.3) can be immersed in plasmid DNA in normal saline overnight and used to inoculate the cutaneous tissue. Although the precise mechanism of antigen presentation and induction of immune responses has not been clearly defined in vivo, DNA immunization clearly elicits potent antibody, T helper (Th) and cytotoxic T lymphocyte (CTL) responses in rodents. The different methods of injection elicit slightly different immune responses and will be discussed further (Table 11.1).

Advantages of DNA Vaccines

DNA vaccines have a number of advantages as well as some disadvantages compared to other forms of immunization such as protein vaccines or viral vector delivery systems (Table 11.2). One of the greatest advantages of genetic vaccines is the relative ease with which they can be constructed. Furthermore, simplicity of molecular biology techniques with which DNA can be manipulated also allows one to change the antigenicity of a protein. For example, certain antigenic epitopes can be re-introduced or deleted from a given gene of interest. Or, antigen proteins may be fused to other biologically active molecules to alter their immunogenicity. In addition, more than one plasmid may be injected at a time to enable the possibility to manipulate the desired immune response to the antigen. For example, a number of cytokines and costimulatory molecules have been

Table 11.1. Immune responses to different methods of DNA immunization

Directly injected intradermal DNA immunization
Th_1 responses:
  IgG_{2a} >IgG_1 production
  $IFN\gamma$ high, low IL-4, IL-5
  Strong CTL

Gene gun-injected intradermal DNA immunization
Th_0 or Th_2 responses (may be antigen-dependent):
  IgG_1 >IgG_{2a} production
  IL-4, sometimes also $IFN\gamma$
  Strong CTL

While direct introduction of plasmid by needle injection or by the Tine device results in strong Th_1 responses with CTL, plasmid delivered by the gene gun generally results in a less polarized response with CTL induction as well as responses associated with Th_1 ($IFN\gamma$) and Th_2 (IL-4) polarization

Table 11.2. Advantages and disadvantages of DNA vaccines

Advantages	Disadvantages
• Strong immune responses in animal models: humoral, CTL, Th_1 • Inherent immunostimulatory properties • Ease of construction, manipulation of antigenicity of protein • Simplicity of synthesis and purification of DNA • Extreme stability for ease of transport and storage • Extended antigen expression • Combined gene delivery with cytokines or costimulatory molecules to direct the immune response • Ease of both MHC class I as well as MHC class II presentation • No risk of infection (compared to live attenuated viruses) • Less potential risk of recombination (compared to viral vector vaccines) • Repeated immunizations are possible (compared to viral vector vaccines)	• Strong Th_1 environment may not always be desired • Questionable efficacy in widely outbred species such as humans • Possible tolerance rather than immunity in some individuals • May trigger autoimmunity although no evidence in animal models • Possible integration into host genome

co-delivered to affect the subsequent immune response (Cohen et al. 1998). This strategy of immunization will be discussed in a later section.

Synthesis and purification of DNA are also relatively simple compared to the conventional vaccines using attenuated pathogens or recombinant proteins. DNA is also a relatively heat stable molecule which is especially beneficial for developing nations where it may be an additional challenge to store the vaccine in a cold environment. Furthermore, unlike protein vaccination, immunization with pDNA provides both an extended period of antigen expression (Wolff et al. 1990) and the adjuvant effects of the immunostimulatory sequences to continuously stimulate the immune system (Fynan et al. 1993). In addition, unlike viral DNA delivery strategies, plasmid DNA immunization has no risk of infection, and there is less potential risk of recombination than with replication-deficient viral vectors. Moreover, repeated immunizations are possible since no other viral proteins or carrier molecules are associated. Most importantly, DNA vaccines induce very strong cell-mediated responses.

While protein vaccines may be degraded or cleared by antibodies, DNA vaccines allow host cells to take up the DNA and synthesize the antigenic protein. Antigens synthesized by host cells via DNA immunization can also be released from cells to be endocytosed by professional antigen-presenting cells and then enter the MHC class II presentation pathway to stimulate $CD4^+$ Th lymphocytes. $CD4^+$ Th lymphocytes which recognize the antigenic peptide bound by MHC class II become activated and then secrete cytokines to aid in the activation of other immune cells, such as B cells and CTL. Unlike standard protein-based vaccines, in addition to being presented on MHC class II, the intracellular source of antigen then has access to the MHC class I antigen presentation pathway. Antigens encoded by pDNA vaccines may utilize this intracellular pathway to subsequently elicit $CD8^+$ CTL responses. However, the mechanisms by which plasmid encoded antigens are presented to naive $CD8^+$ T lymphocytes via MHC class I molecules may be more complex.

Disadvantages of DNA Vaccines

One concern with the use of DNA vaccines, as with viral vector vaccines, is the possibility of integration into the host genome and, depending on the site of integration, the risk of affecting the expression of genes controlling cell growth, hence the potential of increasing the risk of malignancy. In addition, the strong Th_1 cytokine milieu induced by DNA vaccines would theoretically be counterproductive in the presence of an ongoing infection in which a Th_2 response could be more effective, such as in helminthic infections. In fact, the vaccination might even induce tolerance to the antigen rather than immunity in some number of individuals depending on the genetic makeup or simply on the maturity of the immune system. For example, DNA immunization against the circumsporozoite protein of *Plasmodium yoelii* in neonatal mice resulted in persistent tolerance (over 9 months), and in aged mice produced significantly lower humoral and cell-mediated immunity (and provided less protection) than in young adult mice (Klinman et al. 1997). However, not all DNA vaccines induce tolerance in neonates (Siegrist and Lambert 1997).

The possibility of DNA vaccines influencing the immune system (either by inducing potent antigen-specific immune responses or through the innate adjuvanticity of the DNA molecule itself) to induce responses to self-antigens and consequently trigger autoimmunity is another potential problem. Studies by Klinman and colleagues demonstrate a threefold rise in the number of splenocytes producing anti-DNA antibodies after DNA booster immunizations compared to mice who only received primary immunizations (Klinman et al. 1997). Despite these increases, in mice prone to spontaneous overproduction of pathogenic IgG anti-DNA antibodies, vaccination did not significantly increase the production of autoantibodies to DNA or myosin. In addition, mice immunized four times with pDNA remained healthy with no signs of glomerulonephritis or myositis throughout the 16-month observation period and kidneys from vaccinated mice showed no evidence of glomerulonephritis or immune complex deposition. Therefore, although the possibility of autoimmune disease induction by DNA vaccination exists, in practice these animal models of DNA vaccination did not reveal any signs of autoimmunity. Lastly, although DNA immunization has been clearly shown to induce potent immune responses in several animal models, plasmid DNA vaccination of humans has not been as effective in clinical trials. Therefore, both the technology and immunization protocols require further improvements. However, the advantages of DNA vaccines outweigh the (at this time mainly theoretical) disadvantages to justify their use in the development of viable immunization protocols for infectious diseases as well as immunotherapy of cancer and allergies.

The Immune Response to DNA Vaccination

An important advantage of DNA vaccination is the type of immune response induced in $CD4^+$ Th cells. Th cells differentiate from Th_0 precursors into two readily discernible populations, Th_1 and Th_2, based on the types of cytokines they produce (Mosman et al. 1986). Th_1 cells produce IL-2, IFNγ, and TNFβ while Th_2 cells produce IL-4, IL-5, IL-6 and IL-13 (Abbas et al. 1996, O'Garra 1998). The dominant factors that determine such differentiation are the cytokines present during the priming period (Seder and Paul 1994; Fig. 11.4). For example, if IFNγ and IL-12 are present, the resulting $CD4^+$ T cells will make IFNγ, but if IL-4 is present the cells will make IL-4. Furthermore, Th_1 and Th_2 clones differ in the type of immune response they stimulate (Fig. 11.4). Th_1 cells mediate delayed type hypersensitivity (DTH) reactions, increase IgG_{2a} and IgG_3 isotype synthesis (in the mouse) via IFNγ secretion (Street and Mosmann 1991), and are associated with a strong CTL response. Th_2 cells activate B cells to produce IgG_1 and IgE subclasses via IL-4 secretion and activate eosinophils via IL-5 (Drazen et al. 1996).

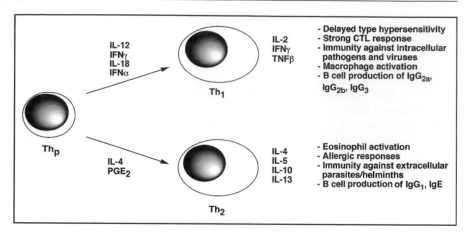

Fig. 11.4. Cytokines induce the differentiation of functionally different subsets of T helper cells. Naive CD4+ T cells can develop into Th_1 cells responsible for cell-mediated immunity in response to Th_1 inducing cytokines such as IFNα, IFNγ, IL-12 or IL-18. Th2 cells implicated in allergic diseases develop in the presence of IL-4 or prostaglandin E_2 (Paul 1999)

Most importantly, the type of Th immune response elicited in the setting of infection can greatly influence its outcome. For example, susceptible strains of mice infected with *Leishmania major* mount a Th_2 response while surviving strains of mice make a Th_1 response and become immune (Heinzel et al. 1989, Scott et al. 1989). Furthermore, in lesions of the resistant tuberculoid form of leprosy, messenger RNAs encoding for IL-2 and IFNγ were most evident, while in the susceptible lepromatous form IL-4, IL-5 and IL-10 predominated (Yamamura et al. 1991). Also it appears that highly resistant tuberculoid patients and healthy individuals exclusively develop Th_1-like responses against mycobacterial antigens (Mutis et al. 1993).

Naked pDNA immunization by direct i.d. injection induces Th cell differentiation to the Th_1 type, which secrete high levels of IFNγ and lead to the production of IgG_{2a} antibodies as well as the activation of strong MHC class I-restricted CTL responses (Ulmer et al. 1993, Manickan et al. 1995, Raz et al. 1996, Feltquate et al. 1997). Not only can an ongoing antigen-specific Th_2 response induced by protein in alum be subsequently "switched" to an antigen-specific Th_1 response by naked pDNA immunization, but the Th_1 response induced by pDNA immunization also prevails over a later attempt to induce a Th_2 response by protein in alum immunization (Raz et al. 1996).

Similarly, DNA vaccination of the skin via the Tine device also results in long lasting CTL responses. Mice immunized with Tine-delivered plasmid DNA encoding the nucleoprotein from the influenza virus made antibody responses which were IgG_{2a} biased, suggesting a Th_1 phenotype (Fig. 11.5a and b). Furthermore, in i.d. naked DNA immunization Th_1 responses are induced by DNA delivery using the Tine device, as demonstrated by IFNγ production (Fig. 11.5c). The long-lasting immunity is demonstrated by mice that mounted

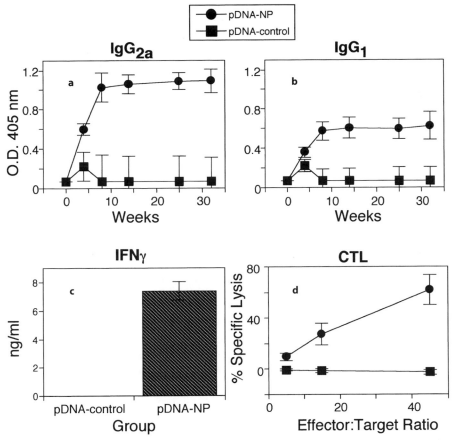

Fig. 11.5. Intradermal immunization by the Tine device results in increased IgG_{2a} (**a**) relative to IgG_1 (**b**), IFNγ production (**c**) and CTL responses (**d**)

an antigen-specific CTL response even after eighteen months after immunization (Fig. 11.5 d).

DNA vaccination administered by gene gun immunization (also termed biolistic DNA injection) results in the induction of antigen-specific humoral and cytotoxic cellular immune responses (Haynes et al. 1994). However, unlike i.d. (or i.m.) delivery by direct injection, the gene gun delivery method gives rise to less clearly polarized Th responses (Pertmer et al. 1996) and Th2 responses (Feltquate et al. 1997). Pertmer and colleagues found that immunization with the gene gun resulted in CTL responses and IFNγ production as well as IgG_1 antibodies. Over time, the IFNγ production waned as the mice showed a marked increase in IL-4 production following repeated immunizations (Pertmer et al. 1996). On the other hand, Feltquate and colleagues performed studies comparing the immune response induced by direct injection and gene gun immunization in skin and muscle. Mice immunized with plasmid encoding the hemagglutinin

(HA) protein via biolistic immunization made Th_2 responses with predominantly IgG_1 and IL-4 production, while the same plasmid in saline injected i.d. gave Th_1 responses with IgG_{2a} and IFNγ. A possible explanation for the Th_2 response in spite of the ISS present in the plasmid DNA is that gene gun immunization requires much less DNA and therefore less ISS is injected into the mice compared to direct needle injected DNA immunization. However, as little as 1 microgram of plasmid DNA delivered by direct injection still resulted in IgG_{2a} antibodies while 1.5 micrograms delivered by gene gun produced mostly IgG_1.

Mechanism of Antigen Presentation and Induction of CTL Response

Classically, $CD8^+$ T cells recognize antigen in the context of major histocompatibility complex (MHC) class I while $CD4^+$ T cells recognize antigen bound by MHC class II. Intracellular sources of antigen are processed through the ubiquitin/proteasome degradation pathway (Paul 1999) and then the resulting peptides are shuttled through the endoplasmic reticulum membrane via the transporter associated with antigen processing proteins (known as TAP1 and 2). In the endoplasmic reticulum, the peptides bind MHC class I molecules and the complex of MHC and peptide is then transported to the cell surface. Antigens presented on MHC class I are classically thought to be intracellular in origin. MHC class I, however, can also present antigens from an exogenous source using a processing pathway that involves the shuttling of extracellularly derived antigens from the endosomal pathway to the cytosol. Several studies have demonstrated exogenous antigens can be presented on MHC class I (Kovacsovics-Bankowski and Rock 1994 and 1995, Martinez-Kinader et al. 1995, Reis e Sousa and Germain 1995, Schirmbeck et al. 1995).

Extracellular sources of antigen are classically presented on MHC class II. The proteins are endocytosed and enter the lysosome/endosomal pathway where they are degraded to peptide fragments and then bind MHC class II in specialized vesicles (Peters et al. 1991 and 1995, Sanderson et al. 1994, Tulp et al. 1994). Since most MHC class II-expressing cells are professional antigen-presenting cells (APC) they are the likely candidates for priming Th cells in DNA vaccination. However, MHC class I molecules are present on all nucleated cells and therefore the possibility that non-professional APC may present antigen to prime $CD8^+$ T cells has been tested. Bone marrow chimera experiments have demonstrated that the CTL induced by i.m. injection of naked plasmid DNA are primed by cells of bone marrow origin, rather than by somatic tissues (Corr et al. 1996, Doe et al. 1996).

"Activation" of the APC is required for CTL priming. The stimulation of a T cell via its antigen receptor in the absence of a second nonspecific costimulatory signal leads to tolerance rather than activation (Schwartz 1992), although the nonspecific signal can be provided by another cell (Kundig et al. 1995). Therefore, in order for a MHC class I-restricted $CD8^+$ T cell to be primed by DNA immunization, a professional APC that expresses costimulatory molecules must be either directly transfected by the plasmid and present the antigen by the intracellular pathway or the APC has to ingest protein produced by another cell. The latter method would require the APC to process and present the antigen by the exogenous pathway (also known as cross priming).

Th cells are generally considered to play a critical role in determining the direction of an immune response. Once activated, $CD4^+$ T cells upregulate CD40 ligand which can stimulate neighboring B cells and antigen-presenting cells to produce various cytokines that recruit and activate non-antigen specific cells such as antigen-presenting cells (Grewal et al. 1996, Yang and Wilson 1996). CD40 stimulation activates antigen-presenting cells and allows them to be potent CTL stimulators (Bennett et al. 1998, Ridge et al. 1998, Schoenberger et al. 1998). However, the fact that CTL responses are impaired in CD4-deficient mice (Maecker et al. 1998), implies that bone marrow-derived APC do not encounter the plasmid DNA sufficiently to bypass the need for $CD4^+$ T cell help in the priming of CTL.

I.d. injection of plasmid DNA results in protein antigen expression in keratinocytes, fibroblasts, and cells with the morphologic appearance of dendritic cells (Raz et al. 1994; Fig. 11.6). Furthermore, pDNA can be detected by PCR in the tail, but not in the draining lymph nodes, spleen or liver three months after a single injection of 100 μg of pDNA (Raz et al. 1994). Although CTL are primed by bone marrow-derived APC (Corr et al. 1996, Doe et al. 1996), whether or not directly transfected APC are required for CTL induction is not clear. Studies by Fu et al. conclude that directly transfected APC are not required (Fu et al. 1997). Furthermore, studies with plasmid DNA encoding antigen under the control of a monocyte/macrophage-specific promoter induced only poor antibody and CTL responses (Corr et al. 1999).

However, directly transfected dendritic cells in both needle injected i.d. immunization (Casares et al. 1997, Akbari et al. 1999) as well as biolistic immunization (Condon et al. 1996, Porgador et al. 1998) have been reported. In fact, studies by Casares et al. demonstrated that dendritic cells from the draining lymph nodes of mice immunized i.m. with pDNA could elicit a cytokine response from an antigen-specific T cell hybridoma. DNA extracted from these purified dendritic cells contained pDNA sequences as detected by PCR (Casares et al. 1997). Similar results were obtained from Langerhans cells (epidermal dendritic cells) which were allowed to emigrate in vitro from the skin of intracutaneously injected mice. However, the direct detection of the protein product in dendritic cells from the skin between 0–5 hours after an i.d. injection was unsuccessful. Additionally, studies of biolistic DNA injection with plasmid encoding the green fluorescent protein (GFP) detected morphologically identified dendritic cells that expressed the marker protein as well as contained gold particles (Condon et al. 1996). Therefore, transfected professional APC can be detected by both needle injection and gene gun injection of plasmid DNA.

Biolistic injection studies reveal the need for the target skin to remain intact for 3–7 days in order for the immune response to reach optimal levels (Torres et al. 1997). In fact, removal of the injected skin up to 24 hours after biolistic injection significantly diminished the antibody and CTL response. In addition, studies using a tetracycline repressible system showed that mice immunized by i.d. needle injection required the injected site to be intact when suppression of anti-

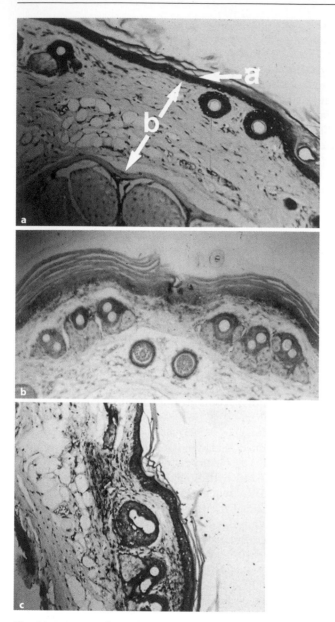

Fig. 11.6. Immunohistochemical analysis of the transgene product (NP) in pCMV-NP-injected tails. **a** The epidermis (*a*) and dermis (*b*) of tail segments taken from a control mouse injected with a single injection of 100 µg of empty vector. No NP staining was observed in these tail segments 3, 10 and 30 days after injection. **b** A tail segment processed 10 days after a single i.d. injection of 100 µg of pCMV-NP showing expression of the NP (*purple-blue*) in the epidermis and dermis (×100). **c** A tail segment processed 30 days after a single i.d. injection of 100 µg of pCMV-NP showing a high level of NP expression in the dermis (×100). Reproduced with permission from Proc Natl Acad Sci USA

gen expression was released (Corr et al. 1999). These studies suggested that the cells at the site of injection in either biolistic or directly injected skin play an important role in DNA-induced immune responses. Furthermore, intraperitoneal injection of allogeneic myoblasts transfected in vitro can elicit a CTL response to the antigen restricted to the host's MHC haplotype (Ulmer et al. 1996). Since the myoblasts did not express the same MHC as the host, this study demonstrated the potential for APC presentation following the protein transfer from somatic cells to APC.

Finally, experiments using chimeric mice with transgenic transcriptional activators in either somatic tissue or bone marrow suggested that CTL priming is dependent on nonlymphoid tissue predominantly expressing antigen encoded by the plasmid DNA (Corr et al. 1999). Since protein immunization alone does not result in comparable CTL responses when compared to DNA injection although protein antigens are taken up by APC to prime the CTL, some component of DNA is still important. One possibility is the stimulation of the microenvironment to stimulate cytokines or cell surface molecules that may then induce the subsequent differentiation of both CTL and Th cells. Furthermore, DNA may stimulate other yet unidentified processes, such as upregulation of the presentation of extracellular protein on MHC class I.

In summary, both non-lymphoid cells and professional antigen-presenting cells have been demonstrated to express the antigen following DNA immunization. Furthermore, experiments using chimeric mice showed that CTL are primed by bone marrow-derived cells. However, the relative roles of somatic tissue compared to lymphoid expression of the plasmid as sources of protein antigen are still not well defined.

Mechanism of Action: Induction of a Th_1 Response

The Th_1 response to genetic vaccination, characterized by increased IgG_{2a} and IFNγ with decreased IgE and IL-4, is largely due to the immunostimulatory effects of sequences present within the pDNA itself. Altering the number of ISS within the pDNA can change the magnitude of the Th_1 response (Sato et al. 1996). In addition, coinjection of protein and oligonucleotides containing the ISS (Roman et al. 1997), or antigen combined with incomplete Freund's adjuvant and ISS containing oligonucleotides (Chu et al. 1997), can also elicit an antigen-specific Th_1 response.

The mechanism by which the ISS within the pDNA induces a Th_1 response is not clearly defined. The fact that fresh human monocytes/macrophages upregulate the expression of IFNα, IFNβ, IL-12 and IL-18 mRNA upon in vitro transfection with the ISS (Roman et al. 1997) suggests a role for soluble factors. All of these cytokines have been established as inducers of IFNγ and promote the differentiation of naive Th_0 cells to Th_1 (Brinkmann et al. 1993, Okamura et al. 1995, Trinchieri 1995, Yaegashi et al. 1995). It has been suggested that the Th_1-inducing cytokines produced upon ISS stimulation may not only directly affect nearby Th_0 cells but may also influence the cells of the innate arm of the immune system to produce IFNγ and to create an overall Th_1-inducing environment (Roman et al. 1997).

However, despite the suggestive in vitro evidence for a role of cytokines from APC such as monocytes/macrophages in the promotion of a Th_1 type differentiation in DNA vaccination, the mechanism by which DNA vaccines induce an antigen-specific Th_1 response in vivo is still not precisely defined. First of all, whether Th cell priming occurs at the site of injection or at a nearby lymphoid organ is not clear. Antigen is expressed at the site of injection in myocytes by i.m. injection (Wolff et al. 1990) and in keratinocytes, fibroblasts, and cells with the morphologic appearance of dendritic cells by i.d. injection (Raz et al. 1994). However, dendritic cells have been detected in the draining lymph nodes of mice immunized with pDNA (see previous section). If the APC are directly transfected, they may be stimulated by ISS, make Th_1-inducing cytokines, and prime naive antigen-specific Th precursor cells to become Th_1 cells. However, if Th priming occurs by a professional APC which takes up protein synthesized by transfected somatic cells, the mechanism for ISS induction of Th_1 differentiation is less clear.

Another less likely mechanism is priming of the Th cell by a non-lymphoid cell. ISS may induce expression of MHC class II and costimulatory molecules on a somatic cell either directly or indirectly by the inflammatory response induced by ISS. This change may allow the somatic cell to become an APC to prime Th cells, at least during secondary immune responses. In addition, ISS-induced cytokine secretion by nearby APCs (or perhaps by other cells) could affect the Th cell differentiation. In this regard, incubation of fresh mouse B cells, peritoneal macrophages or bone-marrow-derived macrophages with ISS oligonucleotides, but not control oligonucleotides has been shown to cause an upregulation of a number of cell surface markers including costimulatory molecules B7-1, B7-2 and CD40, which can influence the subsequent Th differentiation (Martin-Drozco et al. 1999).

A critical aspect of DNA immunization is the intracellular synthesis of antigen, which potentially affords direct access to the MHC class I presentation pathway. An attractive hypothesis to explain the Th_1-biased immune response in DNA immunization is the readily available presentation of antigenic epitopes on MHC class I and the subsequent stimulation of $CD8^+$ T cells. Since $CD8^+$ T cells make $IFN\gamma$ that can influence a naive $CD4^+$ T cell to differentiate to the Th_1 phenotype, the $CD8^+$ T cells may be important. However, CD8-deficient mice still make antigen-specific IgG_{2a} and $IFN\gamma$ comparable to wild type mice in response to DNA immunization (Lee 1999). Lastly, $\gamma\delta$ T cells have also been implicated in the regulation of Th_1/Th_2 development (McMenamin et al. 1994, Ferrick et al. 1995). However, both wild type and mice with a disrupted δ chain gene made comparable levels of antigen-specific IgG_{2a} and $IFN\gamma$ following DNA immunization (Lee 1999).

In summary, the mechanisms of Th_1 induction by DNA immunization are apparently complex. APCs such as monocytes/macrophages do make several Th_1-inducing cytokines and upregulate several costimulators in response to the ISS present in the pDNA. However, direct evidence of these increased cell surface molecules and cytokines released by the APCs has not yet been provided. Perhaps ISS affect the APC in its ability to process extracellular antigens in a more efficient manner leading to presentation in conjunction with MHC class I and II, or the ISS may change the overall environment of the somatic tissue at the site of injection to promote Th$_1$ differentiation.

Cellular Roles of Th$_1$ Memory in DNA Vaccination

Mice previously immunized with plasmid DNA encoding β-galactosidase suppress antigen-specific IgE production in a subsequent immunization with the protein in alum, which normally results in high IgE and Th$_2$ responses (Raz et al. 1996). The Th$_1$ response induced by pDNA immunization can be transferred to recipient mice by either CD4$^+$- or CD8$^+$-enriched T cells from DNA immunized mice (Lee et al. 1997). Mice which had received these cells showed a suppression of IgE production when immunized with protein in alum. Furthermore, adoptive transfer of CD4$^+$-enriched and a to a lesser extent CD8$^+$-enriched splenocytes augment the IgG$_{2a}$ response to a subsequent immunization with β-galactosidase in alum, while recipients of CD4$^+$- or CD8$^+$-enriched cells from naive mice made primarily IgG$_1$ (Lee 1999). In addition, $\gamma\delta$ T cells have been implicated to play a role in the memory response to DNA immunization in experiments showing that donor CD4 cells from $\gamma\delta$ deficient mice do not transfer Th$_1$ memory to naive recipient mice as well as wild type donor mice (D. J. Lee, in preparation).

Studies by others using DNA immunization to prevent the induction of IgE synthesis showed that passive transfer of CD4$^+$-depleted splenocytes but not CD8$^+$-depleted splenocytes were able to suppress the IgE response in rats (Hsu et al. 1996). Interestingly, in these studies, the IgG$_{2a}$ response was unchanged regardless of CD4$^+$ or CD8$^+$ cell depletion. Furthermore, Manickan and others demonstrated that the Th$_1$ protective immune response to herpes simplex virus induced by DNA immunization was mediated by CD4$^+$ cells (Manickan et al. 1995). These differences may be due to the experimental model, design and/or the time points at which the animals were tested. Nevertheless, all data show that the dominance of a Th$_1$ response induced by DNA immunization prevails in subsequent protein immunizations, and can be transferred by T cells.

Applications

The ease with which antigens can be manipulated by altering constructs allows the use of different forms such as secreted, membrane bound antigens, or even ones with deleted sequences to avoid the expression of unwanted antigenic epitopes. Furthermore, while immunization by standard protein injections allows the cells of the immune system to take up and present the foreign protein, genetic immunization gives the added advantage of ectopically expressing membrane bound molecules such as potential antigen-presenting molecules or costimulatory ligands which may alter the overall immune response. In studies with two separate antigen systems (ovalbumin or β-galactosidase), genetic immunization with a combination of the plasmids expressing antigen and costimulators has proven to be effective in enhancing different arms of the immune system. These experiments found B7.1 to be useful for CTL priming and B7.2 to enhance antibody responses (Corr et al. 1997, Iwasaki et al. 1997a, Kim et al. 1997). Other studies have also shown enhanced immune responses using colinear expression of costimulatory molecules (Iwasaki et al. 1997a). The expression of the costimulatory ligand appears to act locally and is dependent on the presence of the plasmid expressing the costimulatory molecule at the same site as the antigen encoding plasmid (Corr et al. 1997). In addition, plasmid encoding the CD40 ligand, a costimulatory molecule upregulated on activated T cells to stimulate APCs, enhances antibody and CTL activity when coimmunized with plasmid encoding antigen (Mendoza et al. 1997, Gurunathan et al. 1998).

The simplicity of mixing different plasmids may also modulate an immune response by coexpressing soluble cytokines to skew a desired immune response. GM-CSF, which may affect antigen presentation, has been shown to stimulate both Th and B cell responses in a number of systems (Xiang and Ertl 1995, Pasquini et al. 1997, Svanholm et al. 1997). Chow and colleagues demonstrated that coimmunization of a hepatitis B virus (HBV) DNA vaccine with the IL-12 or IFN-γ gene exhibited a significant enhancement of Th_1 responses while maintaining inhibition of Th_2 responses. On the other hand, coinjection with the IL-4 gene significantly enhanced the development of specific Th_2 cells while a Th_1 differentiation was suppressed. IL-2 or GM-CSF enhanced the development of Th_1 without affecting the development of Th_2 cells (Chow et al. 1998). Cytokine injection may also be used to alter the normal physiology of the skin. Ectopic IL-8 expression achieved by injection of plasmid DNA into porcine skin resulted in neutrophil recruitment (Hengge et al. 1995). Kim and co-workers explored the induction and regulation of immune responses following the co-delivery of a number of cytokine genes (Kim et al. 1998). Enhancement of antigen-specific humoral responses has been reported with the co-delivery of Th_2 cytokine genes (IL-4, IL-5, and IL-10) as well as those of IL-2 and IL-18. Co-administration of TNF-a and IL-15 genes with HIV-1 DNA immunogens was shown to enhance CTL responses. Antigen genes may also be fused to biologically active proteins such as cytokines to enhance or alter immune responses (Maecker et al. 1997).

Using DNA immunization, immune responses can not only be augmented but also skewed. A coinjection strategy can be used to ectopically express the antigen-presenting molecule of interest (CD1d) as well as the antigen (Lee et al. 1998). By using a combination of plasmids, DNA vaccination can therefore be used as a tool to prime a specific response not only to the antigen of interest, but also allows one to restrict the immune response to the desired antigen-presenting molecule. For example, antigen specific, murine CD1-restricted lymphocytes can be generated in vivo by DNA immunization of normal mice with a combination of plasmids encoding chicken ovalbumin, murine CD1d, and costimulatory molecules.

Infectious Diseases

Although antibodies may be helpful in neutralization of extracellular pathogens, cell-mediated immunity is needed to detect and destroy cells infected with viruses or intracellular bacteria. For example, influenza viruses mutate envelope genes (e.g. hemagglutinin) and as a result are able to evade the previous year's vaccine containing protein subunits that are directed at the envelope glycoprotein. The nucleoprotein of influenza is an internal viral protein and is less susceptible to the antibody-induced antigenic drift than the surface glycoproteins. Early studies of naked DNA vaccine applications utilized plasmids encoding the influenza internal core proteins and/or the surface glycoproteins in several animal models including mice (Ulmer et al. 1993, Justewicz et al. 1995), chicken (Fynan et al. 1993) and ferrets (Donnelly et al. 1995), and have demonstrated protection among different viral strains with varying degrees of efficacy.

DNA vaccines have also been developed for the production of in vivo immunity against HIV-1 (Cohen et al. 1998). Chimpanzees can maintain protective immune responses to HIV-1 up to 48 weeks after challenge (Boyer et al. 1997); however other challenge models in macaques have produced partial protection at best (Kim and Weiner 1997). Preliminary studies from the first DNA vaccine human clinical studies reveal little clinical or laboratory adverse events, and weak antibody responses as well as some increased cellular responses were observed (Kim and Weiner 1997). Recently, studies were performed in rhesus macaques comparing various vaccination protocols including direct i.d. injection or gene gun injection followed by various methods of boosting. The most effective method to protect from subsequent challenge infections with immunodeficiency virus was direct i.d. injection followed by recombinant pox virus boosters (Robinson et al. 1999).

A few examples of infectious diseases for which DNA vaccines are being developed include malaria (Hedstrom et al. 1997), tuberculosis (Tascon et al. 1996, Lowrie et al. 1997), hepatitis B virus (Davis and Brazolot Millan 1997, Prince et al. 1997) and hepatitis C virus (Inchauspe 1997). In addition, a number of other preclinical animal models have demonstrated protective immune responses to viruses such as bovine herpes virus (Cox et al. 1993), herpes simplex virus in rodents (Manickan et al. 1995, Bourne et al. 1996, McClements et al. 1996 and 1997), rabies virus (Xiang et al. 1994, Lodmell et al. 1998), lymphocytic choriomeningitis virus (Martins et al. 1995, Yokoyama et al. 1995), and cottontail rabbit papilloma virus (Donnelly et al. 1996). In fact, immunization of genetically susceptible BALB/c mice using naked DNA protected virtually all of the mice against progressive, nonhealing infections with *L. major* (Gurunathan et al. 1997, Walker et al. 1998).

Allergic Diseases

Allergic diseases are the result of an enhanced Th_2 response to the allergens (Wierenga et al. 1990, Parronchi et al. 1991). The deleterious response is triggered by allergen-specific IgE antibodies bound to IgE receptors at the surface of mast cells and basophils. The presence of allergen causes crosslinking of the bound IgE and results in the immediate release of histamine, IL-4 and IL-5 (Mygind and Dahl 1996) as well as the subsequent production of proinflammatory leukotrienes and platelet-activating factor. Since antigen-encoding pDNA injected i.m. or i.d. into mice elicits a long lasting antigen-specific cellular and humoral response with a Th_1 phenotype (Manickan et al. 1995, Raz et al. 1996), this may provide a novel method of immunotherapy for the treatment of allergic diseases. In fact, plasmid DNA encoding the major allergen of birch pollen has been used to immunize mice (Hartl et al. 1999). These studies showed that DNA immunization induces a strong Th_1 immune response against a relevant inhalant allergen.

Cancer Immunotherapy

The main premise behind immunotherapy for cancer is based on the idea that tumor cells express unique antigens or overexpress normal differentiation proteins that allow them to be recognized by the adaptive immune system as foreign (Durrant 1997, Conry et al. 1995). Mutations in oncogenes or suppressor genes which lead to malignant transformation may also be recognized as "foreign" tumor-specific antigens. Studies by Conry and colleagues have demonstrated the induction of a human carcinoembryonic antigen (CEA) response by the injection of pDNA encoding CEA and the subsequent protection of mice from syngeneic CEA-expressing tumor cell lines (Conry et al. 1995). CEA is expressed at high levels in human colon, breast and non-small cell lung cancers. Likewise, studies by Graham et al. using pDNA encoding the polymorphic epithelial mucin (PEM) associated with breast, pancreatic, and colon cancers, protected mice from challenge with syngeneic PEM-expressing tumor cells (Graham et al. 1996).

Another possible use of gene injection involves the direct transfection of cytokine genes in vivo. Sun and colleagues inhibited the growth of a renal carcinoma tumor model with a combination of murine tumor necrosis factor a and interferon-γ genes via biolistic injection (Sun et al. 1995). In addition, treatment with murine interleukin-2 and interferon-γ genes prolonged the survival of tumor-bearing mice and resulted in tumor eradication in 25% of the test animals. The development of DNA vaccines which can elicit an inflammatory response with Th_1-inducing cytokines from cells of the innate immune system, along with a strong cell-mediated immune response to a specific tumor antigen, offers great potential for the future.

Conclusion

The relative ease of development and production as well as their efficacy in animal models make DNA vaccines an attractive mode of treatment and investigation. While not all safety concerns have been completely addressed, human trials such as the studies in HIV patients are encouraging. In summary, DNA vaccination shows promise in a number of areas including infectious diseases, allergy and cancer immunotherapy. Future improvements in gene expression technology and in enhancing various aspects of adjuvant effects may make this investigational tool a practical one in our daily lives.

Acknowledgements. The work was supported in part by grants AI-40682, AR40770, and AR44850 from the National Institutes of Health. We would like to thank N. Noon and J. Uhle for their assistance. D. J. Lee is supported in part by grants from the National Institute of General Medical Sciences grant GM07198.

References

Abbas AK, Murphy KM, Sher A (1996) Functional diversity of helper T lymphocytes. Nature 383:787–793

Akbari O, Panjwani N, Garcia S, Tascon R, Lowrie D, Stockinger B (1999) DNA vaccination: transfection and activation of dendritic cells as key events for immunity. J Exp Med 189:169–178

Bennett SR, Carbone FR, Karamalis F, Flavell RA, Miller JF, Heath WR (1998) Help for cytotoxic-T-cell responses is mediated by CD40 signalling. Nature 393:478–480

Bourne N, Stanberry LR, Bernstein DI, Lew D (1996) DNA immunization against experimental genital herpes simplex virus infection. J Infect Dis 173:800–807

Boyer JD, Ugen KE, Wang B, Agadjanyan M, Gilbert L, Bagarazzi ML, Chattergoon M, Frost P, Javadian A, Williams WV, Refaeli Y, Ciccarelli RB, McCallus D, Coney L, Weiner DB (1997) Protection of chimpanzees from high-dose heterologous HIV-1 challenge by DNA vaccination. Nat Med 3:526–532

Brinkmann V, Geiger T, Alkan S, Heusser CH (1993) Interferon α increases the frequency of interferon-γ-producing human CD4+ T cells. J Exp Med 178:1655–1663

Casares S, Inaba K, Brumeanu TD, Steinman RM, Bona CA (1997) Antigen presentation by dendritic cells after immunization with DNA encoding a major histocompatibility complex class II-restricted viral epitope. J Exp Med 186:1481–1486

Chow YH, Chiang BL, Lee YL, Chi WK, Lin WC, Chen YT, Tao MH (1998) Development of Th1 and Th2 populations and the nature of immune responses to hepatitis B virus DNA vaccines can be modulated by co-delivery of various cytokine genes. J Immunol 160:1320–1329

Chu RS, Targoni OS, Krieg AM, Lehmann PV, Harding CV (1997) CpG oligodeoxynucleotides act as adjuvants that switch on T helper 1 (Th$_1$) immunity. J Exp Med 186:1623–1631

Cohen AD, Boyer JD, Weiner DB (1998) Modulating the immune response to genetic immunization. FASEB J 12:1611–1626

Condon C, Watkins SC, Celluzzi CM, Thompson K, Falo LD Jr (1996) DNA-based immunization by in vivo transfection of dendritic cells. Nat Med 2:1122–1128

Conry RM, LoBuglio AF, Loechel F, Moore SE, Sumerel LA, Barlow DL, Pike J, Curiel DT (1995) A carcinoembryonic antigen polynucleotide vaccine for human clinical use. Cancer Gene Ther 2:33–38

Corr M, Lee DJ, Carson DA, Tighe H (1996) Gene vaccination with naked plasmid DNA: mechanism of CTL priming. J Exp Med 184:1555–1560

Corr M, Tighe H, Lee D, Dudler J, Trieu M, Brinson DC, Carson DA (1997) Costimulation provided by DNA immunization enhances antitumor immunity. J Immunol 159:4999–5004

Corr M, von Damm A, Lee DJ, Tighe H (1999) In vivo priming by DNA injection occurs predominantly by antigen transfer. J Immunol 163:4721–4727

Cox GJ, Zamb TJ, Babiuk LA (1993) Bovine herpesvirus 1: immune responses in mice and cattle injected with plasmid DNA. J Virol 67:5664–5667

Davis HL, Brazolot Millan CL (1997) DNA-based immunization against hepatitis B virus. Springer Semin Immunopathol 19:195–209

Doe B, Selby M, Barnett S, Baenziger J, Walker CM (1996) Induction of cytotoxic T lymphocytes by intramuscular immunization with plasmid DNA is facilitated by bone marrow-derived cells. Proc Natl Acad Sci USA 93:8578–8583

Donnelly JJ, Friedman A, Martinez D, Montgomery DL, Shiver JW, Motzel SL, Ulmer JB, Liu MA (1995) Preclinical efficacy of a prototype DNA vaccine: enhanced protection against antigenic drift in influenza virus. Nat Med 1:583–587

Donnelly JJ, Martinez D, Jansen KU, Ellis RW, Montgomery DL, Liu MA (1996) Protection against papillomavirus with a polynucleotide vaccine. J Infect Dis 173:314–320

Drazen JM, Arm JP, Austen KF (1996) Sorting out the cytokines of asthma. J Exp Med 183:1–5

Durrant LG (1997) Cancer vaccines. Anticancer Drugs 8:727–733

Feltquate DM, Heaney S, Webster RG, Robinson HL (1997) Different T helper cell types and antibody isotypes generated by saline and gene gun DNA immunization. J Immunol 158:2278–2284

Ferrick DA, Schrenzel MD, Mulvania T, Hsieh B, Ferlin WG, Lepper H (1995) Differential production of interferon-γ and interleukin-4 in response to Th1- and Th2-stimulating pathogens by $\gamma\delta$ T cells in vivo. Nature 373:255–257

Fu TM, Ulmer JB, Caulfield MJ, Deck RR, Friedman A, Wang S, Liu X, Donnelly JJ, Liu MA (1997) Priming of cytotoxic T lymphocytes by DNA vaccines: requirement for professional antigen presenting cells and evidence for antigen transfer from myocytes. Mol Med 3:362–371

Fynan EF, Webster RG, Fuller DH, Haynes JR, Santoro JC, Robinson HL (1993) DNA vaccines: protective immunizations by parenteral, mucosal, and gene-gun inoculations. Proc Natl Acad Sci USA 90:11478–11482

Graham RA, Burchell JM, Beverley P, Taylor-Papadimitriou J (1996) Intramuscular immunisation with MUC1 cDNA can protect C57 mice challenged with MUC1-expressing syngeneic mouse tumour cells. Int J Cancer 65:664–670

Grewal IS, Foellmer HG, Grewal KD, Xu J, Hardardottir F, Baron JL, Janeway CA Jr, Flavell RA (1996) Requirement for CD40 ligand in costimulation induction, T cell activation, and experimental allergic encephalomyelitis. Science 273:1864–1867

Gurunathan S, Sacks DL, Brown DR, Reiner SL, Charest H, Glaichenhaus N, Seder RA (1997) Vaccination with DNA encoding the immunodominant LACK parasite antigen confers protective immunity to mice infected with Leishmania major. J Exp Med 186:1137–1147

Gurunathan S, Irvine KR, Wu CY, Cohen JI, Thomas E, Prussin C, Restifo NP, Seder RA (1998) CD40 ligand/trimer DNA enhances both humoral and cellular immune responses and induces protective immunity to infectious and tumor challenge. J Immunol 161:4563–4571

Hartl A, Kiesslich J, Weiss R, Bernhaupt A, Mostbock S, Scheiblhofer S, Ebner C, Ferreira F, Thalhamer J (1999) Immune responses after immunization with plasmid DNA encoding Bet v 1, the major allergen of birch pollen. J Allergy Clin Immunol 103:107–113

Haynes JR, Fuller DH, Eisenbraun MD, Ford MJ, Pertmer TM (1994) Accell particle-mediated DNA immunization elicits humoral, cytotoxic, and protective immune responses. AIDS Res Hum Retroviruses 10:S43–S45

Hedstrom RC, Doolan DL, Wang R, Gardner MJ, Kumar A, Sedegah M, Gramzinski RA, Sacci JB Jr, Charoenvit Y, Weiss WR, Margalith M, Norman JA, Hobart P, Hoffman SL

(1997) The development of a multivalent DNA vaccine for malaria. Springer Semin Immunopathol 19:147–159

Heinzel FP, Sadick MD, Holaday BJ, Coffman RL, Locksley RM (1989) Reciprocal expression of interferon-γ or interleukin 4 during the resolution or progression of murine leishmaniasis. Evidence for expansion of distinct helper T cell subsets. J Exp Med 169:59–72

Hengge UR, Chan EF, Foster RA, Walker PS, Vogel JC (1995) Cytokine expression in epidermis with biological effects following injection of naked DNA. Nat Genet 10:161–166

Hsu CH, Chua KY, Tao MH, Lai YL, Wu HD, Huang SK, Hsieh KH (1996) Immunoprophylaxis of allergen-induced immunoglobulin E synthesis and airway hyperresponsiveness in vivo by genetic immunization. Nat Med 2:540–544

Hui KM, Sabapathy TK, Oei AA, Chia TF (1994) Generation of allo-reactive cytotoxic T lymphocytes by particle bombardment-mediated gene transfer. J Immunol Methods 171:147–155

Inchauspe G (1997) Gene vaccination for hepatitis C. Springer Semin Immunopathol 19:211–221

Iwasaki A, Stiernholm BJ, Chan AK, Berinstein NL, Barber BH (1997a) Enhanced CTL responses mediated by plasmid DNA immunogens encoding costimulatory molecules and cytokines. J Immunol 158:4591–4601

Iwasaki A, Torres CA, Ohashi PS, Robinson HL, Barber BH (1997b) The dominant role of bone marrow-derived cells in CTL induction following plasmid DNA immunization at different sites. J Immunol 159:11–14

Johnston SA, Tang DC (1994) Gene gun transfection of animal cells and genetic immunization. Methods Cell Biol 43:353–365

Justewicz DM, Morin MJ, Robinson HL, Webster RG (1995) Antibody-forming cell response to virus challenge in mice immunized with DNA encoding the influenza virus hemagglutinin. J Virol 69:7712–7717

Kim JJ, Weiner DB (1997) DNA gene vaccination for HIV. Springer Semin Immunopathol 19:175–194

Kim JJ, Bagarazzi ML, Trivedi N, Hu Y, Kazahaya K, Wilson DM, Ciccarelli R, Chattergoon MA, Dang K, Mahalingam S, Chalian AA, Agadjanyan MG, Boyer JD, Wang B, Weiner DB (1997) Engineering of in vivo immune responses to DNA immunization via co-delivery of costimulatory molecule genes. Nat Biotechnol 15:641–646

Kim JJ, Trivedi NN, Nottingham LK, Morrison L, Tsai A, Hu Y, Mahalingam S, Dang K, Ahn L, Doyle NK, Wilson DM, Chattergoon MA, Chalian AA, Boyer JD, Agadjanyan MG, Weiner DB (1998) Modulation of amplitude and direction of in vivo immune responses by co-administration of cytokine gene expression cassettes with DNA immunogens. Eur J Immunol 28:1089–1103

Klinman DM, Takeno M, Ichino M, Gu M, Yamshchikov G, Mor G, Conover J (1997) DNA vaccines: safety and efficacy issues. Springer Semin Immunopathol 19:245–256

Kovacsovics-Bankowski M, Rock KL (1994) Presentation of exogenous antigens by macrophages: analysis of major histocompatibility complex class I and II presentation and regulation by cytokines. Eur J Immunol 24:2421–2428

Kovacsovics-Bankowski M, Rock KL (1995) A phagosome-to-cytosol pathway for exogenous antigens presented on MHC class I molecules. Science 267:243–246

Kundig TM, Bachmann MF, DiPaolo C, Simard JJ, Battegay M, Lother H, Gessner A, Kuhlcke K, Ohashi PS, Hengartner H, Zinkernagel RM (1995) Fibroblasts as efficient antigen-presenting cells in lymphoid organs. Science 268:1343–1347

Lee DJ (1999) "Naked" plasmid DNA Vaccines: Cellular Roles and Applications. Ph.D. Dissertation, University of California, San Diego

Lee DJ, Tighe H, Corr M, Roman M, Carson DA, Spiegelberg HL, Raz E (1997) Inhibition of IgE antibody formation by plasmid DNA immunization is mediated by both CD4+ and CD8+ T cells. Int Arch Allergy Immunol 113:227–230

Lee DJ, Abeyratne A, Carson DA, Corr M (1998) Induction of an antigen-specific, CD1-restricted cytotoxic T lymphocyte response in vivo. J Exp Med 187:433–438

Lodmell DL, Ray NB, Parnell MJ, Ewalt LC, Hanlon CA, Shaddock JH, Sanderlin DS, Rupprecht CE (1998) DNA immunization protects nonhuman primates against rabies virus. Nat Med 4:949–952

Lowrie DB, Silva CL, Tascon RE (1997) Genetic vaccination against tuberculosis. Springer Semin Immunopathol 19:161–173

Maecker HT, Umetsu DT, DeKruyff RH, Levy S (1997) DNA vaccination with cytokine fusion constructs biases the immune response to ovalbumin. Vaccine 15:1687–1696

Maecker HT, Umetsu DT, DeKruyff RH, Levy S (1998) Cytotoxic T cell responses to DNA vaccination: dependence on antigen presentation via class II MHC. J Immunol 161:6532–6536

Manickan E, Rouse RJ, Yu Z, Wire WS, Rouse BT (1995) Genetic immunization against herpes simplex virus. Protection is mediated by CD4+ T lymphocytes. J Immunol 155:259–265

Martinez-Kinader B, Lipford GB, Wagner H, Heeg K (1995) Sensitization of MHC class I-restricted T cells to exogenous proteins: evidence for an alternative class I-restricted antigen presentation pathway. Immunology 86:287–295

Martin-Orozco E, Kobayashi H, Van Uden J, Nguyen MD, Kornbluth RS, Raz E (1999) Enhancement of antigen-presenting cell surface molecules involved in cognate interactions by immunostimulatory DNA sequences. Int Immunol 11:1111–1118

Martins LP, Lau LL, Asano MS, Ahmed R (1995) DNA vaccination against persistent viral infection. J Virol 69:2574–2582

McClements WL, Armstrong ME, Keys RD, Liu MA (1996) Immunization with DNA vaccines encoding glycoprotein D or glycoprotein B, alone or in combination, induces protective immunity in animal models of herpes simplex virus-2 disease. Proc Natl Acad Sci USA 93:11414–11420

McClements WL, Armstrong ME, Keys RD, Liu MA (1997) The prophylactic effect of immunization with DNA encoding herpes simplex virus glycoproteins on HSV-induced disease in guinea pigs. Vaccine 15:857–860

McMenamin C, Pimm C, McKersey M, Holt PG (1994) Regulation of IgE responses to inhaled antigen in mice by antigen-specific $\gamma\delta$ T cells. Science 265:1869–1871

Mendoza RB, Cantwell MJ, Kipps TJ (1997) Immunostimulatory effects of a plasmid expressing CD40 ligand (CD154) on gene immunization. J Immunol 159:5777–5781

Mosmann TR, Cherwinski H, Bond MW, Giedlin MA, Coffman RL (1986) Two types of murine helper T cell clone. I. Definition according to profiles of lymphokine activities and secreted proteins. J Immunol 136:2348–2357

Mutis T, Kraakman EM, Cornelisse YE, Haanen JB, Spits H, De Vries RR, Ottenhoff TH (1993) Analysis of cytokine production by Mycobacterium-reactive T cells. Failure to explain Mycobacterium leprae-specific nonresponsiveness of peripheral blood T cells from lepromatous leprosy patients. J Immunol 150:4641–4651

Mygind N, Dahl R (1996) Challenge tests in nose and bronchi: pharmacological modulation of rhinitis and asthma. Clin Exp Allergy 3:395–435

Nickoloff B (1993) Dermal Immune System. CRC Press, Ann Arbor, MI

O'Garra A (1998) Cytokines induce the development of functionally heterogeneous T helper cell subsets. Immunity 8:275–283

Okamura H, Tsutsi H, Komatsu T, Yutsudo M, Hakura A, Tanimoto T, Torigoe K, Okura T, Nukada Y, Hattori K, Akita K, Namba M, Tanabe F, Konishi K, Fukuda S, Kurimoto M (1995) Cloning of a new cytokine that induces IFN-γ production by T cells. Nature 378:88–91

Parronchi P, Macchia D, Piccinni MP, Biswas P, Simonelli C, Maggi E, Ricci M, Ansari AA, Romagnani S (1991) Allergen- and bacterial antigen-specific T-cell clones established from atopic donors show a different profile of cytokine production. Proc Natl Acad Sci USA 88:4538–4542

Pasquini S, Xiang Z, Wang Y, He Z, Deng H, Blaszczyk-Thurin M, Ertl HC (1997) Cytokines and costimulatory molecules as genetic adjuvants. Immunol Cell Biol 75:397–401

Paul W (1999) Fundamental Immunology. 4th ed. Lippincott-Raven Publishers, New York

Pertmer TM, Eisenbraun MD, McCabe D, Prayaga SK, Fuller DH, Haynes JR (1995) Gene gun-based nucleic acid immunization: elicitation of humoral and cytotoxic T lymphocyte responses following epidermal delivery of nanogram quantities of DNA. Vaccine 13:1427–1430

Pertmer TM, Roberts TR, Haynes JR (1996) Influenza virus nucleoprotein-specific immunoglobulin G subclass and cytokine responses elicited by DNA vaccination are dependent on the route of vector DNA delivery. J Virol 70:6119–6125

Peters PJ, Raposo G, Neefjes JJ, Oorschot V, Leijendekker RL, Geuze HJ, Ploegh HL (1991) Segregation of MHC class II molecules from MHC class I molecules in the Golgi complex for transport to lysosomal compartments. Nature 349:669–676

Peters PJ, Raposo G, Neefjes JJ, Oorschot V, Leijendekker R, Geuze HJ, Ploegh HL (1995) Major histocompatibility complex class II compartments in human B lymphoblastoid cells are distinct from early endosomes. J Exp Med 182:325–334

Porgador A, Irvine KR, Iwasaki A, Barber BH, Restifo NP, Germain RN (1998) Predominant role for directly transfected dendritic cells in antigen presentation to CD8+ T cells after gene gun immunization. J Exp Med 188:1075–1082

Prince AM, Whalen R, Brotman B (1997) Successful nucleic acid based immunization of newborn chimpanzees against hepatitis B virus. Vaccine 15:916–919

Raz E, Carson DA, Parker SE, Parr TB, Abai AM, Aichinger G, Gromkowski SH, Singh M, Lew D, Yankauckas MA (1994) Intradermal gene immunization: the possible role of DNA uptake in the induction of cellular immunity to viruses. Proc Natl Acad Sci USA 91:9519–9523

Raz E, Tighe H, Sato Y, Corr M, Dudler JA, Roman M, Swain SL, Spiegelberg HL, Carson DA (1996) Preferential induction of a Th1 immune response and inhibition of specific IgE antibody formation by plasmid DNA immunization. Proc Natl Acad Sci USA 93:5141–5145

Reis e Sousa C, Germain RN (1995) Major histocompatibility complex class I presentation of peptides derived from soluble exogenous antigen by a subset of cells engaged in phagocytosis. J Exp Med 182:841–851

Ridge JP, Di Rosa F, Matzinger P (1998) A conditioned dendritic cell can be a temporal bridge between a CD4+ T-helper and a T-killer cell. Nature 393:474–478

Robinson HL, Montefiori DC, Johnson RP, Manson KH, Kalish ML, Lifson JD, Rizvi TA, Lu S, Hu SL, Mazzara GP, Panicali DL, Herndon JG, Glickman R, Candido MA, Lydy SL, Wyand MS, McClure HM (1999) Neutralizing antibody-independent containment of immunodeficiency virus challenges by DNA priming and recombinant pox virus booster immunizations. Nat Med 5:526–534

Roman M, Martin-Orozco E, Goodman JS, Nguyen MD, Sato Y, Ronaghy A, Kornbluth RS, Richman DD, Carson DA, Raz E (1997) Immunostimulatory DNA sequences function as T helper-1-promoting adjuvants. Nat Med 3:849–854

Sanderson F, Kleijmeer MJ, Kelly A, Verwoerd D, Tulp A, Neefjes JJ, Geuze HJ, Trowsdale J (1994) Accumulation of HLA-DM, a regulator of antigen presentation, in MHC class II compartments. Science 266:1566–1569

Sato Y, Roman M, Tighe H, Lee D, Corr M, Nguyen MD, Silverman GJ, Lotz M, Carson DA, Raz E (1996) Immunostimulatory DNA sequences necessary for effective intradermal gene immunization. Science 273:352–354

Schirmbeck R, Melber K, Reimann J (1995) Hepatitis B virus small surface antigen particles are processed in a novel endosomal pathway for major histocompatibility complex class I-restricted epitope presentation. Eur J Immunol 25:1063–1070

Schoenberger SP, Toes RE, van der Voort EI, Offringa R, Melief CJ (1998) T-cell help for cytotoxic T lymphocytes is mediated by CD40-CD40L interactions. Nature 393:480–483

Schwartz RH (1992) Costimulation of T lymphocytes: the role of CD28, CTLA-4, and B7/BB1 in interleukin-2 production and immunotherpay. Cell 71:1068–1076

Scott P, Pearce E, Cheever AW, Coffman RL, Sher A (1989) Role of cytokines and CD4+ T-cell subsets in the regulation of parasite immunity and disease. Immunol Rev 112:161–182

Seder RA, Paul WE (1994) Acquisition of lymphokine-producing phenotype by CD4+ T cells. Annu Rev Immunol 12:635–673

Siegrist CA, Lambert PH (1997) Immunization with DNA vaccines in early life: advantages and limitations as compared to conventional vaccines. Springer Semin Immunopathol 19:233–243

Street NE, Mosmann TR (1991) Functional diversity of T lymphocytes due to secretion of different cytokine patterns. FASEB J 5:171–177

Sun WH, Burkholder JK, Sun J, Culp J, Turner J, Lu XG, Pugh TD, Ershler WB, Yang NS
(1995) In vivo cytokine gene transfer by gene gun reduces tumor growth in mice. Proc
Natl Acad Sci USA 92:2889–2893

Svanholm C, Lowenadler B, Wigzell H (1997) Amplification of T-cell and antibody responses in DNA-based immunization with HIV-1 Nef by co-injection with a GM-CSF
expression vector. Scand J Immunol 46:298–303

Tascon RE, Colston MJ, Ragno S, Stavropoulos E, Gregory D, Lowrie DB (1996) Vaccination against tuberculosis by DNA injection. Nat Med 2:888–892

Torres CA, Iwasaki A, Barber BH, Robinson HL (1997) Differential dependence on target
site tissue for gene gun and intramuscular DNA immunizations. J Immunol 158:4529–
4532

Trinchieri G (1995) Interleukin-12: a proinflammatory cytokine with immunoregulatory
functions that bridge innate resistance and antigen-specific adaptive immunity. Annu
Rev Immunol 13:251–276

Tse Y, Cooper KD (1990) Cutaneous dermal Ia+ cells are capable of initiating delayed
type hypersensitivity responses. J Invest Dermatol 94:267–272

Tulp A, Verwoerd D, Dobberstein B, Ploegh HL, Pieters J (1994) Isolation and characterization of the intracellular MHC class II compartment. Nature 369:120–126

Ulmer JB, Donnelly JJ, Parker SE, Rhodes GH, Felgner PL, Dwarki VJ, Gromkowski SH,
Deck RR, DeWitt CM, Friedman A, et al. (1993) Heterologous protection against influenza by injection of DNA encoding a viral protein. Science 259:1745–1749

Ulmer JB, Deck RR, Dewitt CM, Donnelly JI, Liu MA (1996) Generation of MHC class I-
restricted cytotoxic T lymphocytes by expression of a viral protein in muscle cells:
antigen presentation by non-muscle cells. Immunology 89:59–67

Walker PS, Scharton-Kersten T, Rowton ED, Hengge UR, Bouloc A, Udey MC, Vogel JC
(1998) Genetic immunization with glycoprotein 63 cDNA results in a helper T cell
type 1 immune response and protection in a murine model of leishmaniasis. Hum
Gene Ther 13:1899–1907

Weber-Matthiesen K, Sterry W (1990) Organization of the monocyte/macrophage system
of normal human skin. J Invest Dermatol 95:83–89

Wierenga EA, Snoek M, de Groot C, Chretien I, Bos JD, Jansen HM, Kapsenberg ML
(1990) Evidence for compartmentalization of functional subsets of CD4+ T lymphocytes in atopic patients. J Immunol 144:4651–4656

Wolff JA, Malone RW, Williams P, Chong W, Acsadi G, Jani A, Felgner PL (1990) Direct
gene transfer into mouse muscle in vivo. Science 247:1465–1468

Xiang Z, Ertl HC (1995) Manipulation of the immune response to a plasmid-encoded viral antigen by coinoculation with plasmids expressing cytokines. Immunity 2:129–135

Xiang ZQ, Spitalnik S, Tran M, Wunner WH, Cheng J, Ertl HC (1994) Vaccination with a
plasmid vector carrying the rabies virus glycoprotein gene induces protective immunity against rabies virus. Virology 199:132–140

Yaegashi Y, Nielsen P, Sing A, Galanos C, Freudenberg MA (1995) Interferon-β, a cofactor
in the interferon-γ production induced by gram-negative bacteria in mice. J Exp Med
181:953–960

Yamamura M, Uyemura K, Deans RJ, Weinberg K, Rea TH, Bloom BR, Modlin RL (1991)
Defining protective responses to pathogens: cytokine profiles in leprosy lesions Science
254:277–279. (Published erratum appears in: Science 1992, 255:12)

Yang, Y, Wilson JM (1996) CD40 ligand-dependent T cell activation: requirement of B7-
CD28 signaling through CD40. Science 273:1862–1864

Yokoyama M, Zhang J Whitton JL (1995) DNA immunization confers protection against
lethal lymphocytic choriomeningitis virus infection. J Virol 69:2684–2688

12 Systematic Modulation of Immune Responses by CpG DNA

A. M. KRIEG

Introduction

In recent years, it has become clear that the innate immune system regulates essentially all immune responses. An extremely important mechanism that controls the induction of innate immune responses is the presence of pattern recognition receptors (PRRs) which bind microbial structures that are not present in host tissues. For example, CD14 appears to function as a PRR for the detection of endotoxins and other PRRs detect high mannose proteins that are commonly present in bacteria. Viral RNA molecules appear to form double stranded structures which are thought to bind a PRR and trigger the activation of the double-stranded RNA-dependent protein kinase (Kumar et al. 1997). Another nucleic acid that now appears to also bind PRRs and activate innate immunity is bacterial DNA (Tokunaga et al. 1984, Yamamoto et al. 1988, Messina et al. 1991). It is now clear that the immune stimulatory effects of bacterial DNA result from its content of unmethylated CpG (cytosine followed by a guanine and linked by a phosphodiester bond) dinucleotides in particular base contexts (Krieg et al. 1995 b). CpG dinucleotides are present at approximately the expected frequency in bacterial DNA and are unmethylated. In contrast, CpG dinucleotides are "suppressed" to about 1/4 of the expected frequency and are heavily methylated in vertebrate DNA (Bird 1987). The immune stimulatory effects of bacterial DNA are abolished by methylation with CpG methylase, confirming that this is the structural difference by which the immune system recognizes bacterial DNA as being foreign (Krieg et al. 1995 b). Furthermore, the immune stimulatory effects can be mimicked by synthetic oligodeoxynucleotides (ODN) bearing unmethylated CpG dinucleotides in particular base contexts, which differ between murine and human cells (Yi et al. 1998 a and b, Hartmann and Krieg 1999, Hartmann et al. 1999). These observations demonstrate that the vertebrate immune system has evolved a defense system for the detection of foreign DNA which is based on the specific ability to detect these CpG motifs. The purpose of this chapter is to review the current level of understanding of the immune effects and mechanisms of CpG motifs with particular attention to their significance for gene therapy. Since essentially all gene therapy techniques involve the introduction or production of CpG motifs in host cells, an understanding of CpG DNA will be important for the further advancement of this field. Recent studies have also suggested significant immunologic consequences from the intracellular introduction of double stranded RNA or DNA through a CpG-independent mechanism (Suzuki 1999), but this potential new immune effect of nucleic acids is not yet well enough understood for inclusion in the present chapter.

If immune recognition of CpG motifs is effective in activating protective innate immune defenses, then it may be expected that pathogens would have evolved counter strategies against CpG DNA, especially those pathogens whose life cycles require intracellular replication, such as intracellular bacteria, viruses, and retroviruses. It is therefore noteworthy that essentially all small DNA viruses and retroviruses have extremely low CpG levels in their genomes, typically around 20% of the expected frequency, but as low as 6% in some cases (Shpaer and Mullins 1990, Karlin et al. 1994). The human immunodeficiency virus (HIV) has only about 14% of the CpGs that would be expected if base utilization were random, and these CpGs are almost exclusively in the long terminal repeats of the retrovirus where they are thought to be required for regulating retroviral transcription (Krieg 1996). Some large DNA viruses have not suppressed their CpG content, but have instead dramatically skewed the bases flanking their CpG motifs so that there is a marked underrepresentation of the immune stimulatory CpG (CpG-S) motifs and a marked excess of a different type of immune neutralizing CpG (CpG-N) motif (Krieg et al. 1998 b).

Identification of Immune Stimulatory CpG DNA (CpG-S)

The first observation of the immune stimulatory effects of bacterial DNA resulted from the efforts of Tokunaga and colleagues to identify the component of *Bacillus Calmette Guerin* (BCG) which was responsible for its immune stimulatory and anti-tumor properties (Tokunaga et al. 1984). BCG extracts were fractionated into the DNA, RNA, protein, and lipid fractions, each of which were tested for immune stimulatory effects. Surprisingly, only the DNA fraction was found to have substantial immune stimulatory activity. Further studies by these investigators led to the conclusion that this immune stimulatory activity, which was shared by other bacterial DNAs but not by vertebrate DNAs, was due to the presence of certain self-complementary palindromic sequences that happened to contain CpG dinucleotides (Kuramoto et al. 1992). However, methylation of the CpGs was not thought to have any influence on the immune stimulatory activities of these palindromes (Kuramoto et al. 1992).

Independently from Tokunaga and colleagues, other investigators using antisense ODN began to report the occurrence of immune stimulatory effects. In some cases, these effects were thought to be due to the nuclease-resistant phosphorothioate backbone, which is commonly used in antisense studies. The interpretation of these findings was further complicated by the tendency of many investigators to conclude that the observed immune stimulatory effects resulted from an antisense mechanism of action, while other investigators concluded that a non-antisense mechanism of action appeared to be responsible (Tanaka et al. 1992, Branda et al. 1993, McIntyre et al. 1993, Pisetsky and Reich 1993, Krieg et al. 1989, Hatzfeld et al. 1991, Mojcik et al. 1993, Fischer et al. 1994, Koike et al. 1995). Since none of these immune stimulatory ODN contained palindromes, no connection was made to the earlier findings of Tokunaga et al. However, once we identified the CpG motif as the actual cause of the immune stimulation and demonstrated that palindromes were not required, it became clear that the immune effects of all of these other ODN could also be accounted for by their presence of CpG motifs (Krieg 1998). Although immune stimulation by CpG motifs does not require the use of the nuclease resistant phosphorothioate backbone, ODN without this modification must be used at higher concentrations or in special culture conditions in order to observe the immune effects (Krieg et al. 1995 b).

Identification of Immune Neutralizing CpG DNA (CpG-N)

Immune stimulation by CpG DNA depends critically on the precise bases flanking the CpG which comprise the CpG motif (Table 12.1). Strong immune stimulatory ODN can have essentially any base preceding the CpG except for a C, and any base following the CpG except for a G, although pyrimidines are preferred at the 3' positions (Table 12.1). In retrospect, it is now clear that these differences in CpG motifs explain some early contradictory results in the observations made by different investigators. For example, one of the groups working with antisense ODN reported immune stimulatory sequences that caused B cell proliferation, but prevented immunoglobulin secretion (Tanaka et al. 1992), but nearly all other investigators found that immune stimulatory ODN also induced B cells to secrete immunoglobulin. With the benefit of hindsight, we can now appreciate that the immunoglobulin-inhibiting CpG motif in the former ODN comprised the sequence CCGCG while the other CpG motifs that stimulated immunoglobulin secretion had more optimal types of CpG motifs.

Other evidence for the existence of immune inhibitory motifs comes from the observation that vertebrate DNA, in which typically 20–30% of the CpG dinucleotides are unmethylated, does not trigger any immune stimulation. In fact, DNA derived from a cell line in which DNA methyltransferase has been deleted, which results in the near complete demethylation of the CpG motifs, lacks immune stimulatory effects (Sun et al. 1997). It is therefore noteworthy, that one can calculate from a published frequency analysis of the hexamers present in the vertebrate genome that the most common base preceding CpG motifs is a C and the most common base following CpG motifs is a G (Han et al. 1994). It appears likely that the failure of vertebrate DNA to cause stimulation may be due to this skewing of the flanking bases of the CpG motifs.

Additional evidence for the existence of the immune inhibitory CpG-N motif comes from our analysis of the immune effects and CpG motifs present in the genomes of adenoviruses, which do not have CpG suppression. To our surprise, genomic DNA from serotype 12 adenovirus, which is associated with a pattern of acute infection, was immune stimulatory, while genomic DNA from serotype 2

Table 12.1. Identification of an optimal stimulatory CpG motif for murine IL-12 production

ODN #	Sequence 5'-3'	IL-12 (pg/ml)
Media		<50 pg/ml
1916	TCCTG A<u>CG</u>TTG A A G T	6211
1929	. . . . . . <u>GC</u>	<50 pg/ml
1936	. . . . . <u>z g</u>	654
1937	. . Z . . . <u>CG</u>	7451
1917	. . . . . T <u>CG</u>	6649
1918	. . . . . G<u>CG</u>	7195
1919	. . . . . C<u>CG</u>	3789
1920	. . . . T . <u>CG</u>	6958
1921	. . . . A . <u>CG</u>	6988
1922	. . . . C . <u>CG</u>	9718
1923	. . . . . . <u>CG</u>A	8965
1924	. . . . . . <u>CG</u>C	8371
1925	. . . . . . <u>CG</u>G	<50 pg/ml
1926	. . . . . . <u>CG</u> . A	8711
1927	. . . . . . <u>CG</u> . C	8865
1928	. . . . . . <u>c g</u> . g	<50 pg/ml
1930	. . . . . . <u>CG</u> . . . GG . G	1694
1931	. . . . . . <u>CG</u> . . CC T TC	10765
1935	. . . . . G<u>CG</u>GG	<50 pg/ml
1938	. . . . A G<u>CG</u>	8686
1939	. . . A . . <u>CG</u>	10006
1940	. . . . . . <u>CG</u>GG	<50 pg/ml
1941	. . . . . G<u>C G</u>G	<50 pg/ml
1626	G<u>CA</u> . . . <u>CG</u> . . . . G C .	8904
E. coli DNA	NA	10907
Calf thymus DNA	NA	<50 pg/ml

Cultures were set up with the monocyte cell line J774, and 24 h supernatants collected. IL-12 levels were measured by ELISA using antibodies from Pharmingen (San Diego, USA)

or 5 adenoviruses, which cause more persistent patterns of infections, were not immune stimulatory (Krieg et al. 1998b). The presence of immune neutralizing motifs in the type 2 and 5 adenoviral DNA was confirmed by its ability to inhibit immune activation by bacterial DNA. These contrasting effects of genomic adenoviral DNAs made sense when we compared the frequency of different CpG motifs in their genomes (Table 12.2). The six most common hexamers in the genomes of type 2 or type 5 adenovirus (GCGCGC, GCGGCG, GGCGGC, CGCGCG, GCCGCC, and CGCCGC) were present 30 times more frequently than

Table 12.2. Genomic frequencies of selected hexamers ($\times 10^{-3}$)

Hexamer	Adenovirus type 2	Adenovirus type 12	E. coli	Human
GCGCGC	1.614	0.498	0.462	0.153
GCGGCG	1.530	0.469	0.745	0.285
GGCGGC	1.419	0.440	0.674	0.388
CGCGCG	1.336	0.322	0.379	0.106
GCCGCC	1.280	0.410	0.466	0.377
CGCCGC	1.252	0.410	0.623	0.274
GACGTT (CpG-S)	0.083	0.234	0.263	0.068
AACGTT (CpG-S)	0.056	0.205	0.347	0.056

The frequencies of hexamers in adenoviral and E. coli genomes are a personal communication from J. Han (University of Alabama, Birmingham). The hexamer frequencies in type 5 adenovirus are essentially identical to those in type 2 and are therefore not shown. The last two hexamers are CpG-S motifs shown for comparison and are the most stimulatory of all tested CpG-S motifs (Yi et al. 1996c).
Note that the expected frequency of a randomly selected hexamer is $1/4096 = 0.244 \times 10^{-3}$

the optimal CpG motifs (Table 12.2). However, there was no marked skewing in the frequency of different CpG motifs in the genome of immune stimulatory type 12 adenoviral DNA. The shared features of these putative CpG-N motifs were the motifs CCG, CGG, or CGCG, which were demonstrated to have immune neutralizing activities by testing of synthetic ODN bearing various combinations of CpG motifs (Krieg et al. 1998b). CpG-N motifs were shown to block the stimulatory effects of CpG-S motifs regardless of whether the different motifs were present in *trans* or *cis*.

Unfortunately, the mechanism through which these inhibitory effects are mediated is not well known, nor is it yet clear whether there may be differential effects of CpG-N motifs on the different types of immune stimulatory activities of CpG-S motifs. Therefore, the remainder of this chapter will focus on the effects and applications of the better-understood CpG-S motifs.

Immune Effects of CpG-S DNA

B Cell Activation

Primary B cells and B cell lines can be strongly stimulated by CpG DNA in the absence of any other cell type. In fact, CpG DNA is the most potent single B cell mitogen that has been described, and is capable of driving more than 95% of B cells into the cell cycle (Krieg et al. 1995b). B cells activated with CpG DNA also

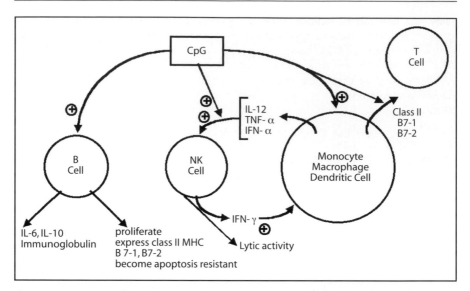

Fig. 12.1. Overview of the cell types that respond to CpG DNA. CpG DNA directly activates B cells and monocytic cells including macrophages and dendritic cells. These cells produce a variety of cytokines, most notably large amounts of Th$_1$-like cytokines such as IL-12. CpG DNA does not directly activate natural killer cells, but enhances their response to proinflammatory cytokines derived from adherent cells. Upon activation, the NK cells have increased lytic activity and secrete IFN-γ that feeds back to further activate the adherent antigen-presenting cells. Like NK cells, T cells are not directly activated by CpG, but are costimulated; T cells that have been presented specific antigen through the T cell receptor are synergistically activated in the presence of CpG DNA

secrete IL-6 and IL-10 within a few hours, followed by the secretion of IgM (Yi et al. 1996 a and c, Redford et al. 1998). The ability of CpG-activated B cells to present antigens is enhanced by increased expression of surface MHC class II molecules and the co-stimulatory molecules B7–1 and B7–2 (Krieg et al. 1995 b, Davis et al. 1998). CpG DNA also prevents both the spontaneous apoptosis of cultured primary B cells as well as experimentally induced apoptosis in B cell lines (Yi et al. 1996 b, Wang et al. 1997, Yi et al. 1998 a). Finally, CpG DNA promotes isotype switching in B cells, which may be important in enhancing the maturation of immune responses (Davis et al. 1998). Human B cells are also strongly stimulated by CpG DNA (Liang et al. 1996, Hartmann and Krieg, manuscript in preparation).

T Cell Activation

CpG DNA does not directly activate highly purified T cells, in contrast to the effects seen on B cells (Lipford et al. 1997 a, Sun et al. 1998 b). Nonetheless, T cells that have been activated through the T cell antigen receptor show very strong costimulatory proliferative responses to CpG DNA, indicating the ability of CpG to drive antigen-specific T cell responses (Bendigs et al. 1999). However, in the presence of adherent cells stimulated by high concentrations of CpG DNA to produce large amounts of type I interferons, CpG can actually inhibit the proliferative response to TCR crosslinking (Sun et al. 1998 b). Nonetheless, these T cells still are activated to express CD69. Thus, the effects of CpG DNA on T cell responses may be highly dependent on the precise characteristics of the experimental system studied.

Natural Killer (NK) Cell Activation

Like T cells, highly purified NK cells are not directly stimulated by CpG DNA (Ballas et al. 1996, Cowdery et al. 1996). However, in the presence of adherent cells that have been stimulated by CpG DNA, NK cells are strongly activated to have enhanced lytic activity and IFN-γ secretion. Studies using purified cell subsets have demonstrated that this interaction requires the secretion of specific cytokines from CpG-activated APCs including IL-12, type I interferons, and/or TNF-α (Ballas et al. 1996, Chace et al. 1997).

Macrophage, Monocyte, and Dendritic Cell Activation

Although the differences among the many subsets of these cells are not yet clear, CpG DNA generally appears to stimulate strong cytokine production. In particular, the cytokines produced by CpG-activated APCs are skewed strongly in the direction of Th$_1$-like responses. For example, dendritic cells activated by CpG secrete large amounts of IL-12 and low amounts of TNF-α. This is in striking contrast to LPS, which induces the opposite pattern of cytokine expression (Jakob et al. 1998). CpG DNA also induces secretion of IL-1, IL-6, and TNF-α as well as the cell surface expression of MHC class II and B7–1 and B7–2 (Stacey et al. 1996, Sparwasser et al. 1997, Sparwasser et al. 1998, Hartmann und Krieg 1999, Hartmann et al. 1999). As with B cells, the effects of CpG DNA on DCs are direct and rapid.

Mechanism of Action of CpG-S DNA

Cell Uptake of DNA

The existence of cell surface proteins that can bind DNA has been recognized for many years (Lerner et al. 1971, Bennett et al. 1985, Loke et al. 1989, Yakubov et al. 1989). These proteins appear to bind DNA in a non-sequence specific fashion. It is not yet clear whether they are actively involved in the cellular uptake of DNA. Nonetheless, it is clear that essentially all subsets of cells actively take up DNA through an energy- and temperature-dependent process which is saturable and appears to lead into and/or through an acidified intracellular endosomal compartment (Bennett et al. 1985, Krieg et al. 1991, Krieg et al. 1993, Tonkinson and Stein 1994, Zhao et al. 1994, Beltinger et al. 1995, Krieg 1995 a, Zhao et al. 1996).

Several lines of evidence argue against the existence of a cell surface receptor for CpG DNA. First of all, there is no difference in the cell surface binding of DNA containing CpG-S motifs compared to DNA without (Yamamoto et al. 1994a, Krieg et al. 1995b). Secondly, CpG-S ODN that have been immobilized on a solid support no longer stimulated B cells, indicating the requirement for cellular uptake (Krieg et al. 1995b). Third, lipofection of CpG-S ODN into spleen cells enhances their immune stimulatory effects, arguing that cell surface signaling is not involved (Yamamoto et al. 1994a). Finally, the fact that compounds such as chloroquine, which interfere with endosomal acidification and maturation, completely inhibit the stimulatory effects of CpG-S DNA yet do not interfere with ODN uptake into cells argues persuasively that some intracellular processing and/or recognition of the CpG-S DNA must occur (Hacker et al. 1998, MacFarlane and Manzel 1998, Yi et al. 1998c).

Against this evidence lies a report that human B cells can be stimulated by immobilized CpG-S ODN, suggesting that activation is mediated through a cell surface receptor (Liang et al. 1996). However, these CpG-S ODN were immobilized on sepharose beads, which have recently been shown by Manzel and MacFarlane to be internalized by cultured B cells (Manzel and MacFarlane 1999). These latter investigators confirmed that CpG-S ODN linked to sepharose beads are stimulatory, but went on to show that linkage to beads that cannot be internalized by cells prevents immune stimulation (Manzel and MacFarlane 1999). Thus, the preponderance of experimental evidence argues for an intracellular receptor for CpG rather than a cell surface receptor. We are currently attempting to identify and characterize such a receptor.

Generation of Reactive Oxygen Species (ROS) by CpG-S DNA

The redox balance of leukocytes is thought to be extremely important because of evidence that binding of several transcription factors to DNA may be altered by changes in the oxidative state of the cell (Sen and Packer 1996, Cotgreave and Gerdes 1998). Several studies have shown the generation of ROS such as superoxide, hydrogen peroxide, or lipid peroxides, that can influence the regulation of stimulation or apoptosis through the B cell antigen receptor or CD40 (Fang et al. 1995 and 1997, Lee and Koretzky 1997). The concentration, type, and intracellular localization of ROS are all likely important in determining the biologic effects of any changes.

By culturing cells in the presence of the ROS-sensitive dye, dihydrorhodamine-123, we showed that CpG DNA triggers the generation of intracellular ROS as early as 5 minutes after stimulation (Yi et al. 1996c). This generation of ROS was specifically blocked by chloroquine, but the generation of ROS in response to other lymphocyte mitogens was not (Yi et al. 1998c). A biologic function for this ROS generation is suggested by the fact that antioxidants prevent the effects of CpG DNA (Yi et al. 1996c). Further studies are underway in order to better define the mechanisms and consequences of ROS generation in response to CpG-S DNA.

Activation of Transcription Factors by CpG-S DNA

Since increases in ROS production have previously been linked to the activation of the transcription factor nuclear factor κB (NFκB), it may not be surprising that CpG triggers the rapid activation of NFκB in both B cells and macrophages (Stacey et al. 1996, Sparwasser et al. 1997, Yi et al. 1996b and 1998c). Specific inhibitors of NFκB activation block the immune stimulatory effects of CpG DNA, arguing that this transcription factor plays a critical role in CpG-induced signal transduction (Yi et al. 1998b). This NFκB activation is associated with the degradation of the inhibitors of κB, IκBα, and IκBβ, and with the nuclear translocation of the p50 and p65 subunits of NFκB.

Another set of signaling pathways activated by CpG DNA is the mitogen-activated protein kinases (MAPKs). CpG DNA activates both the p38 and c-Jun NH$_2$-terminal kinase or JNK pathways in both B cells and macrophages within 7 minutes after addition of CpG-S DNA (Hacker et al. 1998, Yi and Krieg 1998). These MAP kinase pathways lead to the phosphorylation of several transcription factors, including ATF-2 and AP-1. The induction of cytokine secretion by CpG-S DNA is prevented by treatment of cells with a specific inhibitor of the p38 kinase indicating a role for this pathway in mediating CpG effects (Hacker et al. 1998, Yi et al. 1998c). Cells treated with CpG-S DNA also have increased levels of mRNA for other transcription factors, including c-myc, ETS-2, C/EBP-β and -δ (K. J. Stacey and D. A. Hume, personal communication; Sweet et al. 1998, Yi et al. 1998a).

Induction of Gene Expression by CpG-S DNA

The activation of multiple transcription factors by CpG DNA leads to enhanced gene transcription, including protooncogenes, cytokines, and early response genes within 30 minutes (Yi et al. 1996b and 1998a). In keeping with its potent Th$_1$-like immune effects, CpG induces high levels of expression of IL-12 (Chace et al. 1997, Lipford et al. 1997b, Jakob et al. 1998, Sparwasser et al. 1998). This IL-12 induction is partially limited in magnitude and duration by the concomitant induction of B cell expression of IL-10 (Anitescu et al. 1997, Redford et al. 1998). Other cytokines whose expression has been reported to be increased in mouse and/or human cells include TNF-α, IFN-γ, IFN-α/β, MIP-1β, MCP-1, IL-1RA, IL-1β, IL-6, and IL-18 (Yamamoto et al. 1988 and 1994b, Klinman et al. 1996, Yi et al. 1996c, Roman et al. 1997, Schwartz et al. 1997, Zhao et al. 1997, Sun et al. 1998b, Hartmann et al. 1999). CpG DNA also induces the expression of several cell cycle regulating protooncogenes and anti-apoptosis genes such as c-myc and bcl-x$_L$ (Yi et al. 1996b and 1998b).

Therapeutic Implications of CpG-S and CpG-N DNA

Gene Therapy

The immune stimulatory effects of CpG-S DNA are of great relevance and concern to the field of gene therapy, since essentially all gene therapy applications necessarily involve the introduction or generation of intracellular DNA, which could contain CpG-S motifs. In the case of viral vectors, the immune effects attributable to CpG-S DNA may be dwarfed by the immune effects of the viral proteins and host immune responses. However, gene therapy applications involving the delivery of non-viral vectors (plasmids) have already demonstrated significant side effects from CpG-S motifs contained within the vectors. A human clinical trial of cystic fibrosis patients administered intrapulmonary cationic lipid-DNA complexes encoding the cystic fibrosis transmembrane receptor resulted in the development of fever, myalgia, and transient reductions in pulmonary function (J. Zabner, personal communication; Alton et al. 1998). The mechanisms of the immune stimulatory effects have been more fully understood through studies in mouse models. Instillation of lipid DNA complexes into mouse lungs triggers acute inflammatory responses that are abolished by treatment of the DNA with CpG methylase (Freimark et al. 1998, Yew et al. 1999). Although in these studies, lipids were necessary for inducing the full inflammatory effect of the plasmids, we have previously reported that even naked bacterial DNA or CpG-S ODN can cause direct pulmonary inflammatory effects (Schwartz et al. 1997).

Based on our current understanding of the biology of CpG-S motifs and the existence of CpG-N motifs, several possibilities for avoidance of this undesirable immune stimulation are apparent. First of all, although an obvious possibility may seem to be treatment of plasmid vectors with CpG methylase, this "solution" to the problem may not be practical because of the suppression of gene expression from methylated DNA (Tate and Bird 1993). One simple approach to avoiding immune stimulation by CpG-S DNA may be pretreatment with drugs such as hydroxychloroquine and quinacrine, which have been shown to completely block the immune stimulatory effects of the DNA (see above). These drugs have been used safely in humans for many years and would be expected to be safe for use in gene therapy trials. A more definitive solution to the problem of immune stimulation would be to redesign plasmid vectors to reduce their content of CpG-S motifs and/or to increase their content of CpG-N motifs. We have recently evaluated the in vitro immune effects of a plasmid vector in which more than 70 CpG-S motifs have been deleted by in situ mutagenesis. These CpG-S-depleted vectors induce only about 30% of the level of cytokine secretion from leukocytes treated with unmodified vectors in in vitro assays (A.M. Krieg et al., manuscript in preparation). Studies are currently underway to determine if this immune stimulatory effect can be further reduced by cloning of CpG-N motifs into the vectors.

Activation of Innate Immune Defenses by CpG-S DNA

Based on the potent immune stimulatory effects of CpG-S DNA and the hypothesis that it evolved to serve as an inducer of protective innate immune responses, we decided to test whether pretreatment of mice with CpG-S DNA could induce non-specific immune resistance against a lethal infectious challenge. Indeed, pretreatment of mice with either bacterial DNA or CpG-S ODN induces a state of remarkable resistance against a lethal challenge with *Listeria monocytogenes* or *Francisella tularensis* (Krieg et al. 1998 a, Elkins et al. 1999). Protection depended on the presence of IFN-γ since it was not seen in mice deficient in this Th$_1$-inducing cytokine. Interestingly, the timing of the CpG administration was critical in determining whether mice would be protected against the challenge. For optimal protection, mice had to be pretreated with CpG-S DNA at least 48 hours prior to the lethal challenge. A single dose of CpG gave sustained protection for at least two weeks. However, this protection is not generalizable against all types of bacteria: CpG-S DNA treatment does not protect against extracellular bacteria such as *E. coli*, or against polymicrobial sepsis.

Vaccination with CpG-S DNA

Several features suggest that CpG-S DNA should be an effective adjuvant for inducing antigen-specific immune responses. First, the costimulatory activity of CpG DNA for activating B cells and T cells through their antigen receptors should have the effect of promoting antigen-specific immune responses rather than acting as a non-specific polyclonal mitogen. Second, the induction of increased levels of costimulatory molecules and MHC class II expression on APCs should enhance the efficiency of antigen presentation. Finally, the induction of a Th$_1$-like cytokine environment in lymphoid tissues should promote the generation of Th$_1$-like T cell responses.

CpG-S ODN have been shown to be effective vaccine adjuvants for several model antigens including hen egg lysozyme (Chu et al. 1997), ovalbumin (Lipford et al. 1997 a), heterologous gammaglobulin (Sun et al. 1998 a), and β-galactosidase (Roman et al. 1997). Several of these investigators directly compared CpG DNA to complete Freund's adjuvant, the gold standard for inducing potent Th$_1$-like immune responses. While CpG-S ODN did not induce any of the undesirable local inflammatory responses seen with Freund's adjuvant, it was actually more potent as an adjuvant for inducing Th$_1$-like T cell responses (Chu et al. 1997). CpG-S ODN have also been shown to be potent adjuvants for infectious disease antigens such as hepatitis B (Davis et al. 1998) and influenza (Moldoveanu et al. 1998). The adjuvant effects of CpG-S ODN are not limited to mice, but have also been seen in Aotus monkeys immunized against a malaria circumsporozoite protein (Jones et al. 1999) and in orangutans immunized against hepatitis B (Davis et al. 2000).

Genetic or DNA vaccines are essentially plasmids encoding an antigen which is expressed under the control of a eukaryotic promoter (Donnelly et al. 1997). The remarkable efficiency of DNA vaccines in driving strong Th$_1$-like immune responses is now known to be due to the fact that the CpG-S motifs within the plasmid backbone act as a built-in adjuvant (Sato et al. 1996, Klinman et al. 1997, Krieg et al. 1998a). We have recently demonstrated that immunization with DNA vaccines can be further enhanced if the CpG-N motifs within the backbone are deleted by in situ mutagenesis and if additional CpG-S motifs are inserted into the plasmid backbone (Krieg et al. 1998b).

Cancer Therapy with CpG-S DNA

Several types of anticancer applications are possible using CpG-S DNA. First, CpG-S ODN are useful adjuvants for tumor vaccination and induce protective immunity against lethal tumor challenge (Sun et al. 1996, Weiner et al. 1997). This induction of anti-tumor immunity is greatly enhanced by using CpG in combination with GM-CSF (Liu et al. 1998). Secondly, CpG-S-mediated immune activation is associated with increased antibody-dependent cellular cytotoxicity (ADCC), which can be used to greatly enhance the response rate to immunotherapy with anti-tumor monoclonal antibodies (Wooldridge et al. 1997). Finally, the potent NK-stimulating activity of CpG DNA can be used for immunotherapy of tumors such as melanoma, which are sensitive to NK-mediated lysis (Ballas and Krieg, manuscript in preparation).

Allergy Therapy with CpG-S DNA

Allergic diseases are characterized by Th_2-like immune responses against harmless environmental antigens. Given the remarkable Th_1-like effects of CpG-S DNA, we considered the possibility that CpG may antagonize the initiation or maintenance of allergic diseases. In order to test this hypothesis, we evaluated the ability of CpG DNA to prevent the sensitization of mice to the potent Th_2 allergen, schistosome eggs. These studies confirmed that CpG-S DNA given in conjunction with a potent allergen completely prevented sensitization to the allergen, and instead drove the induction of a Th_1-like immune response (Kline et al. 1998). More significantly, even in mice that had already been sensitized to an allergen, treatment with CpG can dramatically reverse the allergic response to allergen exposure (Kline et al. 1998). Although it is in some way easiest to reverse allergic responses by giving CpG together with the allergen, it is also possible to prevent allergic responses in mice by using the CpG as a single agent depending on the timing of administration of CpG-S ODN compared to the allergen exposure (Broide et al. 1998, Sur et al. 1999).

Conclusion

In recent years, the immune stimulatory effects of CpG-S DNA have become widely recognized. While this DNA may have many therapeutic applications, it is more of a nuisance to the field of gene therapy. Nonetheless, there appear to be several ways in which these effects may be minimized or avoided including the intentional use of opposing motifs, termed CpG-N motifs, which neutralize the immune stimulatory activities. Further studies will be required in order to understand the complexities of these different and unexpected immune effects of DNA.

Acknowledgements. The author thanks Tilese Arrington for secretarial assistance. Financial support was provided through a Career Development Award from the Department of Veterans Affairs and grants from the National Institutes of Health and Coley Pharmaceutical Group.

References

Alton EWFW, Geddes DM, Gill DR, Higgins CF, Hyde SC, Innes JA, Porteous DJ (1998) Towards gene therapy for cystic fibrosis: A clinical progress report. Gene Ther 5:291–292

Anitescu M, Chace JH, Tuetken R, Yi A-K, Berg DJ, Krieg AM, Cowdery JS (1997) Interleukin-10 functions in vitro and in vivo to inhibit bacterial DNA-induced secretion of interleukin-12. J Interferon Cytokine Res 17:781–788

Ballas ZK, Rasmussen WL, Krieg AM (1996) Induction of natural killer activity in murine and human cells by CpG motifs in oligodeoxynucleotides and bacterial DNA. J Immunol 157:1840–1845

Beltinger C, Saragovi HU, Smith RM, LeSauteur L, Shah N, DeDionisio L, Christensen L, Raible A, Jarett L, Gewirtz AM (1995) Binding, uptake, and intracellular trafficking of phosphorothioate-modified oligodeoxynucleotides. J Clin Invest 95:1814–18123

Bendigs S, Salzer U, Lipford GB, Wagner H, Heeg K (1999) CpG-oligodeoxynucleotides co-stimulate primary T cells in the absence of antigen-presenting cells. Eur J Immunol 29:1209–1218

Bennett RM, Gabor GT, Merritt MM (1985) DNA binding to human leukocytes. Evidence for a receptor-mediated association, internalization, and degradation of DNA. J Clin Invest 76:2182–2190

Bird AP (1987) CpG islands as gene markers in the vertebrate nucleus. Trends Genet 3:342–347

Branda RF, Moore AL, Mathews L, McCormack JJ, Zon G (1993) Immune stimulation by an antisense oligomer complementary to the rev gene of HIV-1. Biochem Pharmacol 45:2037–2043

Broide D, Schwarze J, Tighe H, Gifford T, Nguyen M-D, Malek S, Van Uden J, Martin-Orozco E, Gelfand EW, Raz E (1998) Immunostimulatory DNA sequences inhibit IL-5, eosinophilic inflammation, and airway hyperresponsiveness in mice. J Immunol 161:7054–7062

Chace JH, Hooker NA, Mildenstein KL, Krieg AM, Cowdery JS (1997) Bacterial DNA-induced NK cell IFN-γ production is dependent on macrophage secretion of IL-12. Clin Immunol Immunopathol 84:185–193

Chu RS, Targoni OS, Krieg AM, Lehmann PV, Harding CV (1997) CpG Oligodeoxynucleotides act as adjuvants that switch on Th_1 immunity. J Exp Med 186:1623–1631

Cotgreave IA, Gerdes RG (1998) Recent trends in glutathione biochemistry – glutathione-protein interactions: A molecular link between oxidative stress and cell proliferation? Biochem Biophys Res Comm 242:1–9

Cowdery JS, Chace JH, Yi A-K, Krieg AM (1996) Bacterial DNA induces NK cells to produce interferon-γ in vivo and increases the toxicity of lipopolysaccharides. J Immunol 156:4570–4575

Davis HL, Weeratna R, Waldschmidt TJ, Tygrett L, Schorr J, Krieg AM (1998) CpG DNA is a potent adjuvant in mice immunized with recombinant hepatitis B surface antigen. J Immunol 160:870–876

Davis HL, Suparto I, Weeratna RR, Jumintarto, Iskandriati DD, Chamzah SS, Ma'ruf AA, Nente CC, Pawitri DD, Krieg AM, Heriyanto, Smits W, Sajuthi DD (2000) CpG DNA overcomes hyporesponsiveness to hepatitis B vaccine in orangutans. Vaccine 18:1920–1924

Donnelly JJ, Ulmer JB, Shiver JW, Liu MA (1997) DNA vaccines. Ann Rev Immunol 15:617–648

Elkins KL, Rhinehart-Jones TR, Stibitz S, Conover JS, Klinman DM (1999) Bacterial DNA containing CpG motifs stimulates lymphocyte-dependent protection of mice against lethal infection with intracellular bacteria. J Immunol 162:2291–2298

Fang W, Rivard JJ, Ganser JA, LeBien TW, Nath KA, Mueller DL, Behrens TW (1995) Bcl-XL rescues WEHI-231 B lymphocytes from oxidant-mediated death following diverse apoptotic stimuli. J Immunol 155:66–75

Fang W, Nath KA, Mackey MF, Noelle RJ, Mueller DL, Behrens TW (1997) CD40 inhibits B cell apoptosis by upregulating bcl-xL expression and blocking oxidant accumulation. Am J Physiol 272:950–956

Fischer G, Kent SC, Joseph L, Green DR, Scott DW (1994) Lymphoma models for B cell activation and tolerance. Anti-mu-mediated growth arrest and apoptosis of murine B cell lymphomas is prevented by the stabilization of myc. J Exp Med 179:221–228

Freimark BD, Blezinger HP, Florack VJ, Nordstrom JL, Long SD, Deshpande DS, Nochumson S, Petrak KL (1998) Cationic lipids enhance cytokine and cell influx levels in the lung following administration of plasmid:cationic lipid complexes. J Immunol 160: 4580–4586

Hacker H, Mischak H, Miethke T, Liptay S, Schmid R, Sparwasser T, Heeg K, Lipford GB, Wagner H (1998) CpG-DNA-specific activation of antigen-presenting cells requires stress kinase activity and is preceded by non-specific endocytosis and endosomal maturation. EMBO J 17:6230–6240

Han J, Zhu Z, Hsu C, Finley WH (1994) Selection of antisense oligonucleotides on the basis of genomic frequency of the target sequence. Antisense Res Devel 4:53–65

Hartmann G, Krieg AM (1999) CpG DNA and LPS induce distinct patterns of activation in human monocytes. Gene Therapy 6:893–903

Hartmann G, Weiner G, Krieg AM (1999) CpG DNA: a potent signal for growth, activation, and maturation of human dendritic cells. Proc Natl Acad Sci USA 96:9305–9310

Hatzfeld J, Li M-L, Brown EL, Sookdeo H, Levesque J-P, O'Toole T, Gurney C, Clark SC, Hatzfeld A (1991) Release of early human hematopoietic progenitors from quiescence by antisense transforming growth factor beta 1 or Rb oligonucleotides. J Exp Med 174:925–929

Jakob T, Walker PS, Krieg AM, Udey MC, Vogel JC (1998) Activation of cutaneous dendritic cells by CpG-containing oligodeoxynucleotides: A role for dendritic cells in the augmentation of Th_1 responses by immunostimulatory DNA. J Immunol 161:3042–3049

Jones TR, Obaldia N, Gramzinski RA, Charoenvit Y, Kolodny N, Kitov S, Davis HL, Krieg AM, Hoffman SL (1999) Synthetic oligodeoxynucleotides containing CpG motifs enhance immunogenicity of a peptide malaria vaccine in Aotus monkeys. Vaccine 17:3065–3071

Karlin S, Doerfler W, Cardon LR (1994) Why is CpG suppressed in the genomes of virtually all small eukaryotic viruses but not in those of large eukaryotic viruses? J Virol 68:2889–2897

Kline JN, Waldschmidt TJ, Businga TR, Lemish JE, Weinstock JV, Thorne PS, Krieg AM (1998) Modulation of airway inflammation by CpG oligodeoxynucleotides in a murine model of asthma. J Immunol 160:2555–2559

Klinman D, Yi A-K, Beaucage SL, Conover J, Krieg AM (1996) CpG motifs expressed by bacterial DNA rapidly induce lymphocytes to secrete IL-6, IL-12 and IFN. Proc Natl Acad Sci USA 93:2879–2883

Klinman DM, Yamshchikov G, Ishigatsubo Y (1997) Contribution of CpG motifs to the immunogenicity of DNA vaccines. J Immunol 158:3635–3639

Koike M, Ishino K, Ikuta T, Huh N, Kuroki T (1995) Growth enhancement of normal human keratinocytes by the antisense oligonucleotide of retinoblastoma susceptibility gene. Oncogene 10:117–122

Krieg AM (1998) Leukocyte stimulation by oligodeoxynucleotides. In: Stein CA, Krieg AM (eds) Applied Oligonucleotide Technology. John Wiley & Sons Inc., New York, NY, p 431–448

Krieg AM, Gause WC, Gourley MF, Steinberg AD (1989) A role for endogenous retroviral sequences in the regulation of lymphocyte activation. J Immunol 143:2448–2451

Krieg AM, Gmelig-Meyling F, Gourley MF, Kisch WJ, Chrisey LA, Steinberg AD (1991) Uptake of oligodeoxyribonucleotides by lymphoid cells is heterogeneous and inducible. Antisense Res Dev 1:161–171

Krieg AM, Tonkinson J, Matson S, Zhao Q, Saxon M, Zhang L-M, Bhanja U, Yakubov L, Stein CA (1993) Modification of antisense phosphodiester oligodeoxynucleotides by a 5' cholesteryl moiety increases cellular association and improves efficacy. Proc Natl Acad Sci USA 90:1048–1052

Krieg AM (1995a) Uptake and localization of phosphodiester and chimeric oligodeoxynucleotides in normal and leukemic primary cells. In: Akhtar S (ed) Delivery Strategies for Antisense Oligonucleotide Therapeutics. CRC Press, Inc., p. 177

Krieg AM, Yi A-K, Matson S, Waldschmidt TJ, Bishop GA, Teasdale R, Koretzky G, Klinman D (1995b) CpG motifs in bacterial DNA trigger direct B-cell activation. Nature 374:546–549

Krieg AM (1996) Lymphocyte activation by CpG dinucleotide motifs in prokaryotic DNA. Trends Microbiol 4:73–76

Krieg AM, Love-Homan L, Yi A-K, Harty JT (1998a) CpG DNA induces sustained IL-12 expression in vivo and resistance to Listeria monocytogenes challenge. J Immunol 161:2428–2434

Krieg AM, Wu T, Weeratna R, Efler SM, Love-Homan L, Zhang L, Yang L, Yi A-K, Short D, Davis H (1998b) Sequence motifs in adenoviral DNA block immune activation by stimulatory CpG motifs. Proc Natl Acad Sci USA 95:12631–12636

Kumar A, Yang YL, Flati V, Der S, Kadereit S, Deb A, Haque J, Reis L, Weissmann C, Williams BR (1997) Deficient cytokine signaling in mouse embryo fibroblasts with a targeted deletion in the PKR gene: Role of IRF-1 and NF-κB. EMBO J 16:406–416

Kuramoto E, Yano O, Kimura Y, Baba M, Makino T, Yamamoto S, Yamamoto T, Kataoka T, Tokunaga T (1992) Oligonucleotide sequences required for natural killer cell activation. Jpn J Cancer Res 83:1128–1131

Lee JR, Koretzky GA (1997) Production of reactive oxygen intermediates following CD40 ligation correlates with c-Jun N-terminal kinase activation and IL-6 secretion in murine B lymphocytes. Eur J Immunol 28:4188–4197

Lerner RA, Meinke W, Goldstein DA (1971) Membrane-associated DNA in the cytoplasm of diploid human lymphocytes. Proc Natl Acad Sci USA 68:1212–1216

Liang H, Nishioka Y, Reich CF, Pisetsky DS, Lipsky PE (1996) Activation of human B cells by phosphorothioate oligodeoxynucleotides. J Clin Invest 98:1119–1129

Lipford GB, Bauer M, Blank C, Reiter R, Wagner H, Heeg K (1997a) CpG-containing synthetic oligonucleotides promote B and cytotoxic T cell responses to protein antigen: a new class of vaccine adjuvants. Eur J Immunol 27:2340–2344

Lipford GB, Sparwasser T, Bauer M, Zimmermann S, Koch E-S, Heeg K, Wagner H (1997b) Immunostimulatory DNA: Sequence-dependent production of potentially harmful or useful cytokines. Eur J Immunol 27:3420–3426

Liu H-M, Newbrough SE, Bhatia SK, Dahle CE, Krieg AM, Weiner GJ (1998) Immuno-stimulatory CpG oligodeoxynucleotides enhance the immune response to vaccine strategies involving granulocyte-macrophage colony-stimulating factor. Blood 92:3730–3736

Loke SL, Stein CA, Zhang XH, Mori K, Nakanishi M, Subasinghe C, Cohen JS, Neckers LM (1989) Characterization of oligonucleotide transport into living cells. Proc Natl Acad Sci USA 86:3474–3478

MacFarlane DE, Manzel L (1998) Antagonism of immunostimulatory CpG-oligodeoxynu-cleotides by quinacrine, chloroquine, and structurally related compounds. J Immunol 160:1122–1131

Manzel L, MacFarlane DE (1999) Immune stimulation by CpG-oligodeoxynucleotide requires internalization. Antisense Nucl Acid Drug Devel 9:459–464

McIntyre KW, Lombard-Gillooly K, Perez JR, Kunsch C, Sarmiento UM, Larigan JD, Land-reth KT, Narayanan R (1993) A sense phosphorothioate oligonucleotide directed to the initiation codon of transcription factor NF-KB p65 causes sequence-specific immune stimulation. Antisense Res Dev 3:309–322

Messina JP, Gilkeson GS, Pisetsky DS (1991) Stimulation of in vitro murine lymphocyte proliferation by bacterial DNA. J Immunol 147:1759–1764

Mojcik C, Gourley MF, Klinman DM, Krieg AM, Gmelig-Meyling F, Steinberg AD (1993) Administration of a phosphorothioate oligonucleotide antisense to murine endogenous retroviral MCF env causes immune effects in vivo in a sequence-specific manner. Clin Immunol Immunopathol 67:130–136

Moldoveanu Z, Love-Homan L, Huang WQ, Krieg AM (1998) CpG DNA, a novel adjuvant for systemic and mucosal immunization with influenza virus. Vaccine 16:1216–1224

Pisetsky DS, Reich CF (1993) Stimulation of murine lymphocyte proliferation by a phos-phorothioate oligonucleotide with antisense activity for herpes simplex virus. Life Sci 54:101–107

Redford TW, Yi A-K, Ward CT, Krieg AM (1998) Cyclosporine A enhances IL-12 production by CpG motifs in bacterial DNA and synthetic oligodeoxynucleotides. J Immunol 161:3930–3935

Roman M, Martin-Orozco E, Goodman JS, Nguyen M-D, Sato Y, Ronaghy A, Kornbluth RS, Richman DD, Carson DA, Raz E (1997) Immunostimulatory DNA sequences function as T helper-1-promoting adjuvants. Nat Med 3:849–854

Sato Y, Roman M, Tighe H, Lee D, Corr M, Nguyen M-D, Silverman GJ, Lotz M, Carson DA, Raz E (1996) Immunostimulatory DNA sequences necessary for effective intrader-mal gene immunization. Science 273:352–354

Schwartz D, Quinn TJ, Thorne PS, Sayeed S, Yi A-K, Krieg AM (1997) CpG motifs in bacterial DNA cause inflammation in the lower respiratory tract. J Clin Invest 100:68–73

Sen CK, Packer L (1996) Antioxidant and redox regulation of gene transcription. FASEB J 10:709–720

Shpaer EG, Mullins JI (1990) Selection against CpG dinucleotides in lentiviral genes: A possible role of methylation in regulation of viral expression. Nucleic Acids Res 18:5793–5797

Sparwasser T, Miethe T, Lipford G, Erdmann A, Hacker H, Heeg K, Wagner H (1997) Macrophages sense pathogens via DNA motifs: Induction of tumor necrosis factor-a-mediated shock. Eur J Immunol 27:1671–1679

Sparwasser T, Koch E-S, Vabulas RM, Heeg K, Lipford GB, Ellwart J, Wagner H (1998) Bacterial DNA and immunostimulatory CpG oligonucleotides trigger maturation and activation of murine dendritic cells. Eur J Immunol 28:2045–2054

Stacey KJ, Sweet MJ, Hume DA (1996) Macrophages ingest and are activated by bacterial DNA. J Immunol 157:2116–2122

Sun S, Cai Z, Langlade-Demoyen P, Kosaka H, Brunmark A, Jackson MR, Peterson PA, Sprent J (1996) Dual function of drosophilia cells as APCs for naive CD8+ T cells: Implications for tumor immunotherapy. Immunity 4:555–564

Sun S, Beard C, Jaenisch R, Jones P, Sprent J (1997) Mitogenicity of DNA from different organisms for murine B cells. J Immunol 159:3119–3125

Sun S, Kishimoto H, Sprent J (1998a) DNA as an adjuvant: Capacity of insect DNA and synthetic oligodeoxynucleotides to augment T cell responses to specific antigen. J Exp Med 187:1145–1150

Sun S, Zhang X, Tough DF, Sprent J (1998b) Type I interferon-mediated stimulation of T cells by CpG DNA. J Exp Med 188:2335–2342

Sur S, Wild JS, Choudhury BK, Sur N, Alam R, Klinman DM (1999) Long term prevention of allergic lung inflammation in a mouse model of asthma by CpG oligodeoxynucleotides. J Immunol 162:6284–6293

Suzuki K, Mori A, Ishii KJ, Saito J, Singer DS, Klinman DM, Krause PR, Kohn LD (1999) Activation of target-tissue immune-recognition molecules by double-stranded polynucleotides. Proc Natl Acad Sci USA 96:2285–2290

Sweet MJ, Stacey KJ, Ross IL (1998) Involvement of Ets, rel and Sp1-like proteins in lipopolysaccharide-mediated activation of the HIV-1 LTR in macrophages. J Inflamm 48:67–83

Tanaka T, Chu CC, Paul WE (1992) An antisense oligonucleotide complementary to a sequence in Ic2b increases c2b germline transcripts, stimulates B cell DNA synthesis, and inhibits immunoglobulin secretion. J Exp Med 175:597–607

Tate PH, Bird AP (1993) Effects of DNA methylation on DNA-binding proteins and gene expression. Curr Opin Genet Dev 3:226–231

Tokunaga T, Yamamoto H, Shimada S, Abe H, Fukuda T, Fujisawa Y, Furutani Y, Yano O, Kataoka T, Sudo T, Makiguchi N, Suganuma T (1984) Antitumor activity of deoxyribonucleic acid fraction from *Mycobacterium bovis* GCG. Isolation, physicochemical characterization, and antitumor activity. J Natl Cancer Inst 72:955–962

Tonkinson JL, Stein CA (1994) Patterns of intracellular compartmentalization, trafficking and acidification of 5′-fluorescein labeled phosphodiester and phosphorothioate oligodeoxynucleotides in HL60 cells. Nucleic Acids Res 22:4268–4275

Wang Z, Karras JG, Colarusso TP, Foote LC, Rothstein TL (1997) Unmethylated CpG motifs protect murine B lymphocytes against Fas-mediated apoptosis. Cell Immunol 180:162–167

Weiner GJ, Liu H-M, Wooldridge JE, Dahle CE, Krieg AM (1997) Immunostimulatory oligodeoxynucleotides containing the CpG motif are effective as immune adjuvants in tumor antigen immunization. Proc Natl Acad Sci USA 94:10833–10837

Wooldridge JE, Ballas Z, Krieg AM, Weiner GJ (1997) Immunostimulatory oligodeoxynucleotides containing CpG motifs enhance the efficacy of monoclonal antibody therapy of lymphoma. Blood 89:2994–2998

Yakubov LA, Deeva EA, Zarytova VF, Ivanova EM, Ryte AS, Yurchenko LV, Vlassov VV (1989) Mechanism of oligonucleotide uptake by cells: Involvement of specific receptors? Proc Natl Acad Sci USA 86:6454–6458

Yamamoto S, Kuramoto E, Shimada S, Tokunaga T (1988) In vitro augmentation of natural killer cell activity and production of interferon-α/β and -γ with deoxyribonucleic acid fraction from *Mycobacterium bovis* BCG. Jpn J Cancer Res 79:866–873

Yamamoto T, Yamamoto S, Kataoka T, Tokunaga T (1994a) Lipofection of synthetic oligodeoxyribonucleotide having a palindromic sequence of AACGTT to murine splenocytes enhances interferon production and natural killer activity. Microbiol Immunol 38:831–836

Yamamoto T, Yamamoto S, Kataoka T, Tokunaga T (1994b) Synthetic oligonucleotides with certain palindromes stimulate interferon production of human peripheral blood lymphocytes in vitro. Jpn J Cancer Res 85:775–779

Yew NS, Wang KX, Przybylska M, Bagley RG, Stedman M, Marshall J, Scheule RK, Cheng SH (1999) Contribution of plasmid DNA to inflammation in the lung after administration of cationic lipid:pDNA complexes. Hum Gene Ther 10:223–234

Yi A-K, Chace JH, Cowdery JS, Krieg AM (1996a) IFN-γ promotes IL-6 and IgM secretion in response to CpG motifs in bacterial DNA and oligodeoxynucleotides. J Immunol 156:558–564

Yi A-K, Hornbeck P, Lafrenz DE, Krieg AM (1996b) CpG DNA rescue of murine B lymphoma cells from anti-IgM induced growth arrest and programmed cell death is associated with increased expression of c-myc and bcl-xL. J Immunol 157:4918–4925

Yi A-K, Klinman DM, Martin TL, Matson S, Krieg AM (1996c) Rapid immune activation by CpG motifs in bacterial DNA: Systemic induction of IL-6 transcription through an antioxidant-sensitive pathway. J Immunol 157:5394–5402

Yi, A-K, Krieg AM (1998) Rapid induction of mitogen activated protein kinases by immune stimulatory CpG DNA. J Immunol 161:4493–4497

Yi A-K, Chang M, Peckham DW, Krieg AM, Ashman RF (1998a) CpG oligodeoxyribonucleotides rescue mature spleen B cells from spontaneous apoptosis and promote cell cycle entry. J Immunol 160:5898–5906

Yi, A-K, Krieg AM (1998b) CpG DNA rescue from anti-IgM induced WEHI-231 B lymphoma apoptosis via modulation of IκBα and IκBβ and sustained activation of nuclear factor-κB/c-Rel. J Immunol 160:1240–1245

Yi A-K, Tuetken R, Redford T, Kirsch J, Krieg AM (1998c) CpG motifs in bacterial DNA activates leukocytes through the pH-dependent generation of reactive oxygen species. J Immunol 160:4755–4761

Zhao Q, Waldschmidt T, Fisher E, Herrera CJ, Krieg AM (1994) Stage specific oligonucleotide uptake in murine bone marrow B cell precursors. Blood 84:3660–3666

Zhao Q, Temsamani J, Iadarola PL, Jiang Z, Agrawal S (1996) Effect of different chemically modified oligodeoxynucleotides on immune stimulation. Biochem Pharmacol 51:173–182

Zhao Q, Temsamani J, Zhou R-Z, Agrawal S (1997) Pattern and kinetics of cytokine production following administration of phosphorothioate oligonucleotides in mice. Antisense Nucleic Acid Drug Dev 7:495–502

13 Genetic and Dendritic Cell Vaccination as a Novel Therapy for Melanoma

D. Schadendorf, A. Paschen, Y. Sun

Melanoma and Tumor Immunology

Melanoma is a malignant tumor of neuroectodermal origin with an increasing incidence and mortality. It needs to be detected and eliminated early, since melanoma is characterized by its high resistance to conventional therapies including surgery and chemotherapy (Ahmann et al. 1989, Garbe 1993, Johnson et al. 1995). On the other hand, melanoma is supposed to be one of the most immunogenic tumors which is demonstrated by tumor infiltrating lymphocytes (TIL) destroying melanoma cells (Oettgen and Old 1991, Parkinson et al. 1992, Dagleish 1996). Its immunogenicity may also be responsible for the occurrence of spontaneous partial or complete melanoma regression and for the concomitant destruction of melanocytes in benign lesions leading to clinical phenomena such as halo nevi, uveitis and vitiligo in melanoma patients.

Nevertheless, it became clear that immune responses to tumor antigens are frequently not observed because of tolerance and immunological non-responsiveness to cancer. In order to overcome this hurdle, cancer vaccines must break tolerance and activate a "cryptic" T cell population that escaped tolerance induction by low affinity binding, which is critically dependent on the proper activation of the encountering antigen-presenting cell (APC). Danger signals will lead to appropriate co-stimulation and T cell activation (reviewed in Bell et al. 1999). The critical role of CD4 cells and CD40/CD40L interaction in delivering help to CD8 cells, and providing an adequate cytokine milieu has been recognized to be of great importance in recent years (Bennett et al. 1997, Mackey et al. 1998). In order to fight cancer, the idea to use the destructive power of the immune system is easily visualized in autoimmune diseases and by the rejection of allografts in transplantation medicine. A number of clinical observations in human malignant melanoma suggest a particularly vigorous immune response (Oettgen and Old 1991, Parkinson et al. 1992, Mackensen et al. 1994, Dagleish 1996). CD8+ T-lymphocytes derived from melanoma lesions, the peripheral blood and tumor tissue were shown to be capable of mediating impressive tumor regressions in vivo (Kawakami et al. 1994, Robbins et al. 1994). The availability and further characterization of such tumor-specific T-cell clones in recent years led to the identification of several melanoma-associated antigens (reviewed in Boon et al. 1997, Rosenberg 1999 and Rosenberg et al. 1999; Table 13.1) providing tools which allow the rationale design of vaccination strategies.

Table 13.1. Melanoma-associated antigens recognized by human T lymphocytes[a]

Target antigen	HLA molecule	Peptides sequence	Amino acids	Reference
MAGE-1	HLA-A1	EADPTGHSY	161–169	van der Bruggen et al. 1991
	HLA-A3	SLFRAVITK	96–104	Chaux et al. 1999a
	HLA-A24	NYKHCFPEI	135–143	Fujie et al. 1999
	HLA-A28	EVYDGREHSA	222–231	Chaux et al. 1999a
	HLA-B37	REPVTKAEML	127–136	Tanzerella et al. 1999
	HLA-B53	DPARYEFLW	258–266	Chaux et al. 1999a
	HLA-Cw2	SAFPTTINF	62–70	Chaux et al. 1999a
	HLA-Cw3/-Cw16	SAYGEPRKL	230–238	van der Bruggen et al. 1994b
	HLA-DR13	LLKYRAREPVTKAE	121–134	Chaux et al. 1999b
MAGE-2	HLA-A2	KMVELVHFL	112–120	Visseren et al. 1997
		YLQLVFGIEV	157–166	Visseren et al. 1997
	HLA-24	EYLQLVFGI	156–164	Tahara et al. 1999
	HLA-B37	REPVTKAEML	127–136	Tanzerella et al. 1999
	HLA-DR13	LLKYRAREPVTKAE	121–134	Chaux et al. 1999b
MAGE-3	HLA-A1	EVDPIGHLY	168–176	Gaugler et al. 1994
	HLA-A2	FLWGPRALV	271–279	van der Bruggen et al. 1994a
		KVAELVHFL	112–120	
	HLA-A24	IMPKAGLLI	195–203	Kawashima et al. 1998
		TFPDLESEF	97–105	Tanaka et al. 1997
	HLA-B37	REPVTKAEML	127–136	Oiso et al. 1999
	HLA-B44	MEVDPIGHLY	167–176	Tanzerella et al. 1999
	HLA-DR13	AELVHFLLLKYRAR	114–127	Herman et al. 1996
		LLKYRAREPVTKAE	121–134	Chaux et al. 1999b
	HLA-DR11	TSYVKVLHHMVKISG	281–295	Chaux et al. 1999b; Manici et al. 1999
MAGE-4	HLA-A2	GVYDGREHTV	230–239	Duffour et al. 1999
MAGE-6	HLA-A34	MVKISGGPR	290–298	Zorn and Hercend 1999a
	HLA-B37	REPVTKAEML	127–136	Tanzerella et al. 1999
	HLA-DR13	LLKYRAREPVTKAE	121–134	Chaux et al. 1999b
MAGE-10	HLA-A2.1	GLYDGMEHL	254–262	Huang et al. 1999
	HLA-B53	DPARYEFLW	290–298	Chaux et al. 1999a
MAGE-12	HLA-Cw7	VRIGHLYIL	170–178	van der Bruggen et al. 1994b
	HLA-DR13	AELVHFLLLKYRAR	114–127	Chaux et al. 1999b
BAGE	HLA-Cw16	AARAVFLAL	2–10	Boel et al. 1995
GAGE-1, 2, 8	HLA-Cw6	YRPRPRRY	9–16	Van den Eynde et al. 1995
GAGE-3 to 7	HLA-A29	YYWPRPRRY	10–18	De Backer et al. 1999
NY-ESO-1/CAG-3/	HLA-A2	QLSLLMWITQC (ORF-1)	155–165	Jäger et al. 1998
	HLA-A31	ASGPGGGAPR (ORF-1)	53–62	Wang et al. 1998b
	HLA-A31	LAAQERRYPR (ORF-2)		Wang et al. 1998a

Table 13.1 (continued)

Target antigen	HLA molecule	Peptides sequence	Amino acids	Reference
LAGE/ CAMEL	HLA-A2	MLMAQEALAFL (ORF-2)		Aarnoudse et al. 1999 Lethe et al. 1998
pMel-34/ Tyrosinase	HLA-A2	YMDGTMSQV	369–377	Skipper et al. 1996a
		YMNGTMSQV	369–377	Wölfel et al. 1994
		MLLAVLYCL	1–9	Wölfel et al. 1994
	HLA-A24	AFLPWHRLF	206–214	Kang et al. 1995
	HLA-B35	LPSSADVEF	312–320	Morel et al. 1999
	HLA-B44	SEIWRDIDF	192–200	Brichard et al. 1996
	HLA-A1	KCDICTDEY	243–251	Kittlesen et al. 1998
		SSDYVIPIGTY	146–156	Kawakami et al. 1998
	HLA-DR4	QNILLSNAPLGPQFP	56–70	Topalian et al. 1996
		DYSYLQDSDPDSFQD	448–462	Topalian et al. 1996
	HLA-DR15	FLLHHAFVDSIFEQWLQ -RHRP	386–406	Kobayashi et al. 1998
TRP-1/ gp75	HLA-A31	MSLQRQFLR (ORF-3)	1–9	Wang et al. 1996b
TRP-2	HLA-A*0201	SVYDFFVWL	180–188	Parkhurst et al. 1998
	HLA-A*0201	SLHNLYHSFL	367–376	Reynolds et al. 1998
	HLA-A31, -A33	LLGPGRPYR	197–205	Wang et al. 1996a and 1998a
	HLA-CW8	ANDPIFVVL	387–395	Castelli et al. 1999
TRP-2 (int2)	HLA-A68011/ -3301	EVISCKLIKR	222–231	Lupetti et al. 1998
pMel-17/ gp100	HLA-A2	VLYRYGSFSV	476–485	Kawakami et al. 1994a
		KTWGQYWQV	154–162	Kawakami et al. 1994a
		YLEPGPVTA	280–288	Kawakami et al. 1994a
		LLDGTATLRL	457–466	Kawakami et al. 1994b
		SLADTNSLAV	570–579	Tsai et al. 1997
		ITDQVPFSV	209–217	Kawakami et al. 1994a
		RLMKQDFSV	619–627	Kawakami et al. 1998
		RLPRIFCSC	639–647	Kawakami et al. 1998
		(A)MLGTHTMEV	177(178)-186	Tsai et al. 1997
	HLA-A3	LIYRRRLMK	614–622	Kawakami et al. 1998
		ALLAVGATK	17–25	Castelli et al. 1998; Skipper et al. 1996b
	HLA-A3, -A11	(I)ALNFPGSQK	86(87)-95	Kawashima et al. 1998
	HLA-Cw8	SNDGPTLI	71–78	Castelli et al. 1999
	HLA(DR1), DR4, (DR3)	WNRQLYPEWTEAQRLD	44–59	Li et al. 1998
gp100 (int-4)	HLA-A24	VYFFLPDHL	170–178	Robbins et al. 1994
Melan-A/ MART-1	HLA-A2	ILTVILGVL	32–40	Castelli et al. 1999
		(E)AAGIGILTV	(26)27–35	Kawakami et al. 1994
		GIGILTVL	29–36	Romero et al. 1997
		GILTVILGV	31–38	
	HLA-B45.1	AEEAAGIGIL(T)	24–33(34)	Schneider et al. 1998

Table 13.1 (continued)

Target antigen	HLA molecule	Peptides sequence	Amino acids	Reference
707-AP	HLA-A2	RVAALARDAP		Takahashi et al. 1997a
N-Acetyl-Gn-Trans-ferase V	HLA-A2	VLPDVFIRC	38–46 (intron sequence)	Guilloux et al. 1996
p15	HLA-A24	AYGLDFYIL		Robbins et al. 1995
Catenin	HLA-A24	SYLDSGIH_F_	29–37	Robbins et al. 1996
SR-2	HLA-A3	KIFSEVT_L_K		
MUM-1	HLA-B44	EEKL_I_VVLF	782–808	Coulie et al. 1995
Myosin class I	HLA-A3	_K_INKNPKYK		Zorn and Hercend 1999b
CDK4	HLA-A2.1	A_C_DPHSGHFV		Wölfel et al. 1995
TPI (treose-phosphat-Isomerase)	HLA-DR1	GELIG_I_LNAAKVPAD	23–37	Pieper et al. 1999
Fusion-protein LDLR/FUT	HLA-DR1	(PVI)WRRAPA(PGA)	315–323	Wang et al. 1999b
CDC27	HLA-DR4	FSWAMDLDPKGA	760–771	Wang et al. 1999a

[a] Modified from Sun et al. (1999b) J Mol Med 77:593–608

In order to fight the melanoma lesions, there are several different approaches currently being explored utilizing the host's immune system. These include 1) augmentation of the immunogenicity of tumor cells by genetic modification with cytokine genes, also known as "gene therapy", and 2) the use of T cell-defined melanoma-associated peptides, either directly for immunization (peptide vaccines) or after loading onto professional antigen-presenting cells such as dendritic cells (dendritic cell-based vaccines).

Cytokine Gene-Modified Tumor Cell Vaccines

Cytokine Gene Transfer – The Rationale and Preclinical Results

In the past decades, the identification and cloning of cytokines provided an important set of tools for the manipulation of immunologic responses. For example, systemic infusions of IL-2 alone or in conjunction with autologous lymphokine-activated killer (LAK) cells into patients with advanced metastatic melanoma were shown to achieve comparable clinical responses as conventional therapies. However, this treatment regimen is sometimes associated with severe side effects (organ dysfunction or even death) related to high-dose cytokine administration (Rosenberg et al. 1985 and 1998). Given that most cytokines act locally whose accumulation in the serum is prevented by virtue of their short half-life, it was suggested that local and paracrine delivery of immunostimulatory cytokines produced and secreted by tumor cells may have a more pronounced therapeutic benefit while avoiding systemic toxicity. This mode of cytokine delivery can be achieved by introduction of cytokine genes into tumor cells.

Starting with the pioneering work of Tepper and co-workers (1989) who showed that J558L plasmocytoma cells were rejected after transfection with the gene coding for IL-4, a large number of immunostimulatory cytokines have been tested in such a mode (reviewed in Vieweg and Gilboa 1995, Schadendorf 1997, Sun et al. 1999a and b). In most cases, the transduction of tumor cells with cytokine genes led to the rejection of the genetically modified cells by syngeneic hosts suggesting enhanced immunogenicity of transduced cells. Of considerable more interest is the fact that tumor cells transduced to express cytokines such as IL-2, IL-4, IL-7, IL-12, IFN-γ, TNF-α, or GM-CSF were capable of inducing a systemic anti-tumor immune memory. Animals vaccinated with cytokine gene-transduced cells rejected a subsequent challenge of non-transduced (wild type) tumor cells at a distant site and, in some cases, eliminated a preexisting tumor. Because several studies have used poorly- or non-immunogenic tumor models, the induced protective anti-tumor immunity could thus be solely attributed to the transduction with a cytokine. Examinations of the cellular mechanisms underlying the protective anti-tumor immunity revealed the uniform dependence on T cells, mostly the subset of CD8$^+$ T cells and in part of the CD4$^+$ T subset (Vieweg and Gilboa 1995, Schadendorf 1997, Sun et al. 1999b). Probably, CD8$^+$ and CD4$^+$ T lymphocytes were directly activated by transfected tumor cells, or more likely indirectly via professional APCs such as DCs that pick up tumor antigens (tumor-cell debris), process and finally present them to both class I-restricted CD8$^+$ T cells and class II-restricted CD4$^+$ T cells (Pardoll and Beckerleg 1995).

In summary, animal studies have clearly demonstrated that genetic modification of tumor cells with cytokine genes can generate potent systemic anti-tumor immunity. However, no conclusive indication was provided as to which cytokine is the best in terms of increasing tumor immunogenicity in a given tumor model. Nevertheless, these preclinical studies have revealed the regulatory mechanistic and functional principles for cytokine gene-modified tumor vaccines.

Cytokine Gene-Modified Tumor Cell Vaccines – Clinical Phase I/II Trials

The successful insertion of cytokine genes into human tumor cell lines and primary tumor explants has made cancer gene therapy enter the clinic. Since the first therapeutic experiments in 1990, more than 250 additional clinical gene therapy trials were approved and more than 2000 patients treated worldwide by the end of 1996 (Marcel and Grausz 1997, Hengge and Schadendorf 2000). Almost 25% of these studies had no therapeutic intent and were gene marking trials. The majority (60%) of the trials aimed to treat cancer and the great majority of investigators used immunization strategies with cytokine-gene modified tumor cells. Melanoma is supposedly one of the most immunogenic human solid tumors and was therefore chosen as a favorable target for gene-modified cancer vaccines (summarized in Schadendorf 1997). In view of the ethical responsibility, phase I clinical trials with gene-modified tumor cell vaccines should only be performed in patients who failed all current therapies. Thus, the major goal of these studies is to assess the safety of this innovative approach, to determine the toxicity caused by locally secreted cytokines, and to evaluate the immunological functions induced by these approaches.

Results of IL-7- or IL-12-Secreting Tumor Cell Vaccines in Melanoma Treatment

We have initiated two clinical phase I studies aiming at the induction of T cell-mediated anti-tumor immune responses by immunizing advanced melanoma patients (Schadendorf et al. 1995, Schadendorf et al. 1996, Möller et al. 1998, Sun et al. 1998). Autologous melanoma cell lines established from metastases were transfected either with both chains of the IL-12 gene (Sun et al. 1998) or with the IL-7-gene (Möller et al. 1998). The transduced autologous tumor cells were subjected to irradiation prior to subcutaneous injection into patients at weeks 1, 2, 3 and 6 at a dose of 5×10^6 to 3×10^7 per patient. In parallel, delayed-type hypersensitivity (DTH)-reactivity and an extensive immunological monitoring including flow cytometry, natural killer (NK)- and LAK-activity as well as cytotoxic lymphocytes (CTL) analysis were performed. The cytokine gene transfer protocol uses a newly developed gene transfer technology that combines ballistic transfer of biological molecules and magnetic cell sorting.

Evaluation of the first 10 patients immunized with autologous IL-7 gene-modified melanoma cells demonstrated the safety, the lack of toxicity and the feasibility of such an approach; however, no major clinical responses were achieved (Möller et al. 1998). 4 patients showed stable disease (SD) and 2 had a mixed response. Eight of 10 patients completed the initial three subcutaneous vaccinations and were eligible for immunological evaluation: four showing an increased NK response and seven showing an increased LAK response upon vaccination. In 3/7 patients, the frequency of tumor-reactive CTL precursors in peripheral blood increased between 2.6- to 28-fold after the third vaccination. Interestingly, all three patients with increased CTL responses were also clinical responders: two with a mixed response and one with a SD, implying a role of $CD8^+$ CTL in controlling tumor growth. The magnitude of the T-cell reactivity induced by the vaccine was found to be highly associated with the patient's Karnofsky score and recall antigen skin reactivity before vaccination. This suggests that patients with minimal tumor load or minimal residual disease may preferentially benefit from such a tumor vaccine.

In a subsequent phase I study, 6 advanced melanoma patients were immunized with IL-12 gene-modified, irradiated, autologous tumor cells (Sun et al. 1998).

Clinically, there was no major toxicity except for mild fever and flu-like symptoms in some patients. All patients completed more than 4 vaccinations and were eligible for evaluation at week 5. No major clinical responses were achieved. 3 patients showed SDs, two of which were alive for more than 10 months. One showed a minor clinical response (MR) with the regression of some cutaneous metastases during the first three months. Post-vaccination two patients developed a DTH reactivity against autologous melanoma cells, one showing a heavy infiltrate of $CD4^+$ and $CD8^+$ T-lymphocytes in regressing metastases. Analysis of the frequency of tumor-reactive CTL precursor in peripheral blood revealed a significant increase (up to 15-fold) in 2 patients after immunization.

Results of GM-CSF- or IFN-γ-Secreting Tumor Cell Vaccines in Melanoma Therapy

Soiffer et al. (1998) have investigated the biologic activity of GM-CSF gene-modified melanoma vaccines in 29 patients with stage IV melanoma. Three successive patient cohorts were immunized intradermally and subcutaneously with 10^7 irradiated tumor cells (each treatment) administered at 28-, 14-, or 7-day intervals for a total of 3, 6, or 12 vaccinations, respectively. One partial response (PR), one mixed response, and 3 MRs were observed. Substantial erythema and induration were induced at the vaccination sites in all patients and Grade 1 fatigue and nasal congestion were occasionally noted; however, no systemic toxicities were recorded. In all patients, an initially negative DTH reaction to irradiated, non-transfected, autologous tumor cells was converted to a strong response after several vaccinations. This conversion could be interpreted as an augmented antitumor cellular immunity against the original tumor. In addition, this immunization scheme also generated enhanced anti-tumor humoral immune responses, as demonstrated by an increased anti-melanoma antibody response (IgG-type) in 7 patients examined. Immunohistological analysis revealed that distant metastases from 11 of 16 patients were largely infiltrated by both T cells ($CD4^+$ and $CD8^+$) and plasma cells after, but not before vaccination, even though these anti-tumor immune responses failed to induce clinical tumor regressions in most cases.

In another phase I clinical trial, Abdel-Wahab et al. (1997) treated 20 stage III-IV melanoma patients with IFN-γ gene-modified irradiated autologous tumor vaccines, in escalating doses once every 2 weeks for a total of 6 injections (i.e. 2 vaccinations with 2×10^6, 6×10^6, and 18×10^6 each). 2 patients showed a complete response and 2 additional patients experienced transient shrinking of subcutaneous nodular disease. No side effects were noted. In this trial, the humoral immune responses of immunized patients were intensively investigated: 8 of 13 evaluable patients showed an increasing anti-melanoma IgG titer during the course of immunization. IgG titers increased with the number of vaccinations and were detected for up to 4 weeks following the last vaccination. The observation that the increased IgG response was dominated by IgG_2 versus IgG_1 isotypes in all 8 responders suggested that T helper type 1 (Th_1) cells were activated in these patients. Most recently, allogenic melanoma cells transduced with the interleukin-4 gene have been clinically evaluated with some success (Arienti et al. 1999).

Results of IL-2 Gene-Transfected Cell-Based Vaccines in the Treatment of Melanoma

Because direct transduction of autologous tumors is highly individualized, expensive and labor intensive, simpler approaches that maintain the immunological activity of paracrine cytokine stimulation are currently also under clinical investigation. These include 1) standardized gene-transduced allogeneic tumor cell lines as vaccines and 2) tumor cells admixed with transduced bystander cells (e.g. fibroblasts). The former approach is based on the idea that some tumor rejection antigens are shared rather than unique, whereas the latter strategy takes advantage of the fact that the cytokine does not need to be produced by the tumor itself, thereby obviating the need for transduction of each patient's tumor cells.

Arienti et al. (1996) and Belli et al. (1997) have used an HLA-A2-matched, Melan-A/Mart-1$^+$, gp100$^+$, tyrosinase$^+$, allogeneic melanoma cell line engineered to secrete IL-2, to immunize 12 stage IV melanoma patients four times at a dose of 5 or 15×10^7 cells. Both local and systemic toxicities were mild. 3 out of 8 evaluable patients showed mixed clinical responses. Two patients showed an increased reactivity of specific CTLs directed against tyrosinase and gp100 melanoma-associated antigens following vaccination. In an additional two patients, the frequency of melanoma-specific CTL precursors in peripheral blood was increased after vaccination. Veelken et al. (1997) applied a vaccine containing IL-2-secreting allogeneic fibroblasts and autologous tumor cells to 15 patients with advanced malignancies including 6 melanoma patients. No major clinical response was observed, nor major side effects attributable to the vaccine. In 2 melanoma patients, a dense infiltrate of both CD4$^+$ and CD8$^+$ T cells at vaccination sites was demonstrated. Analysis of the variability of the TCR in infiltrating lymphocytes from the vaccination or tumor sites of one patient revealed the identical V-D-J junctional sequence of CTL indicating that the same CTL clone had infiltrated the tumor, was circulating in peripheral blood, and was present at the vaccination site (Mackensen et al. 1997).

Limitations and Remaining Questions

The above studies demonstrated the feasibility, apparent safety and low toxicity of cytokine gene-modified tumor cell vaccines and suggested the potential of this approach to boost host anti-tumor immunity even in far-advanced melanoma patients. However, it must be realized that ex vivo genetic modification for vaccination is still at the beginning of its development, and it is still far away from providing a *curative* T-cell response. A number of questions remain open which have only partly been addressed in animal studies:

1. The immunogenicity of gene-modified tumor cell preparations used for vaccinations might be crucially affected by irradiation or mitomycin treatment, since animal studies by Hock and co-workers (1993) suggested a dramatic decrease in protection after tumor cell inactivation.

2. The dose of gene-modified cells necessary for vaccinations is presently unclear.
3. The level of cytokines produced by genetically altered tumor cells needed to effectively stimulate the immune system is not known. The first animal studies addressing this question suggest that different cytokines have different optimal concentrations which further differ in the animal tumor model tested. Furthermore, in certain instances, a bell-shaped response curve has been observed with a dramatic decrease in vaccination efficacy after passing a certain cytokine level (Schmidt et al. 1995).
4. The mechanisms involved in tumor suppression are not well understood possibly interfering with the vaccination effects at distant sites of the metastatic disease or in mounting an immune response including the immunological memory.
5. The optimal immunization schedule and route have not been systematically explored.
6. The mechanism of action of gene-modified tumor cells in causing tumor immunity and tumor regression is still under discussion.
7. Furthermore, the evaluation of immunological endpoints (analysis of precursor frequency, CTL, DTH etc.) is difficult to compare, since methodology, reliability and reproducibility to evaluate such parameters are still under debate.

Defined Antigen Vaccines

A number of antigens present on melanoma cells that could potentially serve as targets for the host T-cell responses has recently been identified (Boon et al. 1997, Rosenberg 1999). Although all of these antigens may not be present on every tumor cell, it becomes more likely that at least one relevant antigenic target can be identified for every patient's melanoma as the number of defined tumor antigens increases. Based on their expression pattern, these T cell-defined melanoma antigens can be categorized into three broad groups: 1) tissue-specific differentiation antigens expressed only in normal melanocytic cells and melanomas, such as tyrosinase, Melan-A/MART-1, gp100, TRP1 and TRP2; 2) tumor-specific shared antigens expressed in various types of human cancers but not in normal tissues except testis, as exemplified by MAGE, BAGE and GAGE gene family; and 3) tumor-specific unique antigens produced by point mutations in genes that are ubiquitously expressed including β-catenin, MUM-1 and CDK4. A summary of presently known T cell-recognized melanoma-associated peptides and their MHC restriction elements is listed in Table 13.1. Since the first two classes of antigens are both expressed in the majority of melanoma, strategies using their antigenic peptides are currently being evaluated.

In a phase I clinical trial, Rosenberg and co-workers (1998) immunized HLA-A2$^+$ patients with stage IV metastatic melanoma using a modified peptide (g209-2M) derived from the gp100 melanoma differentiation antigen. Immunological assays of peripheral blood mononuclear cells from patients after treatment showed that 91% of the patients were successfully immunized with this synthetic peptide. In another cohort of patients who received the peptide vaccine plus adjuvant IL-2, 13 of 31 patients (42%) had an objective tumor regression (Rosenberg et al. 1998). Similarly, Marchand et al. (1999) in another clinical trial examined the therapeutic MAGE-3 peptide in HLA-A1$^+$ patients with metastatic melanoma. Of 25 immunized patients eligible for evaluation, 7 showed objective clinical responses, although in this study the effectors mediating tumor regression have yet to be identified. Taken together, these results suggest that peptide immunization may represent a potentially effective tool for the treatment of melanoma.

Dendritic Cell-based Vaccines

Dendritic cells (DC) are commonly viewed as important professional APCs. They capture antigens, migrate to appropriate lymphoid organs and initiate an antigen-specific CD4- and CD8-T cell response. The growing knowledge of DC physiology and the capability to culture, maintain and expand DC from different human sources including hematopoietic progenitors in bone marrow and peripheral blood combined with the detection of an increasing number of tumor-associated antigens and T cell-recognized peptide epitopes have generated enthusiasm in the field of tumor immunotherapy and various clinical applications in phase I/II studies of different malignancies.

DC and the Control of Immunity

Basic immunology demonstrates the pivotal role of DC in generating an immune response. DC are specialized for the induction of a primary T cell response (Banchereau and Steinman 1998, Bell et al. 1999). DC derived from various sources such as bone marrow or peripheral blood are responsible for initiating T-cell responses in vivo, including CD4 and CD8 responses by their unique capability to present antigens to naive T-cells (reviewed in Banchereau and Steinman 1998, Bell et al. 1999). Differentiation of monocytes into DC was shown to be accelerated by contact to endothelium and phagocytosis (Randolph et al. 1998).

Since DC can now easily be generated from different sources including peripheral blood (Romani et al. 1994, Sallusto and Lanzavecchia 1994), these cells can either be used after pulsing with peptides or after transfection with a tumor antigen for vaccination of cancer patients (Alijagic et al. 1995, Mayordomo et al. 1995 and 1996, Celuzzi et al. 1996, Paglia et al. 1996, Porgador et al. 1996). The implication for vaccine design is that DC would be more potent than tumor cells as immunogens. Alternative approaches to stimulate the immune system such as immunization with naked DNA depend on DC (Pardoll and Beckerleg 1995, Casares et al. 1997).

CTL and NK cells, are both essential effectors of anti-tumor immunity. DC were shown not only to prime antigen-specific T-cells but also to trigger innate, NK cell-mediated anti-tumor immunity via cell-to-cell contact by DC and resting NK cells (Fernandez et al. 1999). Furthermore, the functional state of DC is critical for the outcome of the immune response. It was not known whether subsets of DC provide different cytokine microenviroments that determine the differentiation of either Th_1- or Th_2-cells. Recently, Rissoan et al. (1999) demonstrated that monocyte-derived DC induce Th_1-differentiation. In addition, the critical role of CD40/CD40L interaction for DC maturation and IL-12 production was pointed out and shown to be crucial for the generation of protective antitumor immunity (Mackey et al. 1998).

DC as Therapeutic Vehicles

Mouse studies have demonstrated the potent capacity of DC to induce anti-tumor immunity (Flamand et al. 1994, Mayordomo et al. 1995 and 1996, Celuzzi et al. 1996, Paglia et al. 1996, Porgador et al. 1996). In a mouse tumor model, systemic administration of IL-2 enhanced the therapeutic efficacy of DC-based tumor vaccines inducing tumor regressions in s.c. tumors and pulmonary micro- and macrometastases (Shimizu et al. 1999). The potency of the DC-based immunization was further documented by the fact that it was capable to break immunodominance against minor histocompatibility and synthetic peptide antigens (Grufman et al. 1999). However, it was pointed out that depending on the nature of the antigen (peptides, RNA or DNA) the optimal sequence of antigen loading is crucial (Morse et al. 1999a).

In the human system, autologous DC were used in vitro to generate CTLs against various targets including p53 and CEA by peptide loading (Alters et al. 1998, Chikamatsu et al. 1999). Besides pulsing DC with known peptides or with unfractionated peptides eluted by mild acid treatment (Storkus et al. 1993) from 10^9 or more tumor cells, tumor lysates prepared from autologous tumor samples were used for DC loading especially in clinical situations where no tumor-associated antigens could be identified. Pulsing of DC with tumor lysates led to an augmented T-cell-restricted, HLA-dependent tumor lysis in various tumor systems in vitro (Abdel-Wahab et al. 1998, Mulders et al. 1999). Recently, it was shown that the physical interaction between DC and tumor cells results in antigen transfer that is sufficient to induce a protective and therapeutic tumor rejection in mice (Celuzzi and Falo 1998). A report by Nair and co-workers (1998) suggests that CTL activity generated after peptide pulsing of DC is comparable to the activity after RNA-loading of DC, opening a new avenue of treatment options.

Of great clinical implications were recent scintigraphic assays demonstrating that intradermally administered immature monocyte-derived DCs had an excellent in vivo migratory capacity. Technetium-labeled, peptide-loaded DC traveled to the draining lymph node within 10 min (Thomas et al. 1999). Similar results were obtained by Morse et al. (1999a) who used indium-111-labeled DC to compare i.v., s.c. and intradermal administration. Whereas after i.v. injection of DC, the cells localized to the lungs and then redistributed to the liver, spleen and bone marrow, no DC were found in lymph nodes or tumors. These results are in agreement with data published by Sozzani et al. (1998) demonstrating that chemokine receptors such as CCR7 might be necessary for extravasation from blood vessels into the tissue and lymph nodes.

Clinical Applications of DC

Results of Vaccination with DC for Melanoma Treatment

In a clinical pilot study, DC were generated in the presence of GM-CSF and IL-4 and were pulsed with tumor lysate or a cocktail of peptides known to be recognized by CTLs depending on the patient's HLA haplotype (Nestle et al. 1998). Almost 50 patients with advanced melanoma have been immunized on an outpatient basis until today. Multiple peptides (MAGE-1 and MAGE-3 for HLA-A1, gp100, tyrosinase and Melan-A-derived peptides for HLA-A2, MAGE-3 and tyrosinase for HLA-B44) were used. Due to the lack of defined tumor helper antigens, we added keyhole limpet haemocyanin (KLH) to all vaccine preparations as adjuvant to induce potent KLH-specific memory T cell responses. KLH also has the advantage to be a neo-antigen and can therefore serve as an immunological tracer molecule. In 11 patients, tumor lysates were used instead of peptides as the source of tumor antigen. Thirty-two patients were eligible for evaluation. Vaccination was well tolerated in all patients. Occasionally, mild fever or swelling of the injected lymph node occurred lasting for one or two days. No physical signs of autoimmune disease were observed in any of the patients. However, in 6 patients anti-TSH receptor antibodies became detectable after initiation of DC vaccination. In 5 patients anti-nuclear antibodies were observed after treatment. In 2 patients, vitiligo was induced, and in another patient an individual melanocytic nevus regressed and lost pigmentation under vaccination. Therefore, we conclude that DC pulsed with antigen can be repeatedly injected into patients without significant toxicity.

We used DTH reactions as a convenient method to detect antigen-specific immunity. Vaccination of patients with DC pulsed with a globular protein antigen (KLH), with peptides binding to the HLA-molecules, or with autologous tumor lysates, respectively, induced significant DTH skin reactions. Significant DTH-reactivity (>10 mm in diameter) against DC pulsed with KLH was observed in 90% of patients. Furthermore, a positive DTH-reaction to peptide-pulsed DC was elicited in two of three patients. DTH-reactivity to peptides alone was only seen in 6 of 21 patients.

Stabilization of disease over 3 months was considered beneficial and was observed in nearly half of the patients. Regression of any metastases was achieved in a total of 8 patients experiencing a major clinical response (3CR, 5PR). Partial responders had a mean response duration of more than 7.3 months. Most interestingly, the three complete responders are still disease-free for up to 38 months until now. Tumor regressions were noted primarily in skin, lungs and soft tissue and in one case simultaneously in lymph node and pancreas. Responders were treated in 6/21 cases with peptides and in 5/11 with lysates suggesting that both techniques can be effective. However, patients expressing HLA-A2 had a much better chance of response than patients carrying the HLA-A1 allel. The number of patients treated with an HLA-B44 phenotype was too small but 2 patients clinically responded to vaccination.

In conclusion, these data indicate that vaccination of advanced melanoma patients with peptide-pulsed as well as tumor lysate-pulsed DC is well tolerated and is able to induce anti-tumor immunity in vivo which is associated with measurable DTH-reactivity and clinical responses. Major clinical responses were seen in about one quarter of patients. Analysis of non-responders revealed several immune escape mechanisms including loss of individual HLA-alleles, loss of tumor antigens and molecules involved in protein transport. Further studies are necessary to demonstrate the clinical effectiveness and impact on the survival of melanoma patients. A prospective randomized clinical trial to compare a standard chemotherapy to vaccination with peptide-pulsed dendritic cells is currently underway.

Further Clinical Studies Addressing Lymphoma and Other Solid Tumors

In an early study, 4 patients with follicular lymphoma were treated with immature DC pulsed with idiotypic proteins (Hsu et al. 1996). However, no further data were reported so far. In a similar approach, idiotypic proteins from multiple myeloma were pulsed onto monocyte-derived, autologous DC in one patient. The induction of an idiotype-specific immune response was documented by the generation of tumor-specific T-cells associated with a transient fall of serum idiotype protein levels (Wen et al. 1998).

Murphy and co-workers (1996) have treated patients with advanced prostate cancer using autologous dendritic cells pulsed with HLA-A2-specific peptides derived from prostate-specific antigen (PSA) with some success. DC pulsed with autologous tumor lysates derived from metastatic renal cell cancer were shown to increase expansion of TIL and to augment T-cell-restricted tumor lysis (Mulders et al. 1999). A first clinical pilot study reported one fourth responding patients (Höltl et al. 1998).

Immunization with tumor cell lysates loaded onto immature autologous APC-based vaccines was done in 17 patients with advanced melanoma. No major clinical responses were observed, but stabilization was seen in 13 patients for more than 30 months. In 5 of 9 patients, TILs were shown to be predominantly CD8+ (Chakraborty et al. 1998). In a pilot study, 9 healthy donors were injected s.c. with mature autologous monocyte-derived DC loaded with KLH, influenza matrix peptide or tetanus toxoid demonstrating priming of CD4$^+$ T cells to KLH (9/9), boosting of tetanus toxoid immunity (5/6), and a several fold increase of influenza matrix peptide T-cell reactivity after a single injection of mature DC (Dhodapkar et al. 1999). More recently, mature antigen-pulsed DCs (cell lysate) were shown to elicit strong cellular and humoral immune responses in patients with metastatic renal cell cancers in a phase I study involving 12 patients (Höltl et al. 1997).

Interestingly, in the only published trial, in which DC were infused i.v., no clinical benefit was detected. In that phase I protocol, patients with advanced CEA-positive malignancies were treated with carcinoembryonic antigen peptide (CAP-1)-loaded onto DC in escalating cell infusions (up to 1×10^8 cells/dose) without major responses (Morse et al. 1999 a).

Whether the route of administration is critical is currently not clear. However, subcutaneous injections were shown to induce antigen-specific T cell responses in several studies.

Bacterial Delivery of Tumor Antigens

Various bacteria have recently been exploited as a vector system for targeting antigens to the immune system. In past years bacteria were shown to be particularly effective as a tumor antigen vector in animal models. Of particular interest are bacteria that infect APCs and have the capacity to present their antigens in a MHC class I-dependent fashion. Especially, bacteria that infect mucosal epithelia such as *Listeria monocytogenes*, *Shigella flexneri* or *Salmonella typhimurium* have attracted major attention. For all these strains invasive, nonreplicating, attenuated and recombinant variants apart from wild type strains are available which are suitable vectors for antigen delivery. Several advantages are associated with the use of bacteria as a vaccine vehicle including low costs, well-known infectivity and defined risk profile of the wild type strains, sensitivity to antibiotics which allows the control of infection in the patient as well as in the environment. Furthermore, a part of the bacterial DNA, CpG, is an excellent adjuvant and danger signal mediating preferentially Th_1-responses (Wagner 1999).

Listeria monocytogenes

L. monocytogenes is an intracelluar pathogen capable of infecting humans and a variety of animal species via the oral route. Extensive in vitro studies have characterized the infection cycle and various virulence factors responsible for penetration of the host cell, and the escape from the phagosomes into the cytoplasm, where it replicates and polymerizes actin to migrate intracellularly and uses several enzymes including listeriolysin to spread from cell to cell (reviewed in Harty et al. 1996). Selective genetic manipulation of the bacterial genome such as the deletion of virulence factors has created a number of attenuated, recombinant variants with several different characteristics. Wild type *L. monocytogenes* manipulated to express some model antigens was shown to protect mice from a lethal tumor cell challenge and to cause tumor regression of established tumors (Paterson and Ikonomidis 1996, Pan et al. 1995 and 1999). In a separate study it was demonstrated that eukaryotic expression vectors can be delivered to macrophages using self-destructing *L. monocytogenes* (Dietrich et al. 1998). Recently, a first report using a defined attenuated *L. monocytogenes* mutant was effective to trigger a long-lasting immune response against a mouse fibrosarcoma (Paglia et al. 1997). Currently, such mutants have been manipulated in our laboratory to express various melanoma-associated antigens in order to be tested for the potential to induce a protective immune response against melanoma.

L. monocytogenes is a promising candidate vaccine vector that possesses the unique ability to target APC in vivo and to deliver antigens that can be processed in both MHC-I- and MHC-II-associated pathways. Furthermore, infection with *L. monocytogenes* always creates a strong release of cytokines such as IL-12 that biases the T-cell response towards Th$_1$ also serving as a perfect adjuvant.

Other Bacteria

Recently *Shigella flexneri* was used as a highly attenuated vector to deliver measle antigens via the intranasal route in order to demonstrate the safety and the efficacy of such a construct (Fennelly et al. 1999). In addition, an invasive but non-replicating strain of *Shigella flexneri* was shown to carry DNA plasmids encoding a model antigen to mammalian cells (Sizemore et al. 1995). Similarly to *Salmonella typhimurium,* antigens were under the control of an eukaryotic promoter (usually CMV) on a separate plasmid and were introduced into *Shigella flexneri* before therapeutic infection. This is in contrast to the above-described experiments using *Listeria* in which the antigens are under the control of prokaryotic promoters. Attenuated *Salmonella typhimurium* strains are registered as oral vaccines against typhus. In recent years, *Salmonella* was used as carrier of eukaryotic plasmids encoding viral, bacterial and other antigens. Antigens expressed by *Salmonella typhimurium* strains stimulate antigen-specific IgG, T-cell responses (CD4, CD8) and mucosal antibody responses (Hormaeche 1991). Recently, *Salmonella typhimurium (SL7207)* was shown to induce protective immunity against a murine fibrosarcoma upon oral vaccination expressing β-gal as a model antigen (Paglia et al. 1998). Vaccine production using bacteria as carriers seems so much easier than conventional approaches. However, several problems need to solved before an infection with gene-modified, attenuated bacteria can be used for the treatment of or protection from melanoma.

Conclusions and Perspectives

Tumor immunology has made great progress in recent years. Several animal studies have indicated that genetic modifications of tumor cells to express cytokines can enhance tumor immunogenicity. A long-lived, systemic anti-tumor immunity can be generated in vivo by immunizations of animals with genetically modified tumor cells secreting either IL-2, IL-4, IL-7, IL-12, IFN-γ, or GM-CSF.

Based on these successful animal studies, a number of phase I clinical trials using cytokine-secreting tumor cell vaccines were initiated in recent years, predominantly in human melanoma. Some of them have been completed. At present, it seems justified to conclude that strategies involving cytokine-secreting tumor vaccines can influence the immunological tumor-host relationship; however, in most cases, the response seems not strong enough to completely eradicate the tumor in highly pretreated and far-advanced patients. It must be realized that the application of gene therapy to the treatment of malignancies is still in the earliest stage of its development. The careful optimization of the most promising strategies, thoughtful selection of patient populations, and proper clinical trial design will accelerate the identification of reproducible clinical benefit from this strategy.

Besides the genetically modified tumor cell vaccines, other innovative approaches to melanoma vaccines are also being tested clinically, including peptide vaccines and dendritic cell vaccines. Recent animal studies have indicated that a potent protective immune response can be generated in vivo by using DC loaded with peptides or tumor lysates which was shown to mediate tumor rejection and long-lived anti-tumor immunity (Flamand et al. 1994, Mayordomo et al. 1995 and 1996, Celuzzi et al. 1996, Paglia et al. 1996, Porgador et al. 1996). Based on these successful animal studies, pilot studies have shown encouraging results, even though the number of treated patients in each clinical trial was small.

It is clear that the definition of tumor-associated antigens – starting a decade ago – has elicited a plethora of novel therapeutic options including peptide vaccination, the use of APC or the utilization of recombinant viruses and bacteria to expose the patient's immune system to tumor antigens. At present, it seems safe to conclude that vaccination with DC can influence the immunological tumor-host relationship. The role of CD4 cells and additional ways to fully activate the anti-tumor immune response including CD40 activation needs more careful attention and will be of particular interest in the near future. Clinical phase I/II studies are still in their beginning but have shown some interesting clinical results, and first phase III trials are being planned. There is still enormous room for improvement including our understanding of inducing a reliable and sufficiently strong immune response and how to maintain it. This is connected to the choice of the right adjuvant, the best dosing schedule and route as well as the boosting scheme. Although there is a lot of enthusiasm, one should keep in mind that standard therapies such as chemotherapy required decades before at least a few cancer entities could be cured.

Acknowledgements. The work was supported by the DFG and would not have been possible without the contributions of Drs. F.O. Nestle, M. Gillet, B. Wittig, P. Möller, B. Henz, and K. Jurgovsky, and without the excellent technical assistance of A. Sucker.

References

Aarnoudse CA, van den Doel PB, Heemskerk B, Schrier PI (1999) Interleukin-2-induced, melanoma-specific T cells recognize CAMEL, an unexpected translation product of LAGE-1. Int J Cancer 82:442–448

Abdel-Wahab Z, Weltz C, Hester D, Pickett N, Vervaert C, Barber JR, Jolly D, Seigler HF (1997) A phase I clinical trial of immunotherapy with interferon-gamma-gene-modified autologous melanoma cells: monitoring the humoral immune response. Cancer 80:401–412

Abdel-Wahab Z, DeMatos P, Hester D, Dong XD, Seigler HF (1998) Human dendritic cells, pulsed with either melanoma tumor cell lysates or the gp100 peptide (280–288), induce pairs of T-cell cultures with similar phenotype and lytic activity. Cell Immunol 186:63–74

Ahmann DL, Creagan ET, Hahn RG, Edmonson JH, Bisel HF, Schaid D (1989) Complete responses and long-term survivals after systemic chemotherapy for patients with advanced malignant melanoma. Cancer 63:224–227

Alijagic S, Moller P, Artuc M, Jurgovsky K, Czarnetzki BM, Schadendorf D (1995) Dendritic cells generated from peripheral blood transfected with human tyrosinase induce specific T cell activation. Eur J Immunol 25:3100–3107

Alters SE, Gadea JR, Sorich M, O'Donoghue G, Talib S, Philip R (1998) Dendritic cells pulsed with CEA peptide induce CEA-specific CTL with restricted TCR repertoire. J Immunother 1:17–26

Arienti F, Sule-Suso J, Belli F, Mascheroni L, Rivoltini L, Melani C, Maio M, Cascinelli N, Colombo MP, Parmiani G (1996) Limited antitumor T cell response in melanoma patients vaccinated with interleukin-2 gene-transduced allogeneic melanoma cells. Hum Gene Ther 7:1955–63.-7

Arienti F, Belli F, Napolitano F, Sule-Suso J, Mazzocchi A, Gallino GF, Cattelan A, Sanantonio C, Rivoltini L, Melani C, Colombo MP, Cascinelli N, Maio M, Parmiani G (1999) Vaccination of melanoma patients with interleukin 4 gene-transduced allogeneic melanoma cells. Hum Gene Ther 10:2907–2916

Banchereau J, Steinman RM (1998) Dendritic cells and the control of immunity. Nature 392:245–252

Bell D, Young JW, Banchereau J (1999) Dendritic cells. Adv Immunol 72:255–324

Belli F, Arienti F, Sule-Suso J, Clemente C, Mascheroni L, Cattelan A, Santantonio C, Gallino GF, Melani C, Rao S, Colombo MP, Maio M, Cascinelli N, Parmiani G (1997) Active immunization of metastatic melanoma patients with interleukin-2-transduced allogeneic melanoma cells: evaluation of efficacy and tolerability. Cancer Immunol Immunother 44:197–203

Bennett SR, Carbone FR, Karamalis F, Miller JF, Heath WR (1997) Induction of a CD8+ cytotoxic T lymphocyte response by cross-priming requires cognate CD4+ help. J Exp Med 186:65–70

Boel P, Wildmann C, Sensi ML, Brasseur R, Renauld JC, Coulie P, Boon T, van der Bruggen P (1995) BAGE: A new gene encoding an antigen recognized on human melanomas by cytolytic T lymphocytes. Immunity 2:167–175

Boon T, Coulie PG, Van den Eynde B (1997) Tumor antigens recognized by T cells. Immunol Today 18:267–268

Brichard VG, Herman J, Van Pel A, Wildmann C, Gaugler B, Wolfel T, Boon T, Lethe B (1996) A tyrosinase nonapeptide presented by HLA-B44 is recognized on a human melanoma by autologous cytolytic T lymphocytes. Eur J Immunol 26:224–230

Bueler H, Mulligan RC (1996) Induction of antigen-specific tumor immunity by genetic and cellular vaccines against MAGE: enhanced tumor protection by coexpression of granulocyte colony-stimulating factor and B7-1. J Mol Med 2:545–555

Casares S, Inaba K, Brumeanu TD, Steinman RM, Bona CA (1997) Antigen presentation by dendritic cells after immunization with DNA encoding a major histocompatibility complex class II-restricted viral epitope. J Exp Med 186:1481–1486

Castelli C, Storkus WJ, Maeurer MJ, Martin DM, Huang EC, Pramanik DN, Nagabhushan TL, Parmiani G, Lotze MT (1998) Immogenicity of the ALLAVGATK (gp100$^{17-25}$) peptide in HLA-A3.1 melanoma patients. Eur J Immunol 28:1143–1154

Castelli C, Tarsini P, Mazzocchi A, Rini F, Rivoltini L, Ravagnani F, Gallino F, Belli F, Parmiani G (1999) Novel HLA-Cw8-restricted T cell epitopes derived from tyrosinase-related protein-2 and gp100 melanoma antigens. J Immunol 162:1739–748

Celluzzi CM and Falo LD (1998) Physical interaction between dendritic cells and tumor cells results in an immunogen that induces protective and therapeutic tumor rejection. J Immunol 160:3081–3085

Celluzzi CM, Mayordomo JI, Storkus WJ, Lotze MT, Falo LD Jr (1996) Peptide-pulsed dendritic cells induce antigen-specific, CTL-mediated protective tumor immunity. J Exp Med 183:283–287

Chaux P, Luiten R, Demotte N, Vantomme V, Stroobant V, Traversari C, Russo V, Schultz E, Cornelis GR, Boon T, van der Bruggen P (1999a) Identification of five MAGE-A1 epitopes recognized by cytolytic T lymphocytes obtained by in vitro stimulation with dendritic cells transduced with MAGE-A1. J Immunol 163:2928–2936

Chaux P, Vantomme V, Stroobant V, Thielemans K, Corthals J, Luiten R, Eggermont AM, Boon T, van der Bruggen (1999b) Identification of MAGE-3 epitopes presented by HLA-DR molecules to CD4(+) T lymphocytes. J Exp Med 189:767–778

Chakraborty NG, Sporn JR, Tortora AF, Kurtzman SH, Yamase H, Ergin MT, Mukherji B (1998) Immunization with a tumor-cell-lysate-loaded autologous-antigen-presenting-cell-based vaccine in melanoma. Cancer Immunol Immunother 47:58–64

Chikamatsu K, Nakano K, Storkus WJ, Appella E, Lotze MT, Whiteside TL, DeLeo AB (1999) Generation of anti-p53 cytotoxic T lymphocytes from human peripheral blood using autologous dendritic cells. Clin Cancer Res 5:1281–1288

Coulie PG, Lehmann F, Lethe B, Herman J, Lurquin C, Andrawiss M, Boon T (1995) A mutated intron sequence codes for an antigenic peptide recognized by cytolytic T lymphocytes on a human melanoma. Proc Natl Acad Sci USA 92:7976–7980

Dagleish A (1996) The case for therapeutic vaccines. Melanoma Res 6:5–10

De Backer O, Arden KC, Boretti M, Vantomme V, De Smet C, Czekay S, Viars CS, De Plaen E, Brasseur F, Chomez P, Van den Eynde B, Boon T, van der Bruggen P (1999) Characterization of the GAGE genes that are expressed in various human cancers and in normal testis. Cancer Res 59:3157–3165

Dhodapkar MV, Steinman RM, Sapp M, Desai H, Fossella C, Krasovsky J, Donahoe SM, Dunbar PR, Cerundolo V, Nixon DF, Bhardwaj N (1999) Rapid generation of broad T-cell immunity in humans after a single injection of mature dendritic cells. J Clin Invest 104:173–180

Dietrich G, Bubert A, Gentschev I, Sokolovic Z, Simm A, Catic A, Kaufmann SH, Hess J, Szalay AA, Goebel W (1998) Delivery of antigen-encoding plasmid DNA into the cytosol of macrophages by attenuated suicide Listeria monocytogenes. Nat Biotechnol 16:181–185

Duffour MT, Chaux P, Lurquin C, Cornelis G, Boon T, van der Bruggen P (1999) MAGE-A4 peptide presented by HLA-A2 is recognised by cytolytic T lymphocytes. Eur J Immunol 29:3329–3337

Fennelly GJ, Khan SA, Abadi MA, Wild TF, Bloom BR (1999) Mucosal DNA vaccine immunization against measles with a highly attenuated Shigella flexneri vector. J Immunol 162:1603–1610

Fernandez NC, Lozier A, Flament C, Ricciardi-Castagnoli P, Bellet D, Suter M, Perricaudet M, Tursz T, Maraskovsky E, Zitvogel L (1999) Dendritic cells directly trigger NK cell function: cross talk relevant in innate anti-tumor immune responses in vivo. Nat Med 5:405–411

Flamand V, Sornasse T, Thielemans K, Demanet C, Bakkus M, Bazin H, Tielemans F, Leo O, Urbain J, Moser M (1994) Murine dendritic cells pulsed in vitro with tumor antigen induce tumor resistance in vivo. Eur J Immunol 24:605–610

Fujie T, Tahara K, Tanaka F, Mori M, Takesako K, Akiyoshi T (1999) A MAGE-1-encoded HLA-A24-binding synthetic peptide induces specific anti-tumor cytotoxic T lymphocytes. Int J Cancer 80:169–172

Garbe C (1993) Chemotherapy and chemoimmunotherapy in disseminated malignant melanoma. Melanoma Res 3:291–299

Gaugler B, Van den Eynde B, van der Bruggen P, Romero P, Gaforio JJ, De Plaen E, Lethe B, Brasseur F, Boon T (1994) Human gene Mage-3 codes for an antigen recognized on a melanoma by autologous cytolytic T lymphocytes. J Exp Med 179:921–930

Grufman P, Sandberg JK, Wolpert EZ, Karre K (1999) Immunization with dendritic cells breaks immunodominance in CTL responses against minor histocompatibility and synthetic peptide antigens. J Leukoc Biol 66:268–721

Guilloux Y, Lucas S, Brichard VG, Van Pel A, Viret C, De Plaen E, Brasseur F, Lethe B, Jotereau F, Boon T (1996) A peptide recognized by human cytolytic T lymphocytes on HLA-A2 melanomas is encoded by an intron sequence of the N-acetylglucosaminyltransferase V gene. J Exp Med 183:1173–1183

Harty JT, Lenz LL, Bevan MJ (1996) Primary and secondary immune responses to Listeria monocytogenes. Curr Opin Immunol 8:526–530

Hengge UR, Schadendorf D (2000) Modification of melanoma cells via ballistic gene delivery for vaccination. In: Lasic, Templeton (eds) Gene Therapy: Therapeutic mechanisms and strategies. Marcel Dekker, New York, pp165–180

Herman J, van der Bruggen P, Luescher IF, Mandruzzato S, Romero P, Thonnard J, Fleischhauer K, Boon T, Coulie PG (1996) A peptide encoded by the human MAGE3 gene and presented by HLA-B44 induces cytolytic T lymphocytes that recognize tumor cells expressing MAGE3. Immunogenetics 43:377–383

Hock H, Dorsch M, Kunzendorf U, Uberla K, Qin Z, Diamantstein T, Blankenstein T (1993) Vaccinations with tumor cells genetically engineered to produce different cytokines: effectivity not superior to a classical adjuvant. Cancer Res, 53:714–716

Höltl L, Rieser C, Papesh C, Ramoner R, Herold M, Klocker H, Radmayr C, Stenzl A, Bartsch G, Thurnher M (1997) Cellular and humoral immune responses in patients with metastatic renal cell carcinoma after vaccination with antigen-pulsed dendritic cells. J Urol 16:777–782

Höltl L, Rieser C, Papesh C, Ramoner R, Bartsch G, Thurnher M (1998) CD83+ blood dendritic cells as a vaccine for immunotherapy of metastatic renal cell cancer. Lancet 352:1358

Hormaeche CE (1991) Live attenuated Salmonella vaccines and their potential as oral combined vaccines carrying heterologous antigens. J Immunol Meth 142:113–120

Hsu FJ, Benike C, Fagnoni F, Liles TM, Czerwinski D, Taidi B, Engleman EG, Levy R (1996) Vaccination of patients with B-cell lymphoma using autologous dendritic cells. Nat Med 2:52–58

Huang LQ, Brasseur F, Serrano A, De Plaen E, van der Bruggen P, Boon T, Van Pel A (1999) Cytolytic T lymphocytes recognize an antigen encoded by MAGE-A10 on a human melanoma. J Immunol 162:6849–6854

Jäger E, Chen YT, Drijfhout JW, Karbach J, Ringhoffer M, Jager D, Arand M, Wada H, Noguchi Y, Stockert E, Old LJ, Knuth A (1998) Simultaneous humoral and cellular immune response against cancer-testis antigen NY-ESO-1: definition of human histocompatibility leukocyte antigen (HLA)-A2-binding peptide epitopes. J Exp Med 187:265–270

Johnson TM, Smith JW 2nd, Nelson BR, Chang A (1995) Current therapy for cutaneous melanoma. J Am Acad Dermatol 32:689–707

Kang X, Kawakami Y, el-Gamil M, Wang R, Sakaguchi K, Yannelli JR, Appella E, Rosenberg SA, Robbins P (1995) Identification of a tyrosinase epitope recognized by HLA-A24-restricted tumor-infiltrating lymphocytes. J Immunol 155:1343–1348

Kawakami Y, Eliyahu S, Delgado CH, Robbins PF, Sakaguchi K, Appella E, Yannelli JR, Adema GJ, Miki T, Rosenberg SA (1994) Identification of a human melanoma antigen recognized by tumor-infiltrating lymphocytes associated with in vivo tumor rejection. Proc Natl Acad Sci U S A 91:6458–6462

Kawakami Y, Robbins PF, Wang X, Tupesis JP, Parkhurst MR, Kang X, Sakaguchi K, Appella E, Rosenberg SA (1998) Identification of new melanoma epitopes on melanosomal proteins recognized by tumor infiltrating T lymphocytes restricted by HLA-A1, -A2 and -A3 alleles. J Immunol 161:6985–6992

Kawakami Y, Eliyahu S, Sakaguchi K, Robbins PF, Rivoltini L, Yannelli JR, Appella E, Rosenberg SA (1999) Identification of the immunodominant peptides of the MART-1 human melanoma antigen recognized by the majority of HLA A2-restricted tumor infiltrating lymphocytes. J Exp Med 180:347–352

Kawashima I, Tsai V, Southwood S, Takesako K, Celis E, Sette A (1998) Identification of gp100-derived, melanoma-specific cytotoxic T-lymphocyte epitopes restricted by HLA-A3 supertype molecules by primary in vitro immunization with peptide-pulsed dendritic cells. Int J Cancer 78:518–524

Kittlesen DJ, Thompson LW, Gulden PH, Skipper JC, Colella TA, Shabanowitz J, Hunt DF, Engelhard VH, Slingluff CL (1998) Human melanoma patients recognize an HLA-A1-restricted CTL epitope from tyrosinase containing two cysteine residues: implications for tumor vaccine development. J Immunol 160:2099–2106

Kobayashi H, Kokubo T, Sato K, Kimura S, Asano K, Takahashi H, Iizuka H, Miyokawa N, Katagiri M (1998) CD4+ T cells from peripheral blood of a melanoma patient recognize peptides derived from nonmutated tyrosinase. Cancer Res 58:296–301

Lethe B, Lucas S, Michaux L, De Smet C, Godelaine D, Serrano A, De Plaen E, Boon T (1998) LAGE-1, a new gene with tumor specificity. Int J Cancer 76:903–908

Li K, Adibzadeh M, Halder T, Kalbacher H, Heinzel S, Muller C, Zeuthen J, Pawelec G (1998) Tumour-specific MHC-class-II-restricted responses after in vitro sensitization to synthetic peptides corresponding to gp 100 and annexin II eluted from melanoma cells. Cancer Immunol Immunother 47:32–38

Lupetti R, Pisarra P, Verrecchia A, Farina C, Nicolini G, Anichini A, Bordignon C, Sensi M, Parmiani G, Traversari C (1998) Translation of a retained intron in tyrosinase-related protein (TRP) 2 mRNA generates a new cytotoxic T lymphocyte (CTL)-defined and shared human melanoma antigen not expressed in normal cells of the melanocytic lineage. J Exp Med 188:1005–1016

Mackensen A, Carcelain G, Viel S, Raynal MC, Michalaki H, Triebel F, Bosq J, Hercend T (1994) Direct evidence to support the immunosurveillance concept in a human regressive melanoma. J Clin Invest 93:1391–1402

Mackensen A, Veelken H, Lahn M, Wittnebel S, Becker D, Kohler G, Kulmburg P, Brennscheidt U, Rosenthal F, Franke B, Mertelsmann R, Lindemann A (1997) Induction of tumor-specific cytotoxic T lymphocytes by immunization with autologous tumor cells and interleukin-2 gene transfected fibroblasts. J Mol Med 75:290–296

Mackey MF, Gunn JR, Maliszewsky C, Kikutani H, Noelle RJ, Barth RJ Jr (1998) Dendritic cells require maturation via CD40 to generate protective antitumor immunity. J Immunol 161:2094–2098

Manici S, Sturniolo T, Imro MA, Hammer J, Sinigaglia F, Noppen C, Spagnoli G, Mazzi B, Bellone M, Dellabona P, Protti M (1999) Melanoma cells present a MAGE-3 epitope to CD4(+) cytotoxic T cells in association with histocompatibility leukocyte antigen DR11. J Exp Med 189:871–876

Marcel T, Grausz JD (1997) The TMC worldwide gene therapy enrollment report, end 1996. Hum Gene Ther, 8:775–800

Marchand M, van Baren N, Weynants P, Brichard V, Dreno B, Tessier MH, Rankin E, Parmiani G, Arienti F, Humblet Y, Bourlond A, Vanwijck R, Lienard D, Beauduin M, Dietrich PY, Russo V, Kerger J, Masucci G, Jager E, De Greve J, Atzpodien J, Brasseur F, Coulie PG, van der Bruggen P, Boon T (1999) Tumor regressions observed in patients with metastatic melanoma treated with an antigenic peptide encoded by gene MAGE-3 and presented by HLA-A1. Int J Cancer 80:219–230

Mayordomo JI, Zorina T, Storkus WJ, Zitvogel L, Celluzzi C, Falo LD, Melief CJ, Ildstad ST, Kast WM, Deleo AB (1995) Bone marrow-derived dendritic cells pulsed with synthetic tumor peptides elicit protective and therapeutic antitumor immunity. Nat Med 1:1297–1302

Mayordomo JI, Loftus DJ, Sakamoto H, De Cesare CM, Appasamy PM, Lotze MT, Storkus WJ, Appella E, DeLeo AB (1996) Therapy of murine tumors with p53 wild-type and mutant sequence peptide-based vaccines. J Exp Med 183:1357–1365

Möller P, Sun Y, Dorbic T, Alijagic S, Makki A, Jurgovsky K, Schroff M, Henz BM, Wittig B, Schadendorf D (1998) Vaccination with IL-7 gene-modified autologous melanoma cells can enhance the anti-melanoma lytic activity in peripheral blood of patients with a good clinical performance status: a clinical phase I study. Brit J Cancer 77:1907–1916

Morel S, Ooms A, Van Pel A, Wolfel T, Brichard VG, van der Bruggen P, Van den Eynde BJ, Degiovanni G (1995) A tyrosinase peptide presented by HLA-B35 is recognized on a human melanoma by autologous cytotoxic T lymphocytes. Int J Cancer 83:755–759

Morse MA, Coleman RE, Akabani G, Niehaus N, Coleman D, Lyerly HK (1999a) Migration of human dendritic cells after injection in patients with metastatic malignancies. Cancer Res 59:56–58

Morse MA, Deng Y, Coleman D, Hull S, Kitrell-Fisher E, Nair S, Schlom J, Ryback ME, Lyerly HK (1999b) A phase I study of active immunotherapy with carcinoembryonic antigen peptide (CAP-1)-pulsed, autologous human cultured dendritic cells in patients with metastatic malignancies expressing carcinoembryonic antigen. Clin Cancer Res 5:1331–1338

Mulders P, Tso CL, Gitlitz B, Kaboo R, Hinkel A, Frand S, Kiertscher S, Roth MD, de Kernion J, Figlin R, Belldegrun A (1999) Presentation of renal tumor antigens by human dendritic cells activates tumor-infiltrating lymphocytes against autologous tumor: implications for live kidney cancer vaccines. Clin Cancer Res 5:445–454

Murphy G, Tjoa B, Ragde H, Kenny G, Boynton A (1996) Phase I clinical trial: T-cell therapy for prostate cancer using autologous dendritic cells pulsed with HLA-A0201-specific peptides from prostate-specific membrane antigen. Prostate 29:371–380

Nair SK, Boczkowski D, Morse M, Cumming RI, Lyerly HK, Gilboa E (1998) Induction of primary carcinoembryonic antigen (CEA)-specific cytotoxic T lymphocytes in vitro using human dendritic cells transfected with RNA. Nat Biotechnol 16:364–369

Nestle FO, Alijagic S, Gilliet M, Sun Y, Grabbe S, Dummer R, Burg G, Schadendorf D (1998) Vaccination of melanoma patients with peptide or tumor lysate pulsed dendritic cells. Nat Med 4:328–332

Oettgen HF, Old LJ (1991) The history of cancer immunotherapy. In: deVita VT, Hellman S and Rosenberg, SA (eds). Biologic Therapy of Cancer, Principles and Practice. Lippincott pp 87

Oiso M, Eura M, Katsura F, Takiguchi M, Sobao Y, Masuyama K, Nakashima M, Itoh K, Ishikawa T (1999) A newly identified MAGE-3-derived epitope recognized by HLA-A24-restricted cytotoxic T lymphocytes. Int J Cancer 81:387–394

Paglia P, Chiodoni C, Rodolfo M, Colombo MP (1996) Murine dendritic cells loaded in vitro with soluble protein prime cytotoxic T lymphocytes against tumor antigen in vivo. J Exp Med 183:317–322

Paglia P, Arioli I, Frahm N, Chakraborty T, Colombo MP, Guzman CA (1997) The defined attenuated Listeria monocytogenes Dmpl2 mutant is an effective oral vaccine carrier to trigger a long-lasting immune response against a mouse fibrosarcoma. Eur J Immunol 27:1570–1575

Paglia P, Medina E, Arioli I, Guzman CA, Colombo MP (1998) Gene transfer in dendritic cells, induced by oral DNA vaccination with Salmonella typhimurium, results in protective immunity against a murine fibrosarcoma. Blood 92:3172–3176

Pan ZK, Ikonomidis G, Lazenby A, Pardoll D, Paterson Y (1995) A recombinant Listeria monocytogenes vaccine expressing a model tumour antigen protects mice against lethal tumour cell challenge and causes regression of established tumours. Nat Med 1:471–477

Pan ZK, Weiskirch LM, Paterson Y (1999) Regression of established B16F10 melanoma with a recombinant Listeria monocytogenes vaccine. Cancer Res 59:5264–5269

Pardoll DM, Beckerleg AM (1995) Exposing the immunology of naked DNA vaccines. Immunity 3:165–169

Parkhurst MR, Fitzgerald EB, Southwood S, Sette A, Rosenberg SA, Kawakami Y (1998) Identification of a shared HLA-A*0201-restricted T-cell epitope from the melanoma antigen tyrosinase-related protein 2 (TRP2) Cancer Res 58:4895–4901

Parkinson DR, Houghton AN, Hersey P, Borden EC (1992) Biologic therapy for melanoma. In: Cutaneous Melanoma. Balch CM, Houghton AN, Milton GW, Sober AJ, Soong SJ (eds), JB Lippincott, Philadelphia, p 522

Paterson Y, Ikonomidis G (1996) Recombinant Listeria monocytogenes cancer vaccine. Curr Opin Immunol 8:664–669

Pieper R, Christian RE, Gonzales MI, Nishimura MI, Gupta G, Settlage RE, Shabanowitz J, Rosenberg SA, Hunt DF, Topalian SL (1999) Biochemical identification of a mutated human melanoma antigen recognized by CD4(+) T cells. J Exp Med 189:757–766

Porgador A, Snyder D, Gilboa E (1996) Induction of antitumor immunity using bone marrow-generated dendritic cells. J Immunol 156:2918–2926

Randolph GJ, Beaulieu S, Lebecque S, Steinman RM, Muller WA (1998) Differentiation of monocytes into dendritic cells in a model of transendothelial trafficking. Science 282:480–483

Reynolds SR, Celis E, Sette A, Oratz R, Shapiro RL, Johnston D, Fotino M, Bystryn JC (1998) HLA-independent heterogeneity of CD8+ T cell responses to MAGE-3, Melan-A/MART-1, gp100, tyrosinase, MC1R, and TRP-2 in vaccine-treated melanoma patients. J Immunol 161:6970–6976

Rissoan MC, Soumelis V, Kadowaki N, Grouard G, Briere F, de Waal Malefyt R, Liu YJ (1999) Reciprocal control of T helper cell and dendritic cell differentiation. Science 283:1183–1186

Robbins PF, el-Gamil M, Kawakami Y, Stevens E, Yannelli JR, Rosenberg SA (1994) Recognition of tyrosinase by tumor-infiltrating lymphocytes from a patient responding to immunotherapy. Cancer Res 54:3124–3126

Robbins PF, el-Gamil M, Li YF, Topalian SL, Rivoltini L, Sakaguchi K, Appella E, Kawakami Y, Rosenberg SA (1995) Cloning of a new gene encoding an antigen recognized by melanoma-specific HLA-A2-restricted tumor-infiltrating lymphocytes. J Immunol 154:5944–5950

Robbins PF, El-Gamil M, Li YF, Kawakami Y, Loftus D, Appella E, Rosenberg SA (1996) A mutated β-catenin gene encodes a melanoma-specific antigen recognized by tumor infiltrating lymphocytes. J Exp Med 183:1185–1192

Romani N, Gruner S, Brang D, Kampgen E, Lenz A, Trockenbacher B, Konwalinka G, Fritsch PO, Steinman RM, Schuler G (1994) Proliferating dendritic cell progenitors in human blood. J Exp Med 180:83–93

Romero P, Gervois N, Schneider J, Escobar P, Valmori D, Pannetier C, Steinle A, Wolfel T, Lienard D, Brichard V, van Pel A, Jotereau F, Cerottini JC (1997) Cytolytic T lymphocyte recognition of the immunodominant HLA-A*0201-restricted Melan-A/MART-1 antigenic peptide in melanoma. J Immunol 159:2366–2374

Rosenberg SA (1999) A new era for cancer immunotherapy based on the genes that encode cancer antigens. Immunity 10:281–287

Rosenberg SA, Lotze MT, Muul LM, Leitman S, Chang AE, Ettinghausen SE, Matory YL, Skibber JM, Shiloni E, Vetto JT (1985) Observation on the systemic administration of autologous lymphokine-activated killer cells and recombinant interleukin-2 to patients with cancer. N Engl J Med 313:1485–1492

Rosenberg SA, Yang JC, Schwartzentruber DJ, Hwu P, Marincola FM, Topalian SL, Restifo NP, Dudley ME, Schwarz SL, Spiess PJ, Wunderlich JR, Parkhurst MR, Kawakami Y, Seipp CA, Einhorn JH, White DE (1998) Immunologic and therapeutic evaluation of a synthetic peptide vaccine for the treatment of patients with metastatic melanoma. Nat Med 4:321–327

Sallusto F and Lanzavecchia A (1994) Efficient presentation of soluble antigen by cultured human dendritic cells is maintained by granulocyte/macrophage colony-stimulating factor plus interleukin-4 and downregulated by tumor necrosis factor-alpha. J Exp Med 179:1109–1111

Schadendorf D (1997) Cytokines, autologous cell immunostimulatory and gene therapy for cancer treatment. In: Skin Immune System 2nd ed., Bos JD (ed) CRC Press Inc., Boca Raton, USA, pp 657–669

Schadendorf D, Czarnetzki BM, Wittig B (1995) Clinical Protocol – Interleukin-7-, interleukin-12-, and GM-CSF gene transfer in patients with metastatic melanoma. J Mol Med 73:473–477

Schadendorf D, Henz BM, Wittig B (1996) Interleukin 7 trials for melanoma treatment. Mol Med Today 2:143–144

Schmidt W, Schweighoffer T, Herbst E, Maass G, Berger M, Schilcher F, Schaffner G, Birnstiel ML (1995) Cancer vaccines: The interleukin 2 dosage effect. Proc Nat Acad Sci USA 92:4711–4715

Schneider J, Brichard V, Boon T, Meyer zum Buschenfelde KH, Wölfel T (1998) Overlapping peptides of melanocyte differentiation antigen melan-A/MART-1 recognized by autologous cytolytic T lymphocytes in association with HLA-B45.1 and HLA-A2.1. Int J Cancer 75:451–458

Shimizu K, Fields RC, Giedlin M, Mule JJ (1999) Systemic administration of interleukin 2 enhances the therapeutic efficacy of dendritic cell-based tumor vaccines. Proc Natl Acad Sci USA 96:2268–2273

Sizemore DR, Branstrom AA, Sadoff JC (1995) Attenuated Shigella as a DNA delivery vehicle for DNA-mediated immunization. Science 270:299–302

Skipper JC, Hendrickson RC, Gulden PH, Brichard V, Van Pel A, Chen Y, Shabanowitz J, Wolfel T, Slingluff CL Jr, Boon T, Hunt DF, Engelhard VH (1996a) An HLA-A2-restricted tyrosinase antigen on melanoma cells results from posttranslational modification and suggests a novel pathway for processing of membrane proteins. J Exp Med 183:527–534

Skipper JC, Kittlesen DJ, Hendrickson RC, Deacon DD, Harthun NL, Wagner SN, Hunt DF, Engelhard VH, Slingluff CL Jr (1996b) Shared epitopes for HLA-A3-restricted melanoma-reactive human CTL include a naturally processed epitope from Pmel-17/gp100. J Immunol 157:5027–5033

Soiffer R, Lynch T, Mihm M, Jung K, Rhuda C, Schmollinger JC, Hodi FS, Liebster L, Lam P, Mentzer S, Singer S, Tanabe KK, Cosimi AB, Duda R, Sober A, Bhan A, Daley J, Neuberg D, Parry G, Rokovich J, Richards L, Drayer J, Berns A, Clift S, Dranoff G (1998) Vaccination with irradiated autologous melanoma cells engineered to secrete human granulocyte-macrophage colony-stimulating factor generates potent antitumor immunity in patients with metastatic melanoma. Proc Natl Acad Sci USA 95:13141–13146

Sozzani S, Allavena P, D'Amico G, Luini W, Bianchi G, Kataura M, Imai T, Yoshie O, Bonecchi R, Mantovani A (1998) Differential regulation of chemokine receptors during dendritic maturation: a model for their trafficking properties. J Immunol 161:1083–1086

Storkus WJ, Zeh HJ 3d, Maeurer MJ, Salter RD, Lotze MT (1993) Identification of T-cell epitopes: rapid isolation of class I-presented peptides from viable cells by mild acid elution. J Immunother 14:94–103

Sun Y, Jurgovsky K, Moller P, Alijagic S, Dorbic T, Georgieva J, Wittig B, Schadendorf D (1998) Vaccination with IL-12-gene modified autologous melanoma cells – preclinical results and a first clinical phase I study. Gene Ther 5:481–490

Sun Y, Moller P, Berking C, Schlupen E, Volkenandt M, Schadendorf D (1999a) In vivo selective expansion of a tumour-specific cytotoxic T-cell clone derived from peripheral blood of a melanoma patient after vaccination with gene-modified autologous tumour cells. Immunology 98:535–540

Sun Y, Paschen A, Schadendorf D (1999b) Cell-based vaccination against melanoma: background, preliminary results, and perspective. J Mol Med 77:593–608

Tahara K, Takesako K, Sette A, Celis E, Kitano S, Akiyoshi T (1999) Identification of a MAGE-2-encoded human leukocyte antigen-A24-binding synthetic peptide that induces specific antitumor cytotoxic T lymphocytes. Clin Cancer Res 5:2236–2241

Takahashi T, Irie RF, Nishinaka Y, Hoon DSB (1997) 707-AP peptide recognized by human antibody induces human leukocyte antigen A2-restricted cytotoxic T lymphocyte killing of melanoma. Clin Cancer Res 3:1363–1370

Tanaka F, Fujie T, Tahara K, Mori M, Takesako K, Sette A, Celis E, Akiyoshi T (1997) Induction of antitumor cytotoxic T lymphocytes with a MAGE-3 encoded synthetic peptide presented by human leukocytes antigen-A24. Cancer Res 57:4465–4458

Tanzarella S, Russo V, Lionello I, Dalerba P, Rigatti D, Bordignon C, Traversari C (1999) Identification of a promiscuous T cell epitope encoded by multiple members of the MAGE family. Cancer Res 59:2668–2674

Tepper RI, Pattengale PK, Leder P (1989) Murine interleukin 4 displays potent anti-tumor activity in vivo. Cell 57:503–512

Thomas R, Chambers M, Boytar R, Barker K, Cavanagh LL, MacFadyen S, Smithers M, Jenkins M, Andersen J (1999) Immature human monocyte-derived dendritic cells migrate rapidly to draining lymph nodes after intradermal injection for melanoma immunotherapy. Melanoma Res 9:474–481

Topalian SL, Gonzales MI, Parkhurst M, Li YF, Southwood S, Sette A, Rosenberg SA, Robbins PF (1996) Melanoma-specific CD4+ T cells recognize nonmutated HLA-DR-restricted tyrosinase epitopes. J Immunol 183:1965–1971

Tsai V, Southwood S, Sidney J, Sakaguchi K, Kawakami Y, Appella E, Sette A, Celis E (1997) Identification of subdominant CTL epitopes of the gp100 melanoma-associated tumor antigen by primary in vitro immunization with peptide-pulsed dendritic cells. J Immunol 158:1796–1802

van der Bruggen P, Traversari C, Chomez P, Lurquin C, De Plaen E, Van den Eynde B, Knuth A, Boon T (1991) A gene encoding an antigen recognized by cytolytic T cells on a human melanoma. Science 254:1643–1647

van der Bruggen P, Bastin J, Gajewski T, Coulie PG, Boel P, De Smet C, Traversari C, Townsend A, Boon T (1994a) A peptide encoded by human gene MAGE-3 and presented by HLA-A2 induces cytolytic T lymphocytes that recognize tumor cells expressing MAGE-3. Eur J Immunol 24:3038–3043

van der Bruggen P, Szikora JP, Boel P, Wildmann C, Somville M, Sensi M, Boon T (1994b) Autologous cytolytic T lymphocytes recognize a MAGE-1 nonapeptide on melanomas expressing HLA Cw*1601. Eur J Immunol 24:2134–2140

van den Eynde B, Peeters O, De Backer O, Gaugler B, Lucas S, Boon T (1995) A new family of genes coding for an antigen recognized by autologous cytolytic T lymphocytes on a human melanoma. J Exp Med 182:689–698

Veelken H, Mackensen A, Lahn M, Kohler G, Becker D, Franke B, Brennscheidt U, Kulmburg P, Rosenthal FM, Keller H, Hasse J, Schultze-Seemann W, Farthmann EH, Mertelsmann R, Lindemann A (1997) A phase-I clinical study of autologous tumor cells plus interleukin-2-gene-transfected allogeneic fibroblasts as a vaccine in patients with cancer. Int J Cancer 70:269–277

Vieweg J and Gilboa E (1995) Considerations for the use of cytokine-secreting tumor cell preparations for cancer treatment. Cancer Invest 13:193–201

Visseren MJ, van der Burg SH, van der Voort EI, Brandt RM, Schrier PI, van der Bruggen P, Boon T, Melief CJ, Kast WM (1997) Identification of HLA-A*0201-restricted CTL epitopes encoded by the tumor-specific MAGE-2 gene product. Int J Cancer 73:125–130

Wagner H (1999) Bacterial CpG DNA activates immune cells to signal infectious danger. Adv Immunol 73:329–368

Wang RF, Appella E, Kawakami Y, Kang X, Rosenberg SA (1996a) Identification of TRP-2 as a human tumor antigen recognized by cytotoxic T lymphocytes. J Exp Med 184:2207–2216

Wang RF, Parkhurst MR, Kawakami Y, Robbins PF, Rosenberg SA (1996b) Utilization of an alternative open reading frame of a normal gene in generating a novel human cancer antigen. J Exp Med 183:1131–1140

Wang RF, Johnston SL, Southwood S, Sette A, Rosenberg SA (1998a) Recognition of an antigenic peptide derived from tyrosinase-related protein-2 by CTL in the context of HLA-A31 and -A33. J Immunol 160:890–897

Wang RF, Johnston SL, Zeng G, Topalian SL, Schwartzentruber DJ, Rosenberg SA (1998b) A breast and melanoma-shared tumor antigen: T cell responses to antigenic peptides translated from different open reading frames. J Immunol 162:3596–3605

Wang RF, Wang X, Atwood AC, Topalian SL, Rosenberg SA (1999a) Cloning genes encoding MHC class II-restricted antigens: mutated CDC27 as a tumor antigen. Science 284:1351–1354

Wang RF, Wang X, Rosenberg SA (1999b) Identification of a novel MHC class II-restricted tumor antigen resulting from a chromosomal rearrangement recognized by CD4+ T cells. J Exp Med 189:1659–1667

Wen YJ, Ling M, Bailey-Wood R, Lim SH (1998) Idiotypic protein-pulsed adherent peripheral blood monouclear cell-derived dendritic cells prime immune immune system in multiple myeloma. Clin Cancer Res 4:957–962

Wölfel T, Van Pel A, Brichard V, Schneider J, Seliger B, Meyer zum Büschenfelde KH, Boon T (1994) Two tyrosinase nonapeptides recognized on HLA-A2 melanomas by autologous cytolytic T lymphocytes. Eur J Immunol 24:759–764

Wölfel T, Hauer M, Schneider J, Serrano M, Wolfel C, Klehmann-Hieb E, De Plaen E, Hankeln T, Meyer zum Büschenfelde KH, Beach D (1995) A p16^{INK4a}-insensitive CDK4 mutant targeted by cytolytic T lymphocytes in a human melanoma. Science 269:1281–1284

Zorn E, Hercend T (1999a) A MAGE-6-encoded peptide is recognized by expanded lymphocytes infiltrating a spontaneously regressing human primary melanoma lesion. Eur J Immunol 29:602–607

Zorn E, Hercend T (1999b) A natural anti-tumor cytotoxic T cell response in a spontaneously regressing human melanoma targets a neoantigen resulting from a somatic point mutation. Eur J Immunol 29:592–601

14 Molecular Strategies
Interfering with Tumor Progression of Melanoma
and Improving Anti-Tumor Immunity

A. Schneeberger, M. Goos, G. Stingl, S. N. Wagner

Introduction

It might have been predicted that somatic cell gene therapy would be directed primarily towards diseases with a single gene deficiency or defect, but, at least at present, the majority of the trials approved worldwide address cancer. This is in part due to the fact that despite major efforts to improve the efficacy of conventional treatment regimens, cancer still remains the second leading cause of death in industrialized countries. Furthermore, recombinant DNA technology offers various promising strategies for the treatment of malignant diseases. The aim of this chapter is to discuss several of these concepts including the inhibition of oncogenes, replacing tumor suppressor genes, the suicide gene approach and the use of DNA technology to enhance tumor-specific immune responses. As melanoma is the leading cause of death from skin cancer and occurs in relatively young people (mean age at diagnosis: 50 yrs., i.e. some 10 yrs. earlier than breast or lung cancer), we focus on studies investigating the potential of genetic approaches for the treatment of this neoplasm.

Melanoma results from the malignant transformation of melanocytes or nevus cells at cutaneous or, much less frequent, mucosal and visceral sites. Its incidence is dramatically increasing. The striking upward trend has been evident for the past several decades and has been accompanied by a constantly increasing degree of recreational sun exposure (Longstreth et al. 1992). While in 1935 only 1 in 1500 Americans suffered from malignant melanoma, this ratio increased to 1 in 250 by 1980, to 1 in 135 by 1987 and, based on current trends, 1 in 75 by 2000 (Rigel et al. 1996). Death rates have also risen over much of the century, but, as a consequence of improved early diagnosis, much slower than their incidence.

Although there are exceptions, melanoma generally metastasizes in a stepwise manner. These steps consist of local recurrences, regional, and, finally, distant metastases. Accordingly, the stage of disease (the staging system reflects this progression pattern) is one of the main factors determining the prognosis of a given patient. Outcome of melanoma patients in stages I and II (localized disease with no evidence of regional or distant metastases using conventional staging methods) is best predicted by the thickness of the primary tumor (Balch 1992) with survival rates decreasing as a function of tumor thickness. Patients with their tumor reaching <0.75 mm [stage IA], 0.76–1.5 mm [stage IB], 1.51–

4.0 [stage IIA] or >4.0 mm [stage IIB] in thickness according to Breslow exhibit 10-year survival rates of 97, 90, 67 and 43%, respectively (Orfanos et al. 1994). Recent studies propose a new parameter, the status of the sentinel lymph node, as being most informative for estimating the survival of stage I/II melanoma patients (Shivers et al. 1998). The 10-year survival rate declines to 19–28% in patients presenting with regional disease (satellite- or in-transit-metastasis [IIIA] and regional lymph node metastasis [IIIB]). Patients with distant metastasis [stage IV] most frequently succumb to their disease within 6–9 months (10-year survival rate: 3%).

While surgical excision of the primary tumor is often curative in patients with stage I/II disease, the therapeutic options for successful combat of clinically detectable regional and, even more importantly, distant metastases are rather limited and very unsatisfactory. These include surgery, hyperthermic perfusion, radiation therapy, cryotherapy, and systemic chemotherapy and are used either alone or in combination (Houghton and Balch 1992). The overall response rate to chemotherapy is low (about 20–25%) and the duration of the response to chemotherapy, radiation or surgery is usually brief with a median survival of patients with metastatic disease being in the range of 7–10 months (Houghton and Balch 1992). Despite several reports on higher response rates as a consequence of combination therapy compared with single agent therapy (Legha et al. 1998), a definitive survival advantage for combination therapy has yet to be demonstrated.

These circumstances enabled the study of innovative approaches such as gene therapy to treat measurable tumors, or to prevent recurrence after surgery. The strategies that have been proposed for gene therapy of cancer can be divided into three broad categories according to whether the aims are to target the tumor itself, to protect the patient's normal cells (e.g. hematopoietic stem cells) against chemotherapeutic drugs, or to stimulate the anti-tumor immune response of a given patient.

Strategies Targeting the Tumor

The goals of strategies targeting the tumor itself are either (i) the genetic correction of the cancer cells, (ii) their destruction by genetic chemosensitization and (iii) the counteraction of the function of genes associated with tumor progression such as angiogenesis, invasion and metastasis.

Corrective Gene Therapy

The malignant phenotype of a given cell results from the accumulation of multiple genetic defects within this cell (Fearon and Vogelstein 1990, Karp and Broder 1995). These include dominantly-acting mutations of proto-oncogenes, loss of functional tumor suppressor genes, and the activation of genes coding for molecules associated with metastatic behavior (Karp and Broder 1995, Fearon and Vogelstein 1990, Crooke 1992). These insights into the molecular basis of tumorigenesis have led to two different concepts for corrective cancer gene therapy.

Interference with Oncogene Expression

One possible strategy aims at the suppression of oncogene expression. Proto-oncogenes are cellular genes that are highly conserved in evolution (examples include epidermal growth factor and thyroid hormone receptor). To date, more than 100 such genes have been identified in humans. Normal cells transiently respond to their products with a G1 to S-phase transition ultimately leading to cell division. When these genes become constitutively turned on (e.g. by a mutation or viral integration), uncontrolled growth occurs as a result of the induction and/or maintenance of cell transformation. Such activated genes are then called oncogenes. The *ras* oncogene family has been analyzed because of the high frequency of activated *ras* genes in UV-induced non-melanoma skin cancer. Whereas Albino et al. have reported that 24% of their human melanoma cell lines express activated *ras* genes, with *N-ras* being activated 10-times more often than *Ha-ras* (Albino et al. 1989), we and others found activating *N-ras* mutations at codon 61 in only 5–15% of primary melanomas (van't Veer et al. 1989, Wagner et al. 1995). However, *ras* mutations appear to be consistently present in a subset of melanomas, most probably in those of the vertical growth phase (Jafari et al. 1995). Other findings supporting a causative role of this oncogene family in the pathogenesis of melanoma include the observation that expression of activated *Ha-ras* transforms human melanocytes (Albino et al. 1992) and the demonstration that INK4a–/– mice engineered to (over)express activated *Ha-ras* under the control of the tyrosinase promoter spontaneously develop melanomas at a high frequency (Chin et al. 1997). Jansen and colleagues are evaluating the possibility of using *ras* oncogenes as therapeutic targets (Jansen et al. 1995). These investigators have chosen antisense technology to suppress the expression of several members of the *ras* family (e.g. *Ha-ras, N-ras*). Antisense oligonucleotides act by specifically hybridizing with complementary mRNA or DNA sequences. This leads to the inhibition of protein expression through a number of mechanisms including degradation of the targeted RNA through RNase H-mediated cleavage (Crooke 1992). Employing this technology, they showed that daily infusions of *Ha–ras*-specific phosphorothiorate oligonucleotides can slow down the growth of human melanoma cells (expressing this oncogene) that had been implanted into SCID mice (Jansen et al. 1995).

Using a human lung tumor xenograft mouse model, Monia and coworkers demonstrated that systemically applied phosphorothiorate antisense oligonucleotides targeting the human oncogene C–*raf*-1 kinase, but not mismatched control oligonucleotides, can significantly inhibit tumor progression (Monia et al. 1996). However, tumor inhibition was only transient and the tumors quickly resumed growth. The transient nature of the inhibition could be due to the rapid clearance of the antisense oligonucleotides. An alternative explanation would be that the interference with a single step in the signaling cascade can certainly dampen the downstream transmission of the signal, but is also likely to activate parallel pathways neutralizing the effect of the initial inhibitory signal. Therefore, these experiments would suggest that for corrective cancer gene therapy to be successful, several genetic defects of a given tumor should be targeted at the same time. Another possibility to explain the limited effect of the antisense approach would be that these oligonucleotides only bind to one transcript, making them unable to completely saturate the transcription/translation processes adequately. To overcome this limitation, catalytic antisense RNAs (ribozymes) that contain both a specific binding domain and a RNA cleaving site have been developed. Ribozymes bind RNA, cleave it and are being released to bind another molecule, thereby creating a more favorable stoichiometric balance for gene ablation (Sullivan 1994).

C-myc is another oncogene that has been implicated in the etiology of melanoma. It codes for a phosphoroprotein involved in cell proliferation and differentiation. C-myc has been found overexpressed in a fraction of primary melanomas, and while some investigators could demonstrate a correlation of c-myc overexpression and survival of the respective patients (Ross and Wilson 1998), others failed to do so (Konstadoulakis et al. 1998). Transfection studies revealed that overexpression of c-myc is able to increase the tumorigenicity and the metastatic potential of melanoma lines (Schlagbauer-Wadl et al. 1999). Moreover, Putney et al. (Putney et al. 1999) provided evidence that c-myc-specific antisense oligonucleotides exhibit significant antitumor activity in vivo. They infused SCID mice bearing human melanomas with phosphorothiorate c-myc antisense oligonucleotides either encapsulated into biodegradable microspheres or unpackaged. Both treatments diminished c-myc expression by the tumors, reduced their growth and the number of metastases. As a consequence, survival of the animals was prolonged upon delivery from sustained release formulations being therapeutically more effective than administration of free antisense molecules (Putney et al. 1999).

Inhibition of the oncogenic function can also be obtained at the transcriptional level. By applying triplex-forming oligonucleotides or DNA sequences interacting with transcriptional start sites one can inhibit oncogene transcription. This mechanism is currently evaluated clinically using the adenoviral E1A gene, that inhibits transcription of the human c-erbB-2 promoter resulting in suppressed tumorigenicity and metastatic potential of tumor cells carrying the activated oncogene c-erbB-2.

Restoration of Tumor Suppressor Gene Function

The second concept in corrective gene therapy of cancer aims at replacing defective tumor suppressor genes. These genes are components of every normal cell's genome. They control cell differentiation and proliferation. The most commonly mutated tumor suppressor gene in human cancer is p53. Under normal circumstances, its protein product functions as a transcription factor and controls the cell cycle at the G1-S checkpoint: if DNA damage occurs, p53 arrests the cell cycle to allow repair; if this cannot be accomplished, the cell will undergo apoptosis. Point mutations of *p53* are rare in melanoma (Akslen et al. 1998) and it remains to be determined whether abrogation of *p53* activity supports melanocyte transformation and/or the malignant potential of melanoma cells (Albino et al. 1994). *p53* might nonetheless represent a useful target as its overexpression resulted in apoptotic death not only of tumor cells which express mutated *p53* but also of those which contain only wild type (Yonish-Rouach et al. 1991). This concept has already been investigated in preclinical melanoma models. Cirielli et al. overexpressed wild-type *p53* in murine B16 and human SK-MEL-24 melanoma cell lines using an adenoviral vector (Cirielli et al. 1995). They found that this treatment resulted in (i) the apoptotic death of the cells and (ii) that it inhibited their growth in nude, athymic animals. Roth et al. tested the hypothesis that restoration of wild-type *p53* gene function would suppress tumor growth in vivo (Roth et al. 1996). They injected retroviral supernatants directly into the lung cancers of nine patients with documented *p53* mutations. Seven of the nine patients completed the protocol and were evaluable. No toxic effects directly attributable to the vector were noted. Three of the patients showed regression of the treated tumors, three stabilization and one progression. *p53*-induced apoptosis appears to be one of the mechanisms responsible for tumor shrinkage as apoptotic cancer cells were more frequent in post-treatment than in pre-treatment biopsies. Eventually, all of the patients succumbed to progressive disease but, with the exception of one patient, not from progression of the treated tumors (Roth et al. 1996). Currently, these investigators try to enhance the clinical efficacy of their approach by increasing the transfection rate. For this purpose, they use adenoviral instead of retroviral vectors.

About 50% of melanoma-prone families and a certain percentage of patients with sporadic melanomas exhibit genetic abnormalities at the 9p21–22 locus. This region spans several genes with tumor suppressor function including INK4a/p16 (Nobori et al. 1994), INK4a/p14ARF (Mao et al. 1995) and INK4b/p15 (Heufler et al. 1996) (Fig. 14.1). INK4a/p16, one of the best characterized genes in the pathogenesis of melanoma, codes for a cyclin-dependent kinase inhibitor. Physiologically, p16 inhibits the kinase activity of CDK4 and CDK6 which, in turn, prevents pRB phosphorylation and thereby progression from G1 to S phase (Lukas et al. 1995). Conversely, the loss of p16 function results in the inability to inhibit CDK4 and therefore in unrestrained cell cycling. Whereas we have observed homozygous co-deletion of the INK4a/p16 and the INK4b/p15 genes in a small subset of sporadic primary nonmetastatic melanoma samples, point mutations, small deletions of INK4a/p16 or repression of INK4a/p16 gene transcription were not demonstrated (Wagner et al. 1998). In view of the frequent loss of heterozygosity on chromosome 9p21 in sporadic melanomas, these results suggest the presence of (an) additional tumor suppressor gene(s) within this chromosomal region. Thus, INK4a/p16 may represent an interesting target in patients with inherited, but probably not in those with sporadic melanoma.

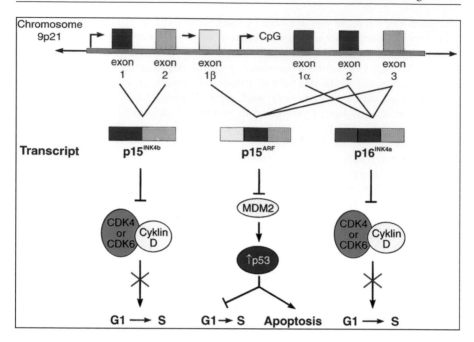

Fig. 14.1. INK4a/ARF locus on chromosome 9p21 p16INK4a is composed of exons 1α, 2, and 3 whereas p19ARF consists of exons 1β, 2, and 3. The resulting transcripts have different reading frames and translate into proteins with different amino acid sequences. p16INK4a blocks CDK4 and CDK6 function which results in G1-phase cell cycle arrest. p19ARF acts on MDM 2, resulting in the stabilization of p53, which, in turn, mediates G1-phase cell cycle arrest or apoptotic cell death. p15INK4b is a CDK inhibitor related to p16INK4a

Molecular Chemotherapy

Molecular Chemosensitization with Drug Susceptibility ("Suicide") Genes

The principle of this strategy is to transduce cancer cells with genes coding for enzymes that are capable of converting a non-toxic prodrug to a toxic agent. Upon administration of the specific prodrug, cancer cells expressing the respective gene trigger will initiate their own demise (Moolten 1994) (Fig. 14.2 a). Because the active agent is produced locally, this approach should allow – in contrast to conventional chemotherapy – to reach the therapeutic threshold at the tumor site whilst minimizing systemic toxicity. One widely studied system involves the herpes simplex virus thymidine kinase (HSVtk) in combination with ganciclovir, a drug often used for the treatment of cytomegalovirus infection in immunocompromised individuals. HSVtk phosphorylates ganciclovir which results in a toxic intermediate product converted to ganciclovir-triphosphate by

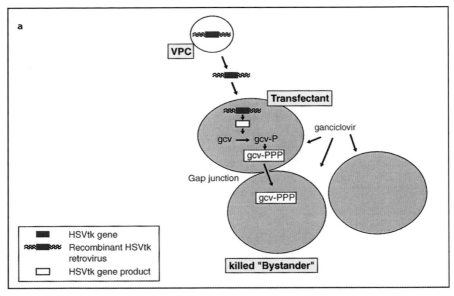

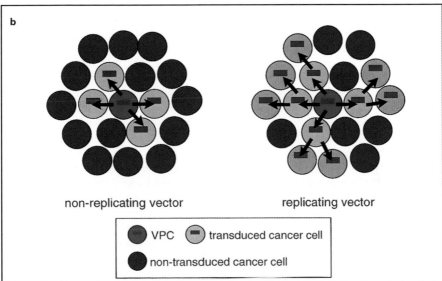

Fig. 14.2 a, b. The suicide gene approach. **a** Illustration of the events leading to suicide gene-mediated tumor cell death. Retroviral vectors produced and released by the implanted vector producing cells (VPC) transduce neighboring cancer cells with the HSVtk gene. Manipulated cancer cells will phosphorylate the systemically administered prodrug ganciclovir (GCV) to its monophosphorylated form, that is then converted by cellular enzymes to ganciclovir triphosphate, a toxic metabolite acting by inhibiting DNA replication. Not only genetically modified cancer cells are killed by the toxic metabolites, but also surrounding tumor cells (bystander effect) **b** Comparison of the mode of action of non-replicating and replicating retroviral vectors

cellular enzymes. This metabolite acts by inhibiting DNA replication (Moolten 1986) and thereby induces apoptotic cell death (Davidson et al. 1981, St. Clair et al. 1987). This strategy has been successfully used in preclinical melanoma models using various gene expression techniques. In a first series of experiments, Vile and Hart could show that the direct injection of naked DNA coding for HSVtk into B16 melanomas resulted in HSVtk gene expression and, after administration of ganciclovir, in a significant reduction of tumor growth (Vile and Hart 1993). As in other suicide gene transfer models, the observed anti-tumor effect appeared to be mediated, at least in part, through a so called "bystander" effect (i.e. killing not only gene-modified cells upon administration of the pro-drug but also surrounding non-transfected tumor cells). This bystander effect is thought to be the result of different mechanisms including the transfer of toxic metabolites to the non-transfected cancer cells via intercellular gap junctions, apoptosis induction through uptake of apoptotic bodies, and an ill-defined immune component (Moolten 1986 and 1994, Gagandeep et al. 1996, Hamel et al. 1996). In a second series of experiments, the same group could show that the intravenous application of the HSVtk gene driven by the tissue-specific tyrosinase promoter followed by ganciclovir treatment led to a considerable reduction of the metastatic burden within the lungs of treated animals. This effect however was highly dependent on an intact immune system (Vile et al. 1994). More recently, Bonnekoh et al. made similar observations in a xenogeneic model for treatment of human melanoma (Bonnekoh et al. 1996). These investigators injected human melanoma cells subcutaneously into nude, athymic animals, allowed the cells to form tumors, and treated them by the intratumoral injection of replication–defective adenoviruses containing an HSVtk gene construct. This treatment significantly reduced the growth of the melanomas and produced an 80% reduction of residual viable tumor (Bonnekoh et al. 1996). Importantly, the human melanomas were more sensitive than the mouse melanoma cells that had been previously studied (Bonnekoh et al. 1995). These studies provided the basis for using this approach to treat stage IV melanoma patients. Klatzman et al. injected metastatic nodules of 8 patients with escalating doses of a murine cell line producing a non-replicating retroviral vector encoding HSVtk and allowed cancer cell transduction for a period of 7 days before administering ganciclovir for 14 days (Klatzmann et al. 1998). The observed treatment-related adverse events were mild and mainly transient, and consisted of inflammatory reactions at the injected nodules and fever upon repeated application. The tumor response was limited, i.e. the size of the injected nodules was only moderately affected, and all patients eventually showed disease progression. Nevertheless, it was noticed that only nodules injected with the vector-producing cells decreased in size during ganciclovir administration while non-injected nodules grew progressively. This speaks in favor of a direct toxic effect of ganciclovir triphosphate, but the authors could not exclude the possibility that the observed clinical effects are due to the (immunological) consequences of injecting murine cells.

Klatzman et al. propose that the only limited tumor response obtained in their study may be the result of poor transduction efficacy of less than 1%, as animal experiments have demonstrated that about 10% of the cancer cells have to express the HSVtk gene for complete elimination of a neoplastic cell popula-

Table 14.1. Improvement of suicide gene therapy

New prodrugs (complementary antitumor mechanisms)
Enzymes (higher activity and specificity)
Vectors (e.g. gene transfer efficiency, targeted delivery/tissue-specific expression)
Immune component (e.g. coexpress cytokines or cell-bound costimulatory molecules)
Increase sensitivity to prodrug/drug (e.g. coexpress tumor suppressor genes)

tion upon GCV administration (Moolten 1986, Culver et al. 1992). Therefore, enhancing the efficiency of gene transfer techniques is one way to increase the clinical efficacy of this treatment (Table 14.1). To this end, Klatzman and colleagues are developing and testing replicating as well as semi-replicating retroviral vectors. The rationale behind these vectors is that the uptake of the retroviral vector would not only lead to transgene expression but also to the replication and release of the vector itself, which could then infect dividing neighboring cells thereby enhancing gene transfer efficiency (Fig. 14.2b). Another possibility to augment the clinical effectiveness of the suicide gene approach lies in the development of new enzyme-prodrug pairs. Some of these new pairs induce toxic effects also in non-dividing cells such as carboxypeptidase G2, nitroreductase or purine nucleoside phosphorylase. Nitroreductase (NTR) and its substrate 5-(aziridin-1-yl)-2,4-dinitrobenzamide (CB1954) are currently being investigated by Ford's group at Glaxo Wellcome. NTR metabolizes CB1954 to produce a highly toxic bi-functional alkylating agent that forms stable inter-strand crosslinks in DNA that kills cells directly through apoptosis (Friedlos et al. 1998). Due to the potent bystander effect of the toxic metabolites, only about 1–5% of a neoplastic cell population has to express the enzyme to kill the whole population upon CB1954 administration as demonstrated by studies in experimental animals. In in vitro studies, the purine nucleoside phosphorylase (PNP) gene, transcriptionally controlled by a dual tandem melanocyte-specific enhancer, also mediated significant cytotoxicity of its corresponding prodrug 6-methyl purine deoxyriboside towards melanoma cells (Park et al. 1999). Together, these results indicate the potential of this strategy for the treatment of solid cancers including melanoma.

Molecular Chemosensitization with Short DNA Sequences

Application of genes such as the tumor suppressor gene *p53* to tumor cells has been shown to facilitate the induction of apoptosis induced by conventional chemotherapeutic agents in vivo (Dorigo et al. 1998). Jansen and colleagues evaluate the potential of *bcl-2*-specific oligonucleotides to chemosensitize melanomas. Treatment with these molecules downregulated the *bcl-2* expression in human melanomas and, as a consequence, led to an increase in their chemosensitivity. This effect was evident after addition of the oligonucleotides to the tumor cell cultures and, more importantly, even when the *bcl-2*-specific antisense oligonucleotides were systemically administered to SCID mice bearing tumors (Jansen et al. 1996 and 1998). Currently, these investigators are testing the feasibility and safety of the *bcl-2*/chemosensitization approach in stage IV melanoma patients. A general problem of this strategy might be that the administration of *bcl-2*-specific oligonucleotides to patients will not only chemosensitize their tumor but also normal cells that rely on *bcl-2* function (e.g. lymphocytes).

Another molecule with chemosensitization potential is *c-myc*. In vitro experiments have shown that treatment with antisense oligonucleotides targeting *c-myc* augments the sensitivity of human melanomas to cisplatin (Leonetti et al. 1999).

Inhibition of Angiogenesis

Neovascularization, changes in the expression pattern of adhesion molecules, activation of proteolytic enzymes and downregulation of molecules inhibiting proteolytic enzymes are processes involved in local tumor growth, invasion and metastasis formation. Our growing understanding of these processes at the molecular level opens novel and specific therapeutic strategies to gene therapy of cancer. Best studied in this regard are the events leading to angiogenesis which are therefore described in more detail.

The growth of tumors beyond a size of 1–2 mm^3 is critically dependent on the formation of new blood vessels. These provide nutrients and, in addition, sustain tumor cell dissemination. Targeting tumor vessels offers a conceptual advantage over strategies addressing tumor cells themselves. Under normal conditions, non-neoplastic cells such as endothelial cells are genetically stable. Therefore, compared to genetically instable cancer cells, they have less possibilities to counteract therapeutic interventions aimed at their destruction. According to the currently accepted view, tumor-induced neovascularization results from an imbalance between molecules stimulating and inhibiting angiogenesis (Folkman 1995). Based on this theory, suppression of angiogenic signals as well as augmentation of angiogenesis inhibitors has been proposed as a potential anti-cancer strategy. Concerning the first approach, vascular endothelial growth factor (VEGF) has been demonstrated to represent a major angiogenic factor. This is a heparin-binding glycoprotein that occurs in four molecular forms (121, 165, 189 or 206 aa), which are derived from the same gene by alternative splicing. The two smaller forms (VEGF-121, VEGF-165) are secreted as disulfide-linked dimers, whereas the larger two remain cell-associated. VEGF became known for its mitogenic effect on endothelial cells (EC) as well as for its capacity to permeabilize the microvasculature, to stimulate EC migration and to produce certain proteinases participating in the degradation of the extracellular matrix. Its expression is upregulated in most human tumors and it has been shown to activate endothelial cells by binding to their high affinity tyrosinase kinase receptors Flt-1 (VEGFR-1) and Flk-1/KDR (VEGFR-2) (Thomas 1996). Interventions targeting the VEGF/VEGFR-1 and VEGFR-2 ligand/receptor system have been tested in preclinical studies. Approaches evaluated thus far include the downregulation of VEGF expression using antisense oligonucleotides (Cheng et al. 1996, Saleh et al. 1996), blockade of VEGFRs by adenoviral delivery of soluble Flt-1 receptor (Kong et al. 1998) and the retroviral delivery of a mutant Flk-1 receptor that acts in a dominant-negative fashion (Millauer et al. 1994, Machein et al. 1999). All these approaches have been shown to effectively inhibit the growth of established tumors in animal models. Similarly, encouraging results were obtained using strategies aimed at augmenting angiogenesis inhibitors. Anti-tumor activity was demonstrated by expressing thrombospondin 1 (Weinstat-Saslow et al. 1994), by in vivo delivery of adeno- and retroviral vectors coding for soluble platelet factor 4 (Tanaka et al. 1997), angiostatin (Griscelli et al. 1998, Tanaka et al. 1998), or angiostatin-endostatin fusion proteins.

However, at present, none of these exciting approaches has been brought into the clinic. This is due to concerns suggesting that in view of the multitude of molecules involved in the regulation of angiogenesis, blocking a single ligand/receptor pair may not be sufficient to inhibit tumor growth in humans. Another limitation is imposed by the currently available gene transfer technologies that do not achieve significant gene expression within tumors/tumor vessels upon intravenous administration.

Chemoprotection

This approach utilizes the introduction of drug resistance genes into hematopoietic precursor cells, thus allowing patients to tolerate higher doses of chemotherapeutic agents. Examples include genes encoding dihydrofolate reductase (DHFR), alkyltransferase, and the multidrug resistance 1 (MDR1) gene, conferring protection against methotrexate, taxol, vinblastine, colchicine, or against a subset of alkylating agents such as MNU and BNU (Connors 1995). The feasibility and safety of this strategy is currently tested in patients bearing cancers with a good response to chemotherapeutic drugs (e.g. breast cancer, ovarian tumors, and lymphoma). However, there are substantial concerns with this regimen. In particular, the presence of contaminating cancer cells within bone marrow samples harvested for genetic modification and the low transduction efficiency achieved with current retroviral vectors are major concerns. In addition, the therapeutic benefit of higher doses of chemotherapeutic agents remains to be demonstrated for melanoma.

Enhancing/Inducing Anti-Tumor Immunity

Most of the gene therapy protocols against cancer initiated so far are dedicated at augmenting the anti-tumor immune response. These trials can be divided into different categories according to the type of targeted cells. Initial studies by Rosenberg and colleagues were focused on the genetic modification of tumor-infiltrating lymphocytes (TILs) (Rosenberg et al. 1988), the idea being that TILs, due to their migration pattern, would be ideal vehicles to locally deliver cytokines with antitumor activity (e.g. TNF-α). By doing so, one should be able to circumvent toxicities associated with the systemic administration of these cytokines. Surprisingly, clinical trials with melanoma-derived TILs genetically engineered to express the neomycin-resistance gene revealed that only few of them localized into tumor foci upon intravenous administration (Rosenberg et al. 1990).

Tumor Cell-Based Vaccines

An alternative to the passive transfer of genetically-modified TILs is the induction and/or augmentation of an existing tumor-specific immune response in a tumor-bearing (or -prone) organism. Initial approaches used inactivated and/or modified, autologous and/or allogeneic cancer cells (Morton et al. 1992). They served as a source of tumor antigens and were modified with the goal of augmenting their immunogenicity. Xenogenization, i.e. the expression of highly antigenic foreign proteins (e.g. histocompatibility antigens, viral proteins) was one of the strategies proposed. This can be accomplished either by infection with non-pathogenic oncolytic viruses (e.g. vaccinia virus, Newcastle disease virus, vesicular stomatitis virus) or by gene transfer technology (Fearon et al. 1988). The immune response against viral antigens associated with the tumor cell membrane is believed to provide helper activity for antibody and T cell responses to adjacent tumor antigens (Lindenmann and Klein 1967, Fujiwara et al. 1984, Shimizu et al. 1984). Since most of the clinical trials using this approach have used historical controls (Hersey et al. 1987, Lehner et al. 1990, Liebrich et al. 1991), the efficacy of this treatment option remains to be determined.

In 1990, two groups of researchers independently reported that the expression of the IL-2 gene in cancer cells abrogates their tumorigenicity upon subcutaneous implantation into syngeneic, euthymic animals (Fearon et al. 1990, Gänsbacher et al. 1990a). They further observed that injection of IL-2-transfected tumor cells protected the animals against a subsequent challenge with the parental, but not with histogenetically unrelated tumor cells (Fearon et al. 1990, Gänsbacher et al. 1990a). The data suggested that (i) the tumor cells themselves interact with the T cells and that (ii) IL-2 functions by bypassing the helper T cell function in the generation of tumor-specific cytotoxic T cells. In keeping with this idea was the finding that cancer cells expressing the costimulatory molecule B7 could be used to induce a protective anti-tumor immune response (for review see Chen et al. 1993). This concept of helper-independent tumor antigen presentation by the cancer cell itself was later questioned when it was found that the protective effect of vaccination with genetically modified cancer cells could not only be accomplished by transfecting the cancer cells with genes encoding typical T cell growth-promoting cytokines, such as IL-2 (Fearon et al. 1990, Gänsbacher et al. 1990a), IL-4 (Golumbek et al. 1991), IL-7 (Aoki et al. 1992, Hock et al. 1993 and 1994), but also when cytokines were expressed in cancer cells which do not primarily act at the T cell level including GM-CSF (Dranoff et al. 1993), IL-6 (Porgador et al. 1992), and IFN-γ (Gänsbacher et al. 1990b, Porgador et al. 1991)).

In order to elucidate the mode of action of IL-2-based cancer vaccines, we have studied the events following the subcutaneous administration of IL-2-transfected, MHC class I$^+$/ MHC class II$^-$ DBA/2-derived M3 melanoma cells (Zatloukal et al. 1995). We have found (i) that IL-2-transfection abrogates the tumorigenicity of M3 cells in both euthymic and athymic mice and (ii) that these IL-2-producing M3 cells can be used to induce a long-lasting, protective anti-tumor immune response in syngeneic euthymic DBA/2 mice, but not in athymic animals. Subsequent studies revealed that these two phenomena are mediated by different effector mechanisms. With regard to tumorigenicity, we could demonstrate that IL-2-transfected cancer cells induce an inflammatory tissue reaction composed of granulocytes, macrophages and NK cells. In vivo cell depletion and cell transfer studies revealed that the NK cell component is critical for the tumoricidal effect (Schneeberger et al. 1999 a). By contrast, the protective effect of IL-2-expressing M3 cells appears to be the result of a specific immune response. Transfer studies with various leukocyte subpopulations of immunized mice into naive animals showed that both CD4$^+$ and CD8$^+$ T cells are needed for optimal protection against a challenge with wild-type M3 cells (Zatloukal et al. 1995). The critical requirement of CD4$^+$ lymphocytes in tumor cell rejection implies that class II-dependent immunity is an important effector mechanism in the M3 model. Because M3 cells are consistently MHC class II negative and cannot be induced to express these molecules (Zatloukal et al. 1995), they do not qualify as antigen-presenting cells for the activation of MHC class II-restricted CD4$^+$ tumor-specific T cells. One must therefore assume that the generation of these CD4$^+$ lymphocytes has occurred as a consequence of tumor antigen presentation by host cells (indirect antigen presentation pathway, Fig. 14.3). The recent demonstration of successful presentation of exogenous antigens in the context of MHC class I molecules (Rock et al. 1990, Pfeifer et al. 1993, Kovacsovics-Bankowski and Rock 1995) opens the possibility that even the generation of MHC class I-restricted, M3-specific CD8$^+$ CTLs did not occur in a direct fashion, i.e. by IL-2-transfected M-3 cells, but rather by host-derived antigen-presenting cells (Steinman 1991). This notion is supported by the virtual absence of T cells from the immunization site and the detection of mRNA indicative of T cell activation and expansion in the draining lymph nodes (Maass et al. 1995). Recently, we generated direct evidence for a critical role of dendritic cells (DC) in the priming events induced by cytokine-based cancer vaccines. Suspecting the regional lymph node as site of T cell activation, we designed experiments to determine the relevant APC. Lymph nodes draining injection sites, where M-3 cells co-expressing the cytokine GM-CSF and the model antigen β-galactosidase had been injected, were assessed for the presence of β-galactosidase epitope-bearing cells using a β-gal-specific T cell clone. Results obtained showed that such cells are present in lymph nodes draining M-3-GM-βgal- but not M-3-GM injection sites and that the antigen presenting activity of such lymph node preparations resides exclusively within the CD11c-positive dendritic cell population (Schneeberger et al. 1999 b). Similar results were obtained by Chiodoni et al. employing CT26 colon carcinoma cells expressing both GM-CSF as well as the cell-bound costimulatory molecule CD40L (Chiodoni et al. 1999).

Nearly one third of the clinical trials devoted to the gene therapy of neoplastic diseases use cancer cells engineered to express immunostimulatory molecules. We have conducted a phase I trial in stage IV melanoma patients using

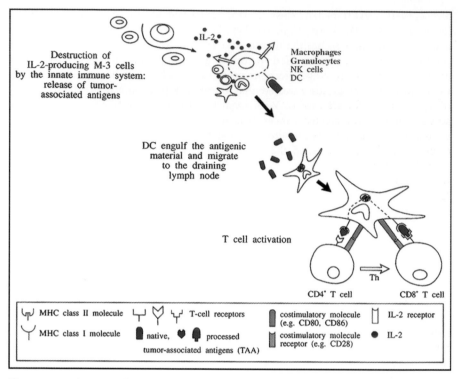

Fig. 14.3. Mechanism of action of IL-2-based cancer vaccines

IL-2-transfected autologous melanoma cells (Stingl et al. 1996). Tumor cell propagation and IL-2 gene transfection employing the adenovirus-enhanced transferrinfection (AVET) system was successful in 54% of our patients. Fifteen patients received 2–8 injections of either 3×10^6 or 1×10^7 transfected melanoma cells. Overall, this treatment was well tolerated. More importantly, findings such as *de novo* or increasing tumor-specific DTH reactions (8/15) as well as the induction of vitiligo (3/15) supported the idea of a vaccine-induced/-amplified melanoma-specific immune response. Although all vaccine recipients ultimately succumbed to their disease, some of our patients exhibited signs of tumor regression and 3 of them experienced a mean survival of 15.7+/–3.5 months as compared to 7.8+/–4.6 months for the entire cohort (Schreiber et al. 1999). Similar results were achieved by various other investigators using a similar strategy (Sato et al. 1996, Abdel-Wahab et al. 1997, Ellem et al. 1997, Soiffer et al. 1998). Difficulties associated with this therapy are the time-consuming and costly vaccine production, the limited success of tumor cell propagation as well as variations in the biological features of the individual vaccines. This led to the development of simpler and better standardized protocols such as the coadministration of inactivated tumor cells and cytokine-releasing agents (e.g. transduced fibroblasts, cytokine-releasing microspheres) (Veelken et al. 1997). Another approach is based on the demonstration that tumor antigens are presented by host-derived APC rather than the cytokine gene-modified tumor cells themselves (Huang et al. 1994, Chiodoni et al. 1999, Schneeberger et al. 1999a) and on the idea of shared tumor antigens. This uses well-defined allogeneic tumor cell lines genetically engineered to express immunostimulatory molecules and is currently under study by us and other investigators (Gänsbacher et al. 1992, Osanto et al. 1993, Cascinelli et al. 1994, Fenton et al. 1995, Arienti et al. 1996, Belli et al. 1997). It allows for standardized vaccine preparation and enables one to immunize patients with a minimal tumor load.

In conclusion, some of these studies provided evidence for an immunological response to the intervention (Nabel et al. 1993, Arienti et al. 1996). To date however, there are only few patients reported with a significant systemic clinical response. One of them is a patient with melanoma who had received his own cancer cells modified to express IFN-γ. He has been described with no evidence of disease for 7 months (Ross et al. 1996).

Antigen-Based Vaccines

The induction of antigen-specific tumor immunity can be accomplished by either peptide-based or nucleic acid-based vaccines. Tumor antigen-derived peptides can either be injected alone (Marchand et al. 1999), together with adjuvant (Rosenberg et al. 1998) or in the context of potent APCs (see below). The first of these strategies bares the theoretical risk of inducing tumor-specific unresponsiveness. A more detailed review of peptide-based vaccines would exceed the scope of this chapter.

Recombinant Viral and Bacterial Vaccines

The molecular definition of tumor antigens recognized by the immune system offers promising avenues for the rational development of cancer vaccines. Most progress in the identification of new tumor antigens has been achieved in the case of melanoma. Many of the melanoma antigens identified so far are non-mutated melanocyte differentiation antigens (e.g. Pmel17/gp100, MART-1/MelanA, tyrosinase, tyrosinase related proteins 1 and 2) which are expressed by virtually all melanomas (Pardoll 1994). While this makes them suitable targets for a common melanoma vaccine, their use may result in the elicitation of autoimmunity (e.g. vitiligo). Other melanoma antigens belong to gene families that are activated in neoplastic, but not in normal tissues except testis (e.g. MAGE, BAGE, GAGE, RAGE, LAGE and NY-ESO-1) or result from mutations of ubiquitously expressed genes (β-catenin, CDK4, FLICE) (Boon and van der Bruggen 1996). The identification of these antigens together with the development of standard techniques to engineer recombinant viruses and bacteria allows the production of novel recombinant vaccines. Viruses employed for this purpose have been selected on the basis of their intrinsic immunogenicity and include vaccinia and other poxviruses as well as adenoviruses. The most compelling feature of anti-gen-based vaccines is the unique possibility to rapidly and accurately evaluate the ability of a given vaccine formulation to induce a specific immune response using novel methods for immunomonitoring such as ELISPOT- or tetramer-technology. This is a critical advantage over cell-based vaccination strategies because it should allow a comparative analysis of the immunological efficacy of various vaccination strategies in relatively few patients. The most promising vaccines can subsequently be tested in prospective, randomized and controlled clinical trials.

Some of these recombinant vaccines have already been successfully applied to animal models of cancer. Toes et al. used the B6 tumor which is transduced with the human adenovirus early region 1 gene (Ad5E1) and generates progressively growing tumors in its syngeneic host (i.e. C57BL/6 mice). In this model, the most efficient vaccination approach was found to involve the injection of a replication-incompetent adenoviral vector containing Ad5E1. This treatment did not only lead to the eradication of established B6 tumors, but also to the induction of a potent and specific CTL memory (Toes et al. 1996). Wang and coworkers demonstrated that vaccination with a fowlpox virus, genetically engineered to encode the model antigen β-galactosidase, protected mice against a challenge with tumor cells expressing this antigen (Wang et al. 1995). Similarly, immunization with a vaccinia-based vector, coding for a MHC class I-restricted ovalbumin epitope, protected syngeneic animals against the growth of ovalbumin-expressing lymphoma cells (McCabe et al. 1995). Besides allowing to optimize factors like route and schedule of administration, these animal models open the possibility to refine many of the recombinant vectors. Ways to augment their immunologic efficacy include the use of minigenes encoding only T cell-defined epitopes (McCabe et al. 1995), string-of-beads minigenes harboring multiple T cell epitopes (Whitton et al. 1993) and the addition of endoplasmatic reticulum insertion signal sequences that bypass TAP transporters and, in some instances, greatly enhance the function of the vaccine (Restifo et al. 1995). Moreover, immunomodulatory molecules (e.g. cytokines like IL-2, IL-12, GM-CSF and/or costimulatory molecules such as B7) can be inserted into the viruses to augment their immunostimulatory potency (Bronte et al. 1995, Chamberlain et al. 1996). Several preclinical studies demonstrated the generation of antigen-specific immunity associated with protection against a subsequent tumor challenge and sometimes rejection of established metastases by recombinant vaccinia or fowlpox constructs encoding melanoma antigens (Bronte et al. 1995, Irvine et al. 1995, McCabe et al. 1995, Restifo et al. 1995, Zhai et al. 1996, Overwijk et al. 1999).

To evaluate the therapeutic potential of this approach in humans, Rosenberg and colleagues constructed replication-deficient adenoviruses encoding either MART-1 or gp100 antigens (Rosenberg et al. 1998). Escalating doses of these recombinant vectors (10^7–10^{11} pfu) were administered alone or in combination with high doses of IL-2 to 54 heavily pretreated stage IV melanoma patients exhibiting progressive disease. The administration of the recombinant virus was well tolerated with no significant side effects seen with up to 4 sequential injections at monthly intervals. Only 1 of 16 patients receiving the MART-1-expressing vector alone achieved a complete response. The response rate in patients treated with MART-1 adenovirus in conjunction with high dose IL-2 was 16%

(2/18) and therefore similar to the 17% response rate these investigators had obtained previously with IL-2 alone (Rosenberg et al. 1994). Comparing the pre- and postvaccination reactivity to the HLA-A2-restricted immunodominant CTL epitopes encoded by MART-1 and gp100, only 5 of 22 patients tested exhibited some evidence of immunization as a result of the adenoviral administration (Rosenberg et al. 1998). The most likely explanation as to the relative lack of immunological and clinical efficacy of these recombinant adenoviruses appears to be the preexisting virus-specific immunity. Humans have high titers of neutralizing antibodies to adenovirus as a result of their ubiquitous presence (and to vaccinia virus due to vaccination campaigns aimed at eradicating smallpox). As a consequence, vectors based on these viruses are cleared by most patients' immune systems making it difficult to use them as backbone of cancer vaccines. Because of this, it is unlikely that recombinant viral vaccines will reach broad clinical application. One way to overcome the limitations imposed by the preexisting immune response to viral proteins may consist in the use of viruses whose natural hosts are non-mammalian as well as the use of bacterial vectors. In this regard, *Listeria monocytogenes* appears to be an interesting candidate (see preceding chapter). Due to its two-phase intracellular life cycle Listeria delivers antigens to the MHC class I and class II presentation pathway. In animal models, a recombinant *Listeria monocytogenes* vaccine encoding a model tumor antigen was potent enough to protect mice against a lethal tumor challenge and to cause regression of established metastases (Pan et al. 1995).

Plasmid ("Naked") DNA-Based Vaccines

The potential of naked DNA to transfect cells upon injection into an organism was first described by Itoh in 1960 (Ito 1960). This finding remained largely unnoticed until 1990 when Wolff et al. demonstrated direct gene transfer into mouse muscle in vivo with reporter gene constructs (Wolff et al. 1990). Numerous subsequent studies have since demonstrated that plasmid DNA can be delivered by various methods such as direct injection, biolistic systems or electroporation and via different routes (e.g. intramuscular, intradermal, mucosal). In addition, these studies have established the potential of naked DNA to reproducibly induce both humoral and cellular responses to the encoded antigens (Ulmer et al. 1993, Rouse et al. 1994, Böhm et al. 1996, McDonnell and Askari 1996, Tascon et al. 1996). Similar to recombinant vectors, plasmid DNA is easy to engineer and to produce in large quantity with great purity but is generally not as potent in eliciting immune responses as viral constructs. Efforts to improve the immunological potency of DNA vaccines include promoter optimization, enhancement of polyadenylation sequences and the use of intronic sequences to improve nuclear transport.

Several investigators have evaluated the ability of plasmid DNA coding for melanoma-associated antigens to protect experimental animals against the growth of syngeneic melanomas. We and Schreurs et al. were able to demonstrate that the i.m. injection of plasmid DNA encoding the human but not the murine form of Pmel17/gp100 protects C57BL/6 mice against the growth of B16 melanoma (Mölling et al. 1997, Schreurs et al. 1998). In this tumor model, the protective effect obtained by immunization with the human homologue is the result of a fortuitous heteroclitic T cell response against the corresponding murine Pmel17/gp100 epitope (Overwijk et al. 1998). Comparable results in the same experimental system have also been reported for human TRP-1, another melanocyte differentiation antigen (Weber et al. 1998). We have tested the potential of naked DNA encoding the murine form of Pmel17/gp100 to induce an antigen-specific and protective immune response in DBA/2 mice. Intradermal administration by direct injection of this construct led to the generation of Pmel17/gp100-specific CTLs. Moreover, this state of immune reactivity was associated with protection against subsequently inoculated M-3 melanoma cells (Wagner et al., submitted). The latter model appears to mimic more closely the aim of inducing an immune response to differentiation antigens, in order to overcome immunological tolerance such as ignorance, anergy or physical deletion. More recently, clinical trials on the safety and efficacy of plasmid DNA-based vaccines have been initiated. One of the trials is run by investigators from the Surgery Branch at the NIH using a plasmid coding for a variant of human Pmel17/gp100 alone and in combination with IL-2. Others are addressing colon cancer, cutaneous T cell lymphoma as well as infectious diseases such as influenza, hepatitis B, AIDS and malaria.

Dendritic Cell Vaccines

DC are bone marrow-derived leukocytes and very potent, if not the most effective, stimulator cells for the induction of primary T cell immune responses (Steinman 1991, Stingl and Bergstresser 1995). The fact that these cells can now be generated in large numbers by in vitro culture of their precursor cells using GM-CSF in combination with other cytokines (TNF-α, IL-4, IL-13, TGF-β, Flt3L) makes them attractive tools for cancer immunotherapy (Caux et al. 1992, Romani et al. 1994, Strobl et al. 1996, Strunk et al. 1996). DC pulsed ex vivo with tumor-antigens (presented to the DC either as whole proteins or as CTL peptide epitopes) have been successfully used in prophylactic as well as in therapeutic mouse models of cancer immunotherapy (Grabbe et al. 1991, Mayordomo et al. 1995, Celluzzi et al. 1996).

More recently, two groups of investigators described their experience with antigen-loaded DC as vaccine for patients with advanced melanoma (Nestle et al. 1998, Thurner et al. 1999). Nestle et al. differentiated adherent PBMC in the presence of GM-CSF and IL-4 to DC, pulsed them – depending on the HLA type of the patient – with tumor lysate or a cocktail of peptides along with KLH as a helper epitope and injected these cells into the lymph nodes of 16 patients with disseminated disease. DC vaccination was well tolerated and induced DTH reactivity towards KLH in all and towards peptide-pulsed DC in 11 patients. Objective responses were seen in 5 patients (2 CR, 3 PR) with regression of metastases in various organs such as skin, soft tissue, lung and pancreas (Nestle et al. 1998 and preceeding chapter). Thurner et al. focused on HLA-A1-positive stage IV melanoma patients who were progressive despite standard chemotherapy

(Thurner et al. 1999). Monocytes from leukapheresis, cultured in the presence of GM-CSF and IL-4 were administered. By day 6, monocyte-conditioned medium was added to mature the DCs. DCs, pulsed with MAGE-3A1 and either tetanus toxoid or tuberculin as recall antigen, were administered at 14 d intervals to 11 patients with the first three vaccinations being applied to the skin (i.d. and s.c.) followed by two intravenous injections. This treatment boosted immunity to recall antigens and led to a significant expansion of MAGE-3-specific pCTLs in 8 out of 11 patients. Two weeks after the fifth vaccination, 6/11 patients had experienced complete regressions of individual metastases in skin, lymph nodes, lung and liver (Thurner et al. 1999). Although these results are quite promising, several obstacles prevent them from being translated to other tumors. These include the fact that only a limited number of T cell-defined antigens are presently characterized. Another hurdle is that T cells do not recognize soluble proteins per se, but antigenic peptides in association with appropriate MHC molecules (Zinkernagel and Doherty 1974). To associate with a given MHC molecule the peptides must display corresponding motifs (Rötzschke et al. 1990, Rammensee et al. 1993). And, as human beings are heterogeneous with regard to the MHC molecules, one would have to determine the MHC haplotype of each patient and then select the ones (from a peptide bank) that fit the respective MHC moieties. It is obvious that such an approach is quite impractical on a routine basis. One possibility to overcome this limitation consists in the expression of the gene of interest in the antigen-presenting cell itself. Then, the "selection" of the appropriate peptide epitopes will be accomplished by the cells' antigen processing and presenting machinery. Currently, many groups of investigators have adopted this strategy and are therefore interested in defining optimal conditions for the transfection of dendritic cells. Some of them could already report at least some success (Alijagic et al. 1996, Boczskowski et al. 1996). Most recently, several groups demonstrated the use of tyrosine-related protein resulting in a protective immune response against B16 melanoma (Kaplan et al. 1999, Steitz et al. 2000). Particularly interesting is the strategy chosen by Gilboa's group. These investigators use RNA-derived from tumor cells as a source of tumor antigen genes and cationic lipids to deliver the RNA into mouse DC. They demonstrated that this procedure enables DC to display the antigenic peptide epitopes on their MHC class I molecules as assessed by their ability to stimulate peptide-specific T cell clones. Even more important was the observation, that vaccination of experimental animals with DC transfected with tumor-derived RNA could significantly reduce the number of melanoma metastases in their lungs (Boczkowski et al. 1996). This strategy offers the unique possibility to generate large amounts of tumor antigen from small tumor samples using PCR amplification techniques. Moreover, tumor-specific RNA can be enriched by subtractive hybridization with RNA from normal tissue which will reduce the content of self-antigens within the preparation and thereby lessen the danger of autoimmunity.

Conclusions

Recent advances in the fields of tumor biology, immunology and molecular biology provided the basis to design therapeutic strategies targeting cancer at the molecular level. Despite their rationale basis and remarkable data achieved in preclinical models, initial enthusiasm has been lowered as principal limitations became apparent when translating these strategies into the clinic, as emphasised by the Orkin-Motulsky report. Limitations in obtaining clinically relevant benefit are due to the inefficiency of current vector systems to obtain quantitative gene transfer, prolonged transgene expression, selectivity or cell-specific targeting. There are several promising approaches to overcome these problems. For example, the development of vector systems with increased in vivo stability and the capacity for conditional replication may help to improve suboptimal tumor transduction and prolong expression of therapeutic genes in vivo. Efforts aimed at augmenting selective targeting, a prerequisite for directly attacking disseminated tumor cells, include the development of specific regulatory sequences, novel strategies to alter the tropism of vector systems (e.g. by incorporation of targeting motifs with specificity for receptors expressed by the tumor or tumor vessels) and the use of cellular vehicles such as the recently described circulating endothelial progenitors that were characterized by the capacity to localize into areas of angiogenesis upon intravenous administration. Lessons learned on how the tumor develops resistance to immune recognition tempered the view that vaccines will quickly revolutionize cancer therapy. The challenges ahead lie in the translation of these advances into reproducible clinical benefit. This will involve thoughtful evaluation of new generation vaccines including selection of the optimal dose, route and schedule of application as well as careful selection of patients.

Acknowledgements. This work was supported by grants from the Industrial Research promotion fund, Vienna, Austria (grant 6/676 to GS), the Austrian Federal Reserve Bank (grant 8264 to AS) and the Deutsche Forschungsgemeinschaft (grant Wa 705/4–1 to SNW).

References

Abdel-Wahab Z, Weltz C, Hester D, Pickett N, Vervaert C, Barber JR, Jolly D, Seigler HF (1997) A phase I trial of immunotherapy with interferon-γ gene-modified autologous melanoma cells. Cancer 80:401–412

Akslen LA, Monstad SE, Larsen B, Straume O, Ogreid D (1998) Frequent mutations of the p53 gene in cutaneous melanoma of the nodular type. Int J Cancer 79:91–95

Albino AP, Nanus DM, Mentle IR, Cordon-Cardo C, McNutt NS, Bressler J, Andreeff M (1989) Analysis of the ras oncogenes in malignant melanoma and precursor lesion: Correlation of point mutations with differentiation phenotype. Oncogene 4:1363–1374

Albino AP, Sozzi G, Nanus DM, Jhanwar SC, Houghton AN (1992) Malignant transformation of human melanocytes: induction of a complete phenotype and genotype. Oncogene 7:3415–3421

Albino AP, Vidal MJ, McNutt NS, Shea CR, Prieto VG, Nanus DM, Palmer JM, Hayward NK (1994) Mutation and expression of the p53 in human malignant melanoma. Melanoma Research 4:35–45

Alijagic S, Moller P, Artuc M, Jurgovsky K, Czarnetzki BM, Schadendorf D (1996) Dendritic cells generated from peripheral blood transfected with human tyrosinase induce specific T cell activation. Eur J Immunol 25:3100–3107

Aoki T, Tashiro K, Miyatake S, Kinashi T, Nakano T, Oda Y, Kikuchi H, Honjo T (1992) Expression of murine interleukin 7 in a murine glioma cell line results in reduced tumorigenicity in vivo. Proc Natl Acad Sci USA 89:3850–3854

Arienti F, Sule-Suso J, Belli F, Mascheroni L, Rivoltini L, Melani C, Maio M, Cascinelli N, Colombo MP, Parmiani G (1996) Limited antitumor T cell response in melanoma patients vaccinated with interleukin-2 gene-transduced allogeneic melanoma cells. Hum Gene Ther 7:1955–1963

Balch CM (1992) Cutaneous melanoma: prognosis and treatment results worldwide. Semin Surg Oncol 8:400–414

Belli F, Arienti F, Sule-Suso J, Clemente C, Mascheroni L, Cattelan A, Santantonio C, Gallino GF, Melani C, Rao S, Colombo MP, Maio M, Cascinelli N, Parmiani G (1997) Active immunization of metastatic melanoma patients with interleukin-2-transduced allogeneic melanoma cells: evaluation of efficacy and tolerability. Cancer Immunol Immunother 44:197–203

Boczkowski D, Nair SK, Snyder D, Gilboa E (1996) Dendritic cells pulsed with RNA are potent antigen-presenting cells in vitro and in vivo. J Exp Med 184:465–472

Böhm W, Kuhrober A, Paier T, Mertens T, Reimann J, Schirmbeck R (1996) DNA vector constructs that prime hepatitis B surface antigen-specific cytotoxic T lymphocyte and antibody responses in mice after intramuscular injection. J Immunol Methods 193:29–40

Bonnekoh B, Greenhalgh DA, Bundman DS, Eckhardt JN, Longley MA, Chen SH, Woo SL, Roop DR (1995) Inhibition of melanoma growth by adenoviral-mediated HSV thymidine kinase gene transfer in vivo. J Invest Dermatol 104:313–317

Bonnekoh B, Greenhalgh DA, Bundman DS, Kosai K, Chen SH, Finegold MJ, Krieg T, Woo SL, Roop R (1996) Adenoviral-mediated herpes simplex virus thymidine kinase gene transfer in vivo for the treatment of experimental human melanoma. J Invest Dermatol 106:1163–1168

Boon T, van der Bruggen P (1996) Human tumor antigens recognized by T lymphocytes. J Exp Med 183:725–729

Bronte V, Tsung K, Rao JB, Chen PW, Wang M, Rosenberg SA, Restifo NP (1995) IL-2 enhances the function of recombinant poxvirus-based vaccines in the treatment of established pulmonary metastases. J Immunol 154:5282–5292

Cascinelli N, Foa R, Parmiani G, Arienti F, Belli F, Bernengo MG, Clemente C, Colombo MP, Guarini A, Illeni MT, et al. (1994) Active immunization of metastatic melanoma patients with interleukin-4 transduced, allogeneic melanoma cells. A phase I–II study. Hum Gene Ther 5:1059–1064

Caux C, Dezutter-Dambuyant C, Schmitt D, Banchereau J (1992) GM-CSF and TNF-α cooperate in the generation of dendritic Langerhans cells. Nature 360:258–261

Celluzzi CM, Mayordomo JI, Storkus WJ, Lotze MT, Falo LD Jr (1996) Peptide-pulsed dendritic cells induce antigen-specific, CTL-mediated protective tumor immunity. J Exp Med 183:283–287

Chamberlain RS, Carroll MW, Bronte V, Hwu P, Warren S, Yang JC, Nishimura M, Moss B, Rosenberg SA, Restifo NP (1996) Costimulation enhances the active immunotherapy effect of recombinant anti-cancer vaccines. Cancer Res 56:2832–2836

Chen L, Linsley PS, Hellstrom KE (1993) Costimulation of T cells for tumor immunity. Immunol Today 14:483–486

Cheng SY, Huang HJ, Nagane M, Ji XD, Wang D, Shih CC, Arap W, Huang CM, Cavenee WK (1996) Suppression of glioblastoma angiogenicity and tumorigenicity by inhibition of endogenous expression of vascular endothelial growth factor. Proc Natl Acad Sci USA 93:8502–8507

Chin L, Pomerantz J, Polsky D, Jacobson M, Cohen C, Cordon-Cardo C, Horner JW 2nd, DePinho RA (1997) Cooperative effects of INK4a and ras in melanoma susceptibility in vivo. Genes Dev 11:2822–2834

Chiodoni C, Paglia P, Stoppacciaro A, Rodolfo M, Parenza M, Colombo MP (1999) Dendritic cells infiltrating tumors cotransduced with granulocyte/macrophage colony-stimulating factor (GM-CSF) and CD40 ligand genes take up and present endogenous tumor-associated antigens and prime naive mice for a cytotoxic T lymphocyte response. J Exp Med 190:125–133

Cirielli C, Riccioni T, Yang C, Pili R, Gloe T, Chang J, Inyaku K, Passaniti A, Capogrossi MC (1995) Adenovirus-mediated gene transfer of wild-type p53 results in melanoma cell apoptosis in vitro and in vivo. Int J Cancer 63:673–679

Connors TA (1995) The choice of prodrugs for gene directed enzyme prodrug therapy of cancer. Gene Ther 2:702–709

Crooke ST (1992) Therapeutic applications of oligonucleotides. Annu Rev Pharmacol Toxicol 32:329–76

Culver KW, Ram Z, Wallbridge S, Ishii H, Oldfield EH, Blaese RM (1992) In vivo gene transfer with retroviral vector-producer cells for treatment of experimental brain tumors. Science 256:1550–1552

Davidson RL, Kaufman ER, Crumpacker CS, Schnipper LE (1981) Inhibition of herpes simplex virus transformed and nontransformed cells by acycloguanosine: Mechanisms of uptake and toxicity. Virology 113:9–19

Dorigo O, Turla ST, Lebedeva S, Gjerset RA (1998) Sensitization of rat glioblastoma multiforme to cisplatin in vivo following restoration of wild-type p53 function. J Neurosurg 88:535–540

Dranoff G, Jaffee E, Lazenby A, Golumbek P, Levitsky H, Brose K, Jackson V, Hamada H, Pardoll D, Mulligan RC (1993) Vaccination with irradiated tumor cells engineered to secrete murine granulocyte-macrophage colony-stimulating factor stimulates potent, specific, and long-lasting anti-tumor immunity. Proc Natl Acad Sci USA 90:3539–3543

Ellem KA, O'Rourke MG, Johnson GR, Parry G, Misko IS, Schmidt CW, Parsons PG, Burrows SR, Cross S, Fell A, Li CL, Bell JR, Dubois PJ, Moss DJ, Good MF, Kelso A, Cohen LK, Dranoff G, Mulligan RC (1997) A case report: Immune response and clinical course of the first human use of granulocyte/macrophage colony-stimulating factor-transduced autologous melanoma cells for immunotherapy. Cancer Immunol Immunother 44:10–20

Fearon ER, Vogelstein B (1990) A genetic model for colorectal tumorgenesis. Cell 61:759–767

Fearon ER, Itaya T, Hunt B, Vogelstein B, Frost P (1988) Induction in a murine tumor of immunogenic tumor variants by transfection with a foreign gene. Cancer Res 48:2975–2980

Fearon ER, Pardoll DM, Itaya T, Golumbek P, Levitsky HI, Simons JW, Karasuyama H, Vogelstein B, Frost P (1990) Interleukin-2 production by tumor cells bypasses T helper function in the generation of an antitumor response. Cell 60:397–403

Fenton RT, Sznol M, Luster DG, Taub DD, Longo DL (1995) A phase 1 trial of B7-transfected or parental lethally irradiated allogeneic melanoma cell lines to induce cell-mediated immunity against tumor-associated antigen presented by HLA-A2 or HLA-A1 in patients with stage lV melanoma. Hum Gene Ther 6:87–106

Folkman J 1995. Angiogenesis in cancer, vascular, rheumatoid and other disease. Nature Med 1:27–31

Friedlos F, Court S, Ford M, Denny WA, Springer C (1998) Gene-directed enzyme prodrug therapy: quantitative bystander cytotoxicity and DNA damage induced by CB1954 in cells expressing bacterial nitroreductase. Gene Ther 5:105–112

Fujiwara H, Shimizu Y, Takai Y, Wakamiya N, Ueda S, Kato S, Hamaoka T (1984) The augmentation of tumor-specific immunity by virus help: I. Demonstration of vaccinia virus-reactive helper T cell activity involved in enhanced induction of cytotoxic T lymphocyte and antibody responses. Eur J Immunol 14:171–175

Gagandeep S, Brew R, Green B, Christmas SE, Klatzmann D, Poston GJ, Kinsella AR (1996) Prodrug-activated gene therapy: Involvement of an immunological component in the bystander effect. Cancer Gene Ther 3:83–88

Gänsbacher B, Zier K, Daniels B, Cronin K, Bannerji R, Gilboa E (1990a) Interleukin 2 gene transfer into tumor cells abrogates tumorigenicity and induces protective immunity. J Exp Med 172:1217–1224

Gänsbacher B, Bannerji R, Daniels B, Zier K, Cronin K, Gilboa E (1990b) Retroviral vector-mediated γ-interferon gene transfer into tumor cells generates potent and long lasting antitumor immunity. Cancer Res 50:7820–7825

Gänsbacher B, Houghton A, Livingston P, Minasian L, Rosenthal F, Gilboa E, Golde D, Oettgen H, Steffens T, Yang SY, Wong G (1992) A pilot study of immunization with HLA-A2 matched allogeneic melanoma cells that secrete interleukin-2 in patients with metastatic melanoma. Hum Gene Ther 3:677–690

Golumbek PT, Lazenby AJ, Levitsky HI, Jaffee LM, Karasuyama H, Baker M, Pardoll DM (1991) Treatment of established renal cancer by tumor cells engineered to secrete interleukin-4. Science 254:713–716

Grabbe S, Bruvers S, Gallo RL, Knisely TL, Nazareno R, Granstein RD (1991) Tumor antigen presentation by murine epidermal cells. J Immunol 146:3656–3661

Griscelli F, Li H, Bennaceur-Griscelli A, Soria J, Opolon P, Soria C, Perricaudet M, Yeh P, Lu H (1998) Angiostatin gene transfer: Inhibition of tumor growth in vivo by blockage of endothelial cell proliferation associated with a mitosis arrest. Proc Natl Acad Sci USA 95:6367–6372

Hamel W, Magnelli L, Chiarugi VP, Israel MA (1996) Herpes simplex virus thymidine kinase/ganciclovir-mediated apoptotic death of bystander cells. Cancer Res 56:2697–2702

Hersey P, Edwards A, Coates A, Shaw H, McCarthy W, Milton G (1987) Evidence that treatment with vaccinia melanoma cell lysates (VMCL) may improve survival of patients with stage II melanoma. Cancer Immunol Immunother 25:257–265

Heufler C, Koch F, Stanzl U, Topar G, Wysocka M, Trinchieri G, Enk A, Steinman RM, Romani N, Schuler G (1996) Interleukin-12 is produced by dendritic cells and mediates T helper 1 development as well as interferon-gamma production by T helper 1 cells. Eur J Immunol. 26:659–668

Hock H, Dorsch M, Kunzendorf U, Qin Z, Diamantstein T, Blankenstein T (1993) Mechanisms of rejection induced by tumor cell-targeted gene transfer of IL-2, IL-4, IL-7, tumor necrosis factor, or interferon-γ. Proc Natl Acad Sci USA 90:2774–2778

Hock H, Dorsch M, Blankenstein T, Diamantstein T (1994) Tumor-cell-targeted interleukin-7 gene transfer reveals T-cell-dependent antitumor activity in vivo. In: Cytokines in cancer therapy. Bergmann L, Mitrou PS (eds). Karger, Basel, p. 277

Houghton AN, Balch CM (1992) Treatment of advanced melanoma. In: Cutaneous melanoma. 2nd ed. Balch CM, Houghton AN, Milton GW, Sober AJ, Soong SJ (eds). J.B. Lippincott Company, Philadelphia, p. 468

Huang AY, Golumbek P, Ahmadzadeh M, Jaffee E, Pardoll D, Levitsky H (1994) Role of bone marrow-derived cells in presenting MHC class I-restricted tumor antigens. Science 264:961–965

Irvine KR, McCabe BJ, Rosenberg SA, Restifo NP (1995) Synthetic oligonucleotide expressed by a recombinant vaccinia virus elicits therapeutic CTL. J Immunol 154:4651–4657

Ito Y (1960) A tumor-producing factor extracted by phenol from papillomatous tissue (Shope) of cottontail rabbits. Virology 12:596

Jafari M, Papp T, Kirchner S, Diener U, Henschler D, Burg G, Schiffmann D (1995) Analysis of ras mutations in human melanomcytic lesions: activation of the ras gene seems to be associated with the nodular type of human malignant melanoma. J Cancer Res Clin Oncol 121:23–30

Jansen B, Wadl H, Inoue SA, Trulzsch B, Selzer E, Duchene M, Eichler HG, Wolff K, Pehamberger H (1995) Phosphorothiorate oligonucleotides reduce melanoma growth in a SCID-hu mouse model by a non-antisense mechanism. Antisense Res Dev 5:271–277

Jansen B, Wadl H, Brown D, Bryan R, Wolff K, Eichler HG, Pehamberger H (1996) Down-regulation of bcl-2 by antisense oligonucleotides reduces tumor size and improves chemosensitivity of human melanoma cells in SCID mice. J Invest Dermatol 107:469

Jansen B, Schlagbauer-Wadl H, Brown BD, Bryan RN, van Elsas A, Muller M, Wolff K, Eichler HG, Pehamberger H (1998) Bcl-2 antisense therapy chemosensitizes human melanoma in SCID mice. Nat Med 4:232–234

Kaplan JM, Yu Q, Piraino ST, Pennington SE, Shankara S, Woodworth LA, Roberts BL (1999) Induction of antitumor immunity with dendritic cells transduced with adenovirus vector-encoding endogenous tumor-associated antigens. J Immunol 163:699–707

Karp JE, Broder S (1995) Molecular foundations of cancer: New targets for intervention. Nature Med 1:309–320

Klatzmann D, Valery CA, Bensimon G, Marro B, Boyer O, Mokhtari K, Diquet B, Salzmann JL, Philippon J (1998) A phase I/II dose-escalation study of herpes simplex virus type 1 thymidine kinase "suicide" gene therapy for metastatic melanoma. Hum Gene Ther 9:2585–2604

Kong HL, Hecht D, Song W, Kovesdi I, Hackett NR, Yayon A, Crystal RG (1998) Regional suppression of tumor growth by in vivo transfer of a cDNA encoding a secreted form of the extracellular domain of flt-1 vascular endothelial growth factor receptor. Hum Gene Ther 9:823–833

Konstadoulakis MM, Vezeridis M, Hatziyianni E, Karakousis CP, Cole B, Bland KI, Wanebo HJ (1998) Molecular oncogene markers and their significance in cutaneous malignant melanoma. Ann Surg Oncol 5:253–260

Kovacsovics-Bankowski M, Rock KL (1995) A phagosome-to-cytosol pathway for exogenous antigens presented on MHC class I molecules. Science 267:243–246

Legha SS, Ring S, Eton O, Bedikian A, Buzaid AC, Plager C, Papadopoulos N (1998) Development of a biochemotherapy regimen with concurrent administration of cisplatin, vinblastine, dacarbazine, interferon-α, and interleukin 2 for patients with metastatic melanoma. J Clin Oncol 16:1752–1759

Lehner B, Schlag P, Liebrich W, Schirrmacher V (1990) Post-operative active specific immunization in curatively resected colorectal cancer patients with a virus-modified autologous tumor cell vaccine. Cancer Immunol Immunother 32:173–178

Leonetti C, Biroccio A, Candiloro A, Citro G, Fornari C, Mottolese M, Del Bufalo D, Zupi G (1999) Increase of cisplatin sensitivity by c-myc antisense oligodeoxynucleotides in a human metastatic melanoma inherently resistant to cisplatin. Clin Cancer Res 5:2588–2595

Liebrich W, Schlag P, Manasterski M, Lehner B, Stohr M, Moller P, Schirrmacher V (1991) In vitro and clinical characterization of a Newcastle disease virus-modified autologous tumor cell vaccine for treatment of colorectal cancer patients. Eur J Cancer 27:703–710

Lindenmann J, Klein PA (1967) Viral oncolysis: Increased immunogenicity of host cell antigen associated with influenza virus. J. Exp. Med. 126:93–108

Longstreth JD, Lea CS, Kripke ML (1992) Ultraviolet radiation and other putative causes of melanoma. In: Cutaneous melanoma, 2nd ed. Balch CM, Houghton AN, Milton GW, Sober AJ, Soong SJ (eds). J.B. Lippincott Company, Philadelphia, p. 46

Lukas J, Parry D, Aagaard L, Mann DJ, Bartkova J, Strauss M, Peters G, Bartek J (1995) Retinoblastoma-protein-dependent cell-cycle inhibition by the tumor suppressor p16. Nature 375:503–506

Maass G, Schmidt W, Berger M, Schilcher F, Koszik F, Schneeberger A, Stingl G, Birnstiel ML, Schweighoffer T (1995) Priming of tumor-specific T cells in the draining lymph nodes after immunization with IL-2-secreting tumor cells: three consecutive stages may be required for successful tumor vaccination. Proc Natl Acad Sci USA 92:5540–5544

Machein MR, Risau W, Plate KH (1999) Antiangiogenic gene therapy in a rat glioma model using a dominant negative vascular endothelial growth factor receptor 2. Hum Gene Ther 10:1117–1128

Mao L, Merlo A, Bedi G, Shapiro GI, Edwards CD, Rollins BJ, Sidransky D (1995) A novel p16 INK4a transcript. Cancer Res 55:2995–2997

Marchand M, van Baren N, Weynants P, Brichard V, Dreno B, Tessier MH, Rankin E, Parmiani G, Arienti F, Humblet Y, Bourlond A, Vanwijck R, Lienard D, Beauduin M, Dietrich PY, Russo V, Kerger J, Masucci G, Jager E, De Greve J, Atzpodien J, Brasseur F, Coulie PG, van der Bruggen P, Boon T (1999) Tumor regressions observed in patients with metastatic melanoma treated with an antigenic peptide encoded by gene MAGE-3 and presented by HLA-A1. Int J Cancer 80:219–230

Mayordomo JI, Zorina T, Storkus WJ, Zitvogel L, Celluzzi C, Falo LD, Melief CJ, Ildstad ST, Kast WM, Deleo AB, Lotze MT (1995) Bone-marrow-derived dendritic cells pulsed with synthetic tumour peptides elicit protective and therapeutic antitumour immunity. Nature Med 1:1297–1302

McCabe BJ, Irvine KR, Nishimura MI, Yang JC, Spiess PJ, Shulman EP, Rosenberg SA, Restifo NP (1995) Minimal determinant expressed by a recombinant vaccinia virus elicits therapeutic antitumor cytolytic T lymphocyte responses. Cancer Res 55:1741–1747

McDonnell WM, Askari FK (1996) DNA Vaccines. N Engl J Med 334:42–45

Millauer B, Shawver LK, Plate KH, Risau W, Ullrich A (1994) Glioblastoma growth inhibited in vivo by a dominant-negative flk-1 mutant. Nature 367:576–579

Mölling K, Strack B, Nawrath M, Heinrich J, Döhring C, Wagner SN, Pavlovic J (1997) Development of a DNA vaccine against malignant melanoma. In: Strategies for Immunointerventions in Dermatology. Burg G, Dummer RG (eds). Springer, Berlin, p. 195

Monia BP, Johnston JF, Geiger T, Muller M, Fabbro D (1996) Antitumor activity of phosphorothiorate antisense oligodeoxynucleotide targeted against C-raf kinase. Nature Med 2:668–675

Moolten FL (1986) Tumor chemosensitivity conferred by inserted herpes simplex thymidine kinase genes: paradigm for a prospective cancer control strategy. Cancer Res. 46:5276–5281

Moolten FL (1994) Drug sensitivity ("suicide") genes for selective cancer chemotherapy. Cancer Gene Ther 1:279–287

Morton DL, Foshag LJ, Hoon DS, Nizze JA, Famatiga E, Wanek LA, Chang C, Davtyan DG, Gupta RK, Elashoff R, Irie RF (1992) Prolongation of survival in metastatic melanoma after specific immunotherapy with a new polyvalent melanoma vaccine. Ann Surg 216:463–482

Nabel GJ, Nabel EG, Yang ZY, Fox BA, Plautz GE, Gao X, Huang L, Shu S, Gordon D, Chang AE (1993) Direct gene-transfer with DNA liposome complexes in melanoma: expression, biologic activity, and lack of toxicity in humans. Proc Natl Acad Sci USA 90:11307–11311

Nestle FO, Alijagic S, Gilliet M, Sun Y, Grabbe S, Dummer R, Burg G, Schadendorf D (1998) Vaccination of melanoma patients with peptide- or tumor lysate-pulsed dendritic cells. Nature Med 4:328–332

Nobori T, Miura K, Wu DJ, Lois A, Takabayashi K, Carson DA (1994) Deletions of the cyclin-dependent kinase-4 inhibitor gene in multiple human cancers. Nature 368:753–756

Orfanos CE, Jung EG, Rassner G, Wolff HH, Garbe C (1994) Position and recommendations of the Malignant Melanoma Committee of the German Society of Dermatology on diagnosis, treatment and after-care of malignant melanoma of the skin. Status 1993/94. Hautarzt 45:285–291

Osanto S, Brouwenstyn N, Vaessen N, Figdor CG, Melief CJ, Schrier PI (1993) Immunization with interleukin-2 transfected melanoma cells. A phase I-II study in patients with metastatic melanoma. Hum Gene Ther 4:323–330

Overwijk WW, Tsung A, Irvine KR, Parkhurst MR, Goletz TJ, Tsung K, Carroll MW, Liu C, Moss B, Rosenberg SA, Restifo NP (1998) gp100/Pmel17 is a murine tumor rejection antigen: induction of self-reactive, tumoricidal T cells using high affinity, altered peptide ligand. J Exp Med 188:277–286

Overwijk WW, Lee DS, Surman DR, Irvine KR, Touloukian CE, Chan CC, Carroll MW, Moss B, Rosenberg SA, Restifo NP (1999) Vaccination with a recombinant vaccinia virus encoding a "self" antigen induces autoimmune vitiligo and tumor cell destruction in mice: requirement for CD4+ T lymphocytes. Proc Natl Acad Sci 96:2982–2987

Pan ZK, Ikonomidis G, Lazenby A, Pardoll D, Paterson Y (1995) A recombinant Listeria monocytogenes vaccine expressing a model tumor antigen protects mice against a lethal tumor challenge and causes regression of established tumors. Nat Med 1:471–477

Pardoll DM (1994) Tumour antigens: A new look for the 1990s. Nature 369:357

Park BJ, Brown CK, Hu Y, Alexander HR, Horti J, Raje S, Figg WD, Bartlett DL (1999) Augmentation of melanoma-specific gene expression using a tandem melanocyte-specific enhancer results in increased cytotoxicity of the purine nucleoside phophorylase gene in melanoma. Hum Gene Ther 10:889–898

Pfeifer JD, Wick MJ, Roberts RL, Findlay K, Normark SJ, Harding CV (1993) Phagocytic processing of bacterial antigens for class I MHC presentation to T cells. Nature 361:359–362

Porgador A, Brenner B, Vadai E, Feldman M, Eisenbach L (1991) Immunization by γ-IFN-treated B16-F10.9 melanoma cells protects against metastatic spread of the parental tumor. Int J Cancer 6:S54–s61

Porgador A, Tzehoval E, Katz A, Vadai E, Revel M, Feldman M, Eisenbach L (1992) Interleukin 6 gene transfection into Lewis lung carcinoma tumor cells suppresses the malignant phenotype and confers immunotherapeutic competence against parental metastatic cells. Cancer Res 52:3679–3686

Putney SD, Brown J, Cucco C, Lee R, Skorski T, Leonetti C, Geiser T, Calabretta B, Zupi G, Zon G (1999) Enhanced anti-tumor effects with microencapsulated c-myc antisense oligonucleotide. Antisense Nucleic Acid Drug Dev 9:451–458

Rammensee HG, Falk K, Rötzschke O (1993) MHC molecules as peptide receptors. Curr Opin Immunol 5:35–44

Restifo NP, Bacik I, Irvine KR, Yewdell JW, McCabe BJ, Anderson RW, Eisenlohr LC, Rosenberg SA, Bennink JR (1995) Antigen processing in vivo and the elicitation of primary CTL responses. J Immunol 154:4414–4422

Rigel DS, Friedman RJ, Kopf AW (1996) The incidence of malignant melanoma in the United States: Issues as we approach the 21st century. J Am Acad Dermatol 34:839–47

Rock KL, Gamble S, Rothstein L (1990) Presentation of exogenous antigen with class I major histocompatibility complex molecules. Science 249:918–921

Romani N, Gruner S, Brang D, Kampgen E, Lenz A, Trockenbacher B, Konwalinka G, Fritsch PO, Steinman RM, Schuler G (1994) Proliferating dendritic cell progenitors in human blood. J Exp Med 180:83–93

Rosenberg SA, Packard BS, Aebersold PM, Solomon D, Topalian SL, Toy ST, Simon P, Lotze MT, Yang JC, Seipp CA, Simpson C, Carter C, Bock S, Schwartzentruber D, Wie JP, White DE (1988) Use of tumor-infiltrating lymphocytes and interleukin-2 in the immunotherapy of patients with metastatic melanoma. N Engl J Med 319:1676–1680

Rosenberg SA, Aebersold P, Cornetta K, Kasid A, Morgan RA, Moen R, Karson EM, Lotze MT, Yang JC, Topalian SL, Merino MJ, Culver K, Miller D, Blaese M, Anderson WF (1990) Gene transfer into humans – immunotherapy of patients with advanced melanoma, using tumor-infiltrating lymphocytes modified by retroviral gene transduction. N Engl J Med 323:570–578

Rosenberg SA, Yang JC, Topalian SL, Schwartzentruber DJ, Weber JS, Parkinson DR, Seipp CA, Einhorn JH, White DE (1994) Treatment of 283 consecutive patients with metastatic melanoma or renal cell cancer using high-dose bolus interleukin 2. JAMA 271:907–913

Rosenberg SA, Zhai Y, Yang JC, Schwartzentruber DJ, Hwu P, Marincola FM, Topalian SL, Restifo NP, Seipp CA, Einhorn JH, Roberts B, White DE (1998) Immunizing patients with metastatic melanoma using recombinant adenoviruses encoding MART-1 or gp100 melanoma antigens. J Natl Cancer Inst 90:1894–1900

Ross DA, Wilson GD (1998) Expression of c-myc oncoprotein represents a new prognostic marker in cutaneous melanoma. Br J Surg 85:46–51

Ross G, Erickson R, Knorr D, Motulsky AG, Parkman R, Samulski J, Straus SE, Smith BR (1996) Gene therapy in the United States: a five-year status report. Hum Gene Ther 7:1781–1790

Roth JA, Nguyen D, Lawrence DD, Kemp BL, Carrasco CH, Ferson DZ, Hong WK, Komaki R, Lee JJ, Nesbitt JC, Pisters KM, Putnam JB, Schea R, Shin DM, Walsh GL, Dolormente MM, Han CI, Martin FD, Yen N, Xu K, Stephens LC, McDonnell TJ, Mukhopadhyay T, Cai D (1996) Retrovirus-mediated wild-type p53 gene transfer to tumors of patients with lung cancer. Nat Med 2:985–991

Rötzschke O, Falk K, Deres K, Schild H, Norda M, Metzger J, Jung G, Rammensee HG (1990) Isolation and analysis of naturally processed viral peptides as recognized by cytotoxic T cells. Nature 348:252–254

Rouse RJ, Nair SK, Lydy SL, Bowen JC, Rouse BT (1994) Induction in vitro of primary cytotoxic T-lymphocyte responses with DNA encoding herpes simplex virus proteins. J Virol 68:5685–5689

Saleh M, Stacker SA, Wilks AF (1996) Inhibition of growth of C6 glioma cells in vivo by expression of antisense vascular endothelial growth factor sequence. Cancer Res 56:393–401

Sato Y, Koshita Y, Hirayama M, Matuyama T, Wakimoto H, Hamada H, Nitsu Y (1996) Augmented antitumor effects of killer cells induced by tumor necrosos factor gene-transduced autologous tumor cells from gastrointestinal cancer patients. Hum Gene Ther 7:1895–1905

Schlagbauer-Wadl H, Griffioen M, van Elsas A, Schrier PI, Pustelnik T, Eichler HG, Wolff K, Pehamberger H, Jansen B (1999) Influence of increased c-myc expression on the growth characteristics of human melanoma. J Invest Dermatol 112:332–336

Schneeberger A, Koszik F, Schmidt W, Kutil R, Stingl G (1999a) The tumorigenicity of IL-2 gene-transfected murine M-3D melanoma cells is determined by the magnitude and quality of the host defense reaction: NK cells play a major role. J Immunol 162:6650–6657

Schneeberger A, Lührs P, Kutil R, Schild H, Steinlein P, Stingl G (1999b) Dendritic cells function as antigen-presenting cells in GM-CSF-based melanoma vaccines. J Invest Dermatol 112:523

Schreiber S, Kampgen E, Wagner E, Pirkhammer D, Trcka J, Korschan H, Lindemann A, Dorffner R, Kittler H, Kasteliz F, Kupcu Z, Sinski A, Zatloukal K, Buschle M, Schmidt W, Birnstiel M, Kempe RE, Voigt T, Weber HA, Pehamberger H, Mertelsmann R, Brocker EB, Wolff K, Stingl G (1999) Immunotherapy of metastatic malignant melanoma by a vaccine consisting of autologous interleukin 2-transfected cancer cells: outcome of a phase I study. Hum Gene Ther 10:983–993

Schreurs MW, de Boer AJ, Figdor CG, Adema GJ (1998) Genetic vaccination against the melanocyte differentiation antigen gp100 induces cytotoxic T lymphocyte-mediated tumor protection. Cancer Res 58:2509–2514

Shimizu Y, Fujiwara H, Ueda S, Wakamiya N, Kato S, Hamaoka T (1984) The augmentation of tumor-specific immunity by virus help: II. Enhanced induction of cytotoxic T lymphocyte and antibody responses to tumor antigens by vaccinia virus-reactive helper T-cells. Eur J Immunol 14:839–843

Shivers SC, Wang X, Li W, Joseph E, Messina J, Glass LF, DeConti R, Cruse CW, Berman C, Fenske NA, Lyman GH, Reintgen DS (1998) Molecular staging of maligant melanoma. Correlation with clinical outcome. JAMA 280:1410–1415

Soiffer R, Lynch T, Mihm M, Jung K, Rhuda C, Schmollinger JC, Hodi FS, Liebster L, Lam P, Mentzer S, Singer S, Tanabe KK, Cosimi AB, Duda R, Sober A, Bhan A, Daley J, Neuberg D, Parry G, Rokovich J, Richards L, Drayer J, Berns A, Clift S, Dranoff G, et al (1998) Vaccination with irradiated autologous melanoma cells engineered to secrete human granulocyte-macrophage colony-stimulating factor generates potent antitumor immunity in patients with metastatic melanoma. Proc Natl Acad Sci USA 95:13141–13146

St Clair MH, Lambe CU, Furman PA (1987) Inhibition by ganciclovir of cell growth and DNA synthesis of cells biochemically transformed with herpesvirus genetic information. Antimicrob Agents Chemother 31:844–849

Steinman RM (1991) The dendritic cell system and its role in immunogenicity. Annu Rev Immunol 9:271–296

Steitz J, Bruck J, Steinbrink K, Enk A, Knop J, Tüting T (2000) Genetic immunization of mice with human tyrosinase-related protein 2: implications for the immunotherapy of melanoma. Int J Cancer 86:89–94

Stingl G, Bergstresser PR (1995) Dendritic cells: A major story unfolds. Immunol Today 16:330–333

Stingl G, Brocker EB, Mertelsmann R, Wolff K, Schreiber S, Kampgen E, Schneeberger A, Dummer W, Brennscheid U, Veelken H, Birnstiel ML, Zatloukal K, Schmidt W, Maass G, Wagner E, Baschle M, Giese M, Kempe ER, Weber HA, Voigt T (1996) Phase I study to the immunotherapy of metastatic malignant melanoma by a cancer vaccine consisting of autologous cancer cells transfected with the human IL-2 gene. Hum Gene Ther 7:551–563

Strobl H, Riedl E, Scheinecker C, Bello-Fernandez C, Pickl WF, Rappersberger K, Majdic O, Knapp W (1996) TGFβ promotes in vitro development of dendritic cells from CD34+ hematopoietic progenitors. J Immunol 157:1499–1507

Strunk D, Rappersberger K, Egger C, Strobl H, Kromer E, Elbe A, Maurer D, Stingl G (1996) Generation of human dendritic cells/Langerhans cells from circulating CD34+ hematopoietic progenitor cells. Blood 87:1292–1302

Sullivan SM (1994) Development of ribozymes for gene therapy. J Invest Dermatol 103:85 S–89 S

Tanaka T, Cao Y, Folkman J, Fine HA (1998) Viral vector-targeted antiangiogenic gene therapy utilizing and angiostatin complementary DNA. Cancer Res. 58:3362–3369

Tanaka T, Manome Y, Wen P, Kufe DW, Fine HA (1997) Viral vector-mediated transduction of a modified platelet factor 4 cDNA inhibits angiogenesis and tumor growth. Nat Med 3:437–442

Tascon RE, Colston MJ, Ragno S, Stavropoulos E, Gregory D, Lowrie DB (1996) Vaccination against tuberculosis by DNA injection. Nat Med 2:888–892

Thomas KA (1996) Vascular endothelial growth factor, a potent and selective angiogenic agent. J Cell Biol 271:603–606

Thurner B, Haendle I, Roder C, Dieckmann D, Keikavoussi P, Jonuleit H, Bender A, Maczek C, Schreiner D, von den Driesch P, Bröcker EB, Steinman RM, Enk A, Kämpgen E, Schuler G (1999) Vaccination with Mage-3A1 peptide-pulsed mature, monocyte-derived dendritic cells expands specific cytotoxic T cells and induces regression of some metastases in advanced stage IV melanoma. J Exp Med 190:1669–1678

Toes RE, Blom RJ, Offringa R, Kast WM, Melief CJ (1996) Functional deletion of tumor-specific CTLs induced by peptide vaccination can lead to the inability to reject tumors. J Immunol 156:3911–3918

Ulmer JB, Donnelly JJ, Parker SE, Rhodes GH, Felgner PL, Dwarki VJ, Gromkowski SH, Deck RR, DeWitt CM, Friedman A, Hawe LA, Leander KR, Martinez D, Perry HC, Shiver JW, Montgomery DL, Liu MA (1993) Heterologous protection against influenza by injection of DNA encoding a viral protein. Science 259:1745–1749

van 't Veer LJ, Burgering BM, Versteeg R, Boot AJ, Ruiter DJ, Osanto S, Schrier PI, Bos JL (1989) N-ras mutations in human cutaneous melanoma from sun-exposed body sites. Mol Cell Biol 9:3114–3116

Veelken H, Mackensen A, Lahn M, Kohler G, Becker D, Franke B, Brennscheidt U, Kulmburg P, Rosenthal FM, Keller H, Hasse J, Schultze-Seemann W, Farthmann EH, Mertelsmann R, Lindemann A (1997) A phase I clinical study of autologous tumor cells plus interleukin-2-gene-transfected allogeneic fibroblasts as a vaccine in patients with cancer. Int J Cancer 70:269–277

Vile RG, Hart IR (1993) Use of tissue-specific expression of the herpes simplex thymidine kinase gene to inhibit growth of established murine melanomas following direct intratumoral injection of DNA. Cancer Res 53:3860–3864

Vile RG, Nelson JA, Castleden S, Chong H, Hart IR (1994) Systemic gene therapy of murine melanoma using tissue specific expression of the HSVtk gene involves an immune component. Cancer Res 54:6628–6634

Wagner SN, Ockenfels HM, Wagner C, Hofler H, Goos M (1995) Ras gene mutations: a rare event in nonmetastatic primary malignant melanoma. J Invest Dermatol 104:868–871

Wagner SN, Wagner C, Briedigkeit L, Goos M (1998) Homozygous deletion of the p16INK4a and the p15INK4b tumour suppressor genes in a subset of human sporadic cutaneous malignant melanoma. Br J Dermatol 138:13–21

Wang M, Bronte V, Chen PW, Gritz L, Panicali D, Rosenberg SA, Restifo NP (1995) Active immunotherapy of cancer with a nonreplicating recombinant fowlpox virus encoding a model tumor-associated antigen. J Immunol 154:4685–4692

Weber LW, Bowne WB, Wolchok JD, Srinivasan R, Qin J, Moroi Y, Clynes R, Song P, Lewis JJ, Houghton AN (1998) Tumor immunity and autoimmunity induced by immunization with homologous DNA. J Clin Invest 102:1258–1264

Weinstat-Saslow DL, Zabrenetzky VS, VanHoutte K, Frazier WA, Roberts DD, Steeg PS (1994) Transfection of thrombospondin 1 complementary DNA into a human breast carcinoma cell line reduces primary tumor growth, metastatic potential, and angiogenesis. Cancer Res 54:6504–6511

Whitton JL, Sheng N, Oldstone MB, McKee TA (1993) A "string-of-beads" vaccine, comprising linked minigenes, confers protection from lethal-dose virus challenge. J Virol 67:348–352

Wolff JA, Malone RW, Williams P, Chong W, Acsadi G, Jani A, Felgner PL (1990) Direct gene transfer into mouse muscle in vivo. Science 247:1465–1468

Yonish-Rouach E, Resnitzky D, Lotem J, Sachs L, Kimchi A, Oren M (1991) Wild-type p53 induces apoptosis of myeloid leukemic cells that is inhibited by interleukin-6. Nature 352:345–347

Zatloukal K, Schneeberger A, Berger M, Schmidt W, Koszik F, Kutil R, Cotten M, Wagner E, Buschle M, Maass G, Payer E, Stingl G, Birnstiel ML (1995) Elicitation of a systemic and protective anti-melanoma immune response by an IL-2-based vaccine: assessment of critical cellular and molecular parameters. J Immunol 154:3406–3419

Zhai Y, Yang JC, Kawakami Y, Spiess P, Wadsworth SC, Cardoza LM, Couture LA, Smith AE, Rosenberg SA (1996) Antigen-specific tumor vaccines. Development and characterization of recombinant adenovirus encoding MART1 or gp100 for cancer therapy. J Immunol 156:700–710

Zinkernagel RM, Doherty PC (1974) Restriction of in vitro T cell-mediated cytotoxicity in lymphocytic choriomeningitis within a syngeneic or semiallogeneic system. Nature 248:701–702

15   Prophylactic and Therapeutic DNA Vaccines Against Infectious Disease

J. E. Kallman, H. C. Maguire Jr, J. S. Yang,
J. J. Kim, D. B. Weiner

Introduction

The skin is the largest as well as the most accessible organ of the human body.
It has a unique population of resident antigen-presenting cells (Langerhans cells)
and, in addition, a specific subset of circulating T cells homes to the skin. The
skin is the target organ for most live attenuated vaccines as well as for the majority of vaccines whose immunogen is based on killed microbes, microbiologi-
cal extracts or recombinant proteins.

DNA vaccines can be delivered to the skin topically, by conventional injection
techniques, or by gene gun (shooting of minute amounts of DNA covered onto
metallic particles into the epidermis and superficial dermis). The field of DNA
vaccination is less than a decade old. Relevant mechanisms are poorly understood and optimum immunization methods remain to be defined. It is the purpose of this chapter to review past and present findings and to indicate likely future directions in the development of DNA vaccines against infectious disease.

Background

Vaccines arguably constitute the greatest achievement of modern medicine. They
have eradicated smallpox, pushed polio to the brink of extinction, and spared
countless people from typhus, tetanus, measles, and many other dangerous infections. However, many deadly or debilitating infectious diseases have evaded successful vaccine development because standard immunization methods targeted
against them work poorly or pose unacceptable risks. These illnesses include
malaria, AIDS, herpes simplex and hepatitis C.

Standard vaccines vary in the kind and duration of protection they provide.
Those based on killed pathogens (such as the hepatitis A and the injected polio
vaccines) or on antigens derived from disease-causing agents (such as the hepatitis B subunit vaccine) generally do not make their way into cells. They give
rise to a predominantly humoral response and do not activate cytotoxic T lymphocytes (CTLs). Such responses are ineffective against many of the microorgan-

isms that act intracellularly. In addition, the protection they confer often diminishes over time, necessitating periodic booster doses. Attenuated live vaccines (such as the measles, mumps, rubella, oral polio, and smallpox vaccines) do enter cells and make antigens that are displayed by the infected cells. Thereby, they stimulate CTL as well as specific antibodies. The dual activity involving the cellular and humoral arms of the immune system is essential for blocking infections by many viruses and for ensuring immunity when an isolated humoral response is insufficient. Live vaccines can frequently confer lifelong immunity, making them a "gold standard" among vaccines. However, they are not without drawbacks: they can induce full-blown infection in immunocompromised patients and can mutate to restore their virulence.

DNA vaccination represents a novel approach for inducing immunity. While it has been known for about a decade that delivery of naked DNA into an animal can lead to in vivo gene expression (Chattergoon et al. 1997), it was not until 1992 that such expression was appreciated as an approach for vaccine development. The concept behind genetic immunization is a simple one: genes encoding an antigen or antigens specific for a particular pathogen are cloned into a DNA plasmid with an appropriate promoter, and the plasmid is administered to the vaccine recipient, typically by intradermal or intramuscular injection. Host cells take up the DNA, the gene is expressed, and the resulting foreign protein is processed and presented to the immune system, inducing a specific immune response. This leads to a CTL response via the MHC class I-restricted pathway. Simultaneously, some of the produced protein is released extracellularly. The exogenously released antigen induces a humoral response; in addition, a helper T lymphocyte (Th) response, via MHC class II-restricted antigen presentation by antigen-presenting cells (APCs) which have taken up the foreign antigen, is also induced. Thus, DNA vaccines elicit protective immunity against a pathogen by both the cellular and humoral arms of the immune system. Successful long-term immunization is associated with the generation of long-lasting B and T cytotoxic memory cells.

DNA vaccination offers the same broad immunologic advantages as immunization with live, attenuated microorganisms, without the accompanying safety concerns associated with live infection: concerns that include vaccine reversion to more virulent forms, aggressive infection in immunocompromised hosts, and spread of the infectious vaccine to unintended populations. DNA vaccines are also attractive from an economic point of view: they are easy and inexpensive to manufacture in large quantities and require no special transportation or storage conditions.

Skin as a Target Organ

While DNA vaccines have been delivered experimentally to a number of target tissues, including mucosa, muscle, lung, and liver, skin remains a particularly attractive target organ. Skin is extremely accessible with a large target area, facilitating the delivery of exogenous DNA. Additionally, the inoculation site can be monitored for adverse reactions and, if necessary, even biopsied or removed in its entirety.

Skin contains specialized cells that enhance immune responses, cells which are notably absent in many other potential target tissues. Keratinocytes, for example, produce interleukin-1 and tumor necrosis factor alpha, factors known to play a role in lymphocyte, macrophage, and dendritic cell activation (Kupper 1990). The Langerhans' cells of the epidermis carry antigens from the skin to the draining regional lymph nodes; antigen-loaded Langerhans' cells are potent activators of naïve T cells. A special subset of circulating T cells homes to the skin and plays a critical role in cutaneous immunity. Dendritic cells and macrophages of the dermis can also take up antigen and initiate an immune response. Thus, in vivo transfection of epidermal and dermal cells provides an efficient means for DNA vaccination.

DNA-transfected cells expressing foreign antigens, whether within the skin or elsewhere in the body, may become targets for immune attack, leading to local inflammation and, potentially, a curtailment of antigen expression. However, the epidermis expresses high levels of lipocortin, a known natural inhibitor of inflammation which may help minimize a local inflammatory response (Raz et al. 1994).

Wounded skin may represent a special case for the delivery of genetic material. Raz and colleagues observed that abrasion of the skin with a plastic tuberculin Tine test coated with free DNA induced "a strong immune response." Eriksson and colleagues utilized a human tattoo device to introduce DNA into intact skin and partial thickness dermal wounds in swine and reported significantly higher levels of gene expression in wounded versus unwounded skin (Eriksson et al. 1998). These observations suggest that cells within the wound environment are more receptive to DNA uptake and expression. Similarly, gene gun mediated DNA transfection efficiencies have been observed by several investigators to be much higher than transfection efficiencies by needle injection, a difference which may be due in part to tissue trauma inflicted by the gene gun. Tissue damage may release mediators that facilitate uptake and expression of exogenous DNA. Alternatively, actively replicating cells within the wound environment may be more receptive to DNA inoculation. The increased gene expression efficiency in wounded versus intact skin remains unexplained: further investigation is required to elucidate possible mechanisms.

Methods of Introducing DNA into the Skin

Several methods have been employed to delivery DNA to the skin. These include topical application (Li and Hoffman, 1995, Fan et al. 1999, Yu et al. 1999), single needle injection (Raz et al. 1994, Hengge et al. 1995), gene gun mediated delivery (Williams et al. 1991, Andree et al. 1994), and microseeding (utilizing a tattoo needle device) (Ciernik et al. 1996, Eriksson et al 1998). In addition, variations on these methods including the supplemental use of pulsed electric fields or liposomes, have been used with varying degrees of success. While certain methods (notably gene gun and microseeding) have shown higher transfection efficiencies it is not clear that higher transfection efficiency results in a more profound immune response.

Topical application of naked DNA to mouse skin has been shown to induce expression and an immune response for both a marker gene, lacZ, and a foreign antigen, hepatitis B surface antigen (HBsAg) (Fan et al. 1999). Importantly, the skin must be stripped off its most superficial layer, the stratum corneum, prior to topical naked DNA application. The immune response induced was found to be 34% of that induced by intramuscular injection. Expression, however, was limited to cells of the hair follicle and no expression or immune response were observed when DNA was topically applied to mice lacking hair.

Zhang and colleagues used pulsed electric fields combined with mild external pressure to augment topical DNA delivery to skin and observed DNA expression at varying depths beneath the *stratum corneum* (Zhang et al. 1996). DNA encoding the reporter gene lacZ was applied topically to hairless mice followed by application of 3 exponential decay pulses of 120 V amplitude with a pulse length of 10 or 20 milliseconds over a period of one minute. After pulsing, pressure was applied for 1 minute or 10 minutes. Increasing pulse length and pressure duration correlated with an increasing depth of penetration of DNA beneath the skin surface. The maximum depth of penetration beneath the skin surface was 370 microns.

Cationic liposomes coated with DNA have been widely used for gene transfer, although primarily in in vitro studies (Felgner and Ringold 1989) This technique exploits the anionic properties of DNA, the character of cationic lipids and the negatively charged cell membrane. Cationic liposomes are prepared by dissolving lipid mixtures in chloroform, evaporating them to dryness, resuspending them in water and sonicating them. The liposomes are mixed with DNA resulting in a non-covalently bound liposome-DNA complex. Gene transfer, termed lipofection in this case, occurs when the liposome-DNA complex is applied topically to target cells. For example, in vivo topical application to mouse skin of liposomes carrying the lacZ reporter gene resulted in gene expression, again limited to the matrix of the hair follicle bulb (Li and Hoffman 1995). Domashenko and Cotsarelis observed expression limited to follicular cells in the anagen phase of the cell cycle following topical liposome-mediated DNA delivery (Domashenko and Cotsarelis 1999), an observation that may partially explain the low efficiencies observed after topical DNA application to normal skin (Fan et al. 1999). Hair plucking prior to application increased the number of follicular cells in anagen phase with a corresponding increase in transfection efficiency (Domashenko and Cotsarelis 1999). The main advantages of liposomes are that there are few constraints to the size of the gene that may be delivered and that liposomes, themselves, are relatively non-toxic. The ability to target liposomes to specific cells is also limited, although recent efforts focusing on the incorporation of tissue specific ligands into the liposomal membrane offers a means to circumvent this limitation.

Injection of plasmid DNA with hypodermic needles has been shown to result in gene expression in murine and porcine skin as well as in human skin grafted onto nude mice (Raz et al. 1994, Hengge et al. 1996). Hengge and colleagues have shown that human skin organ cultures and human skin grafts express injected DNA in the epidermis in a histological pattern similar to injected pig skin and pig skin organ culture (Hengge et al. 1996). In contrast to human and pig skin, where injected genes are expressed predominantly in the epidermis, mouse skin appears to take up and express injected naked plasmid DNA at multiple sites in the epidermis as well as in the underlying dermal fat, and muscle layers (Hengge et al. 1996). These results indicate that organ cultures can take-up and express injected DNA similar to skin injected in vivo. Furthermore, human skin expresses naked DNA after local injection in a pattern similar to that in pig skin, namely in the epidermis.

Gene gun mediated particle bombardment of the skin is a well established and highly efficient approach of DNA delivery to the skin. Microparticles made of gold or tungsten coated with DNA are accelerated by a force (e.g. electromagnetic field, pressurized helium) to penetrate cells and deliver the DNA. Many microparticles wind up in the extracellular space where they may be phagocytosed, but a significant number are delivered intracellularly. Bombardment of many tissues including skin, liver, pancreas, kidney, and muscle has resulted in detectable levels of gene product (Cheng et al. 1993). Multiple studies have reported that gene gun-mediated immunization is more efficient than needle injection, eliciting similar levels of antibody and cellular responses with 100 to 5000 times less DNA in mice (Wang et al. 1993, Pertmer et al. 1995, Feltquate et al. 1997). Pertmer and colleagues reported that as little as 16 ng of plasmid DNA delivered epidermally via gene gun could induce antibody and CTL responses in mice, while intradermal or intramuscular injection of the same plasmids required 10–100 μg of DNA to elicit comparable responses (Pertmer et al. 1995). Some investigators have raised concerns regarding the fate of the metallic particles, pointing out that recipient cells may have shortened lifespans, thus potentially limiting the effectiveness of inoculation (Ciernik et al. 1996).

Another, but less popular, approach for introducing naked DNA into skin is the use of the tattoo needle, termed microseeding. High frequency puncturing of the skin with fine short tattoo needles allows gene transfer of naked plasmid DNA and expression of reporter genes as well as induction of CTL. Ciernik and colleagues used the tattoo device to inoculate the skin of mice and showed significantly more efficient transfer when compared to topical application or single needle injection. In addition, they were able to stimulate a CTL immune response (Ciernik et al. 1996). The tattoo device has been used in intact skin as well as in wounds by Eriksson and colleagues who found the device giving higher expression levels when compared to single needle injection or particle-mediated bombardment. Additionally, they observed significantly higher expression in partial thickness skin wounds compared to intact skin, again suggesting that the wound environment represents a special case for the delivery of DNA. Human skin, while structurally similar to that of swine, differs from that of mice and the ability to deliver DNA using the tattoo device in humans remains untested (Eriksson ct al. 1998). A device providing better control of the frequency of the oscillating needles and optimization of needle length, diameter, and spacing might well yield even more efficient gene transfer. In addition, while Ciernik used sterile water as a solvent and Eriksson used saline, it is possible that other solvents or solvent additives, such as bupivicaine might further improve DNA delivery efficiency (Ciernik et al. 1996).

Mechanisms of Action

While the ability of DNA vaccination to induce immune responses has been well documented, the exact mechanism by which these responses occur is less clear. To be activated, each of the three arms of the immune system needs to encounter foreign protein in a different context: antibodies usually must bind to epitopes on protein molecules; CD4+ T cells primarily recognize peptide-MHC class II complexes on the surface of APCs that have endocytosed and processed exogenous foreign antigens; and CD8+ T cells are generally restricted to peptide-MHC class I complexes derived from endogenously produced protein which has undergone proteasome-dependent intracellular processing.

Pardoll and Beckerleg hypothesize two mechanisms by which DNA vaccines might induce an immune response: the first hypothesis proposes that antigen produced by inoculated cells such as myocytes in intramuscular inoculation is transferred to bone marrow-derived APCs which have infiltrated the inoculated tissue as part of an inflammatory response to the immunization procedure; the second hypothesis presumes that a small number of cells which express high levels of MHC class I and II molecules as well as costimulatory molecules, so-called "professional" APCs, are directly transfected with the inoculated DNA – these cells then migrate to regional lymphoid tissue, where they activate CD4+ T cells, B cells, and CD8+ T cells (Pardoll and Beckerleg 1995).

Corr and colleagues showed that responses to influenza nucleoprotein DNA vaccines were restricted to bone marrow-derived APCs (Corr et al. 1996). Similar findings using chimeric mice were reported for intramuscular immunization (Doe et al. 1996), and for epidermal gene gun immunization (Iwasaki et al. 1997b). These studies strongly suggested that bone marrow-derived cells are responsible for antigen presentation following genetic immunization, and that non-hematopoetic cells such as myocytes do not function as APCs.

More recent studies lend additional support to the "professional" APC hypothesis. For example, it has been shown that after intramuscular or intradermal immunization in mice, only dendritic cells derived from regional lymph nodes are capable of presenting antigenic epitopes to antigen-specific T cells. Injected plasmid DNA can be isolated from lymph node-derived and skin-derived dendritic cells following intramuscular and intradermal inoculation, showing that direct transfection of APCs does occur (Casares et al. 1997). In agreement with these findings, Weiner and colleagues have shown that mice inoculated intramuscularly with green fluorescent protein (GFP)-encoding plasmids produce green macrophages in the peripheral circulation but not in the spleen; the staining pattern was consistent with intracellular GFP expression, rather than phagocytosis of exogenous GFP. Furthermore, the transfected macrophages expressed high levels of CD86 (B7.2), indicating their activated state (Chattergoon et al. 1998). Another intriguing finding is that complete surgical ablation of injected muscle as soon as ten minutes after DNA immunization did not prevent the induction of antigen-specific antibody or CTL responses, and that these responses were no different in magnitude or longevity than those in mice whose muscle was not ablated (Torres et al. 1997). This result suggests that the injected myocytes play almost no role in inducing the immune response, not even as an "antigen factory" for antibody induction. However, this was not the case with epidermal gene gun immunization, where it was necessary for the inoculated skin to be intact for at least 72 hours in order to generate antibody and CTL responses comparable to those in mice whose skin was not removed. These findings suggest not only that different types of immune responses may be generated by immunization at different sites, but also that, at least in intramuscular immunization, some of the DNA itself may be rapidly carried by blood or lymph to distant sites, where the induction of an immune response can occur.

Means to Modulate Immune Responses

The immune response to a DNA vaccine can be manipulated by altering the conditions under which the vaccine is administered. These conditions include the presence or absence of immunostimulatory sequences, the method and route of immunization, the form of the immunogen, the immunization regimen, and the presence or absence of coadministered cytokines or costimulatory molecules. By modifying one or more of these conditions, investigators have been able to alter both the magnitude and orientation of the immune response, selectively enhancing antibody or cell-mediated responses by steering the Th response towards a particular subtype (Table 15.1). This susceptibility of DNA vaccine-induced immunity to manipulation is likely to play an important role in the rational design of DNA-based prophylactic vaccines.

Immunostimulatory Sequences

One aspect of genetic immunization that has recently received attention is the immunostimulatory activity of DNA itself (see also Chapter 11). It has been observed that DNA from bacteria, but not from vertebrates, can induce a nonspecific immune response, possibly due to differences in the frequency of unmethylated CpG dinucleotide complexes found in the two genomes. Krieg and colleagues showed in mice that oligonucleotides containing one or more CpG dinucleotides could trigger B cell proliferation and immunoglobulin secretion (Krieg 1996). These CpG dinucleotide sequences have been termed CpG motifs or immunostimulatory sequences (ISS). The relevance of these findings for genetic

Table 15.1. Comparison of Th_1 and Th_2 subtypes

	Th_1 subtype	Th_2 subtype
Associated cytokines	IL-2, IFN-γ	IL-4, IL-5, IL-10
Predominant isotype	IgG_1 (mouse)	IgG_2 (mouse)
Representative diseases	juvenile diabetes mellitus, contact dermatitis	Leishmaniasis, atopic dermatitis

immunization became clear when it was reported that a DNA vaccine whose plasmid backbone contained a CpG motif induced a more vigorous antibody and CTL response than an otherwise-identical vaccine which did not contain the same motif (Sato et al. 1996). The response to the vaccine lacking the ISS could be restored to normal levels by coinjecting it with noncoding plasmid containing ISS. Subsequent studies have confirmed that CpG motifs can enhance immunity following genetic immunization and can qualitatively modify the immune response by preferentially inducing a Th_1 response (Sato et al. 1996, Klinman et al. 1997, LeClerc et al. 1997, Roman et al. 1997, Horner et al. 1998, Hartmann et al. 1999, Krieg 1999, Pisetsky 1999). This phenomenon may be one reason why most DNA vaccines studied to date induce a predominantly Th_1 response when injected intramuscularly or intradermally. To date, these studies have been reported in small animal species; extension of these findings to larger animals, including primates, will provide important information for further development of this approach.

Method and Site of Immunization

A growing body of evidence suggests that both the site of inoculation and the method of plasmid delivery can affect the nature and degree of induced immunity in mice. Successful DNA vaccination has been demonstrated via a number of different routes, including intravenous, intramuscular, intranasal, intradermal, intravaginal (Fynan et al. 1993, Ulmer et al. 1993, Wang et al. 1993, Davis et al. 1994, Agadjanyan et al. 1997, Bagarazzi et al. 1997, Wang et al. 1997) and more recently, intrasplenic (Wolff 1997), and intrahepatic (Gerloni et al. 1997). The majority of DNA vaccine studies to date, however, have utilized either skin or muscle as their immunization targets. Plasmid delivery is usually accomplished by one of two methods: needle injection of DNA suspended in saline or in a saline mixture containing a facilitator, such as bupivacaine, designed to enhance DNA uptake; or gene gun mediated acceleration of DNA-coated microprojectiles directly into the cells of the target tissue. Both of these methods have been used in skin and muscle, although the gene gun has been more commonly used for epidermal rather than intramuscular administration. As previously mentioned, gene gun mediated DNA delivery has been shown to result in more efficient transfer of DNA to target tissues and enhanced immune response induction.

In addition to the quantitative differences in the responses induced by these different routes of immunization, there is growing evidence that the way a DNA vaccine is administered can also affect the Th cell profile that is generated. Upon activation, $CD4^+$ Th lymphocytes differentiate from precursor Th_0 cells into two functionally distinct subsets. Th_1 cells activate macrophages and induce cell-mediated immunity, including CTL responses, while Th_2 cells primarily induce humoral immunity. Intramuscular needle injection of DNA induces a predominantly Th_1-type response, with an elevated IgG_{2a}:IgG_1 ratio, IFN-γ production, and little IL-4 production (Xiang et al. 1995, Pertmer et al. 1996, Feltquate et al. 1997, Haensler et al. 1999). In contrast, epidermal gene gun inoculation generally induces a Th_2 phenotype with successive immunizations, generating mainly

IgG$_1$ antibodies, less IFN-γ, and more IL-4 (Fuller and Haynes 1994, Pertmer et al 1996, Feltquate et al. 1997). Intradermal injections of DNA have been reported to induce both, Th$_1$ and Th$_2$ profiles, while intramuscular gene gun inoculation seems to generate a profile similar to epidermal gene gun inoculation (Feltquate et al. 1997). The CTL response to both intramuscular and intradermal DNA vaccination is highly dependent upon the generation of CD4$^+$ T cell help via a class II MHC-dependent pathway (Maecker et al. 1999).

The primary immunization mode in some cases appears to irreversibly determine the profile produced, as subsequent DNA immunizations using the alternative method, subsequent immunizations using the protein encoded by the genetic vaccine, or even subsequent viral challenge were all unable to cause a shift from the originally induced Th profile (Pertmer et al. 1996, Raz et al. 1996, Feltquate et al. 1997). This profile can be shifted, however, through the coadministration of genes encoding various cytokines, a topic discussed in detail in the next section. Prayaga and colleagues demonstrated that the Th profile induced following epidermal gene gun immunization with a plasmid encoding HIV-1 gp120 or influenza nucleoprotein, normally of the Th$_2$ type, became more Th$_1$-like when mice were coimmunized with plasmids encoding IL-2, IL-7, or IL-12 (Prayaga et al. 1997). This suggests that the inherent bias of a particular immunization method can be overcome under certain conditions, allowing for greater manipulation of vaccines or immunotherapeutics towards whatever type of immune response is desired.

Cytoplasmic or Membrane-Bound Form of the Encoded Antigen

Genetic vaccination has successfully produced immune responses to proteins that are cytoplasmically sequestered (e.g. β-galactosidase), membrane-bound (e.g. rabies G protein), and secreted (e.g. hepatitis B surface antigen). It is possible that one form of a protein may be better at inducing an immune response than another: for example, a secreted antigen may be more effective at generating antibody and CD4$^+$ Th lymphocyte responses than one which is not secreted. This hypothesis, however, has so far not been borne out in experimental studies. Secreted forms of rabies G protein and HBsAg were no better at inducing humoral and cellular immunity than their membrane-bound counterparts in murine studies (Xiang et al. 1995, Chow et al. 1997), and the plasmid encoding the secreted rabies protein conferred less protection against lethal viral challenge than did the one encoding a membrane-bound antigen (Xiang et al. 1994). Though studies with other antigens are needed, it has not been shown that the form of the plasmid-encoded protein plays a critical role in DNA vaccine-induced immune responses.

Immunization Regimen

The optimal regimen for administering a DNA vaccine, especially the dose, number, and frequency of immunizations, is a subject of considerable debate. While most researchers would agree that multiple immunizations will likely be necessary to maximize immune responses, the exact dosing regimen has yet to be determined. These are important questions, however, as these factors have been shown to have an impact on the nature of the resulting immune response.

In a study using gene gun mediated delivery, immunization of mice with an HIV-1 env DNA vaccine induced strong CTL and weak antibody responses when one, two, or three immunizations were given, but a drop in CTL activity and a marked rise in antibody titers after a fourth immunization. This shift in the nature of the immune response was accompanied by a shift in cytokine production by antigen-stimulated splenocytes with declining IFN-γ and increasing IL-4 production (Fuller and Haynes 1994). A decline in IFN-γ production with successive immunizations has also been reported with an influenza nucleoprotein-encoding plasmid (Pertmer et al. 1996).

The timing of the immunizations may also affect the subsequent immune response: mice vaccinated twice with three months between injections generated much higher antibody titers and cytokine production than mice vaccinated two or three times at monthly intervals, suggesting that a longer rest period between immunizations enhances the response (Prayaga et al. 1997). Whether these findings will hold true for different disease models or different species remains to be seen.

Another way to modulate the immune response may be to use a regimen that combines genetic immunization with other, more traditional, types of immunization. For example, combining a DNA vaccine with a recombinant protein vaccine in a prime-boost regimen may elicit both a Th$_1$ and Th$_2$-type profile, thereby maximizing both cellular and humoral immunity to induce more complete protection. Weiner and colleagues have examined such a regimen in mice with a HIV-2 envelope DNA construct, and found that priming with DNA and boosting with protein significantly enhanced antibody and T cell proliferative responses and increased antibody neutralization activity compared with either approach alone (Agadjanyan et al. 1997). A prime-boost regimen using multiple doses of a HIV-1 env plasmid followed by a boost of HIV-1 env plasmid plus HIV-1 env protein has been evaluated in rhesus monkeys. This protocol induced strong CTL and neutralizing antibody activity in vaccinated animals and completely protected the animals from intravenous challenge with a chimeric SHIV virus expressing an HIV-1 envelope on a SIV backbone. Animals receiving either DNA or protein vaccination alone were not protected (Letvin et al. 1997). While this study used a large number of vaccinations (10) and a small number of animals, and therefore requires repeating, it nonetheless provides a glimpse of the potential power of DNA-protein vaccine combinations.

Cytokines

Of the different ways to modulate the immune response to DNA immunization, the most promising may be through the coadministration of biological adjuvants such as cytokines. Cytokines are molecules secreted mainly by bone marrow-derived cells that act in an autocrine or paracrine manner to induce a specific response in cells expressing the appropriate cytokine receptor. A number of laboratories have reported that coinjection of plasmids encoding cytokines can have a substantial effect on the immune response to plasmid-encoded antigen (Chattergoon et al. 1997).

IL-2 is a potent stimulator of cellular immunity which induces proliferation and differentiation of T cells and induces B cell and NK cell growth (Smith 1988, Janeway and Travers 1994). Chow and colleagues demonstrated that injection of a vector which encoded HBsAg and IL-2 on the same plasmid induced marked increases of antibody responses and T cell proliferation compared to a plasmid encoding HBsAg alone, and led to enhanced T cell production of IL-2 and IFN-γ (Chow et al. 1997). Similar results were reported for the HCV core protein by Geissler and colleagues who also showed augmented CTL responses with IL-2 gene coinjection (Geissler et al. 1997). Taken together, these results suggest that IL-2 gene coadministration can increase both humoral and cellular immunity to a plasmid-encoded antigen and enhance Th$_1$ cytokine production.

IL-4 induces differentiation of Th cells into the Th$_2$ subtype, enhances B cell growth, and mediates Ig class switching (Smith 1988, Swain et al. 1991). Injection of plasmid encoding IL-4 three days prior to immunization with a protein antigen increased antigen-specific antibody levels compared to protein immunization alone, but had no effect on the DTH response in antigen-challenged animals (Raz et al. 1993). Co-inoculation of mice with plasmids encoding IL-4 and the HCV core protein resulted in augmented antibody and T cell proliferation responses, but decreased specific CTL responses compared to HCV plasmid alone (Geissler et al. 1997). Likewise, intranasal administration of plasmids encoding HIV-1 env/rev and IL-4 in liposomes resulted in higher antibody responses but diminished DTH and CTL responses in mice (Okada et al. 1997). In a tumor challenge model, mice with established pulmonary metastases who received recombinant IL-4 protein following gene gun administration of a DNA vaccine encoding the appropriate tumor-associated antigen failed to demonstrate any reduction in the number of metastases, whereas mice who received recombinant IL-2, IL-6, IL-7, or IL-12 all had significant improvement in their respective tumor burden (Irvine et al. 1996). Thus, while IL-4 may enhance the humoral response following genetic immunization, its relative inhibition of Th$_1$-mediated responses may limit its usefulness as an adjuvant in viral or tumor immunotherapy.

Other cytokines that have been studied in concert with genetic immunization include GM-CSF and IL-12. GM-CSF increases the production of granulocytes and macrophages, and induces the maturation and activation of APCs such as dendritic cells (Morrissey et al. 1987, Heufler et al. 1988, Janeway and Travers 1994). In theory, co-expression of GM-CSF and a plasmid-encoded antigen could augment the host's immune response against the antigen by expanding the pool of activated APCs at the injection site. Xiang and Ertl tested this in vivo by co-inoculating mice with plasmids encoding GM-CSF and rabies glycoprotein (Xiang and Ertl 1995). Co-expression of GM-CSF increased antibody responses to rabies glycoprotein in a dose-dependent manner and enhanced Th cell responses compared with injection of rabies glycoprotein vector alone, whereas co-injection of the IFN-γ gene had no enhancing effect. GM-CSF also improved the efficacy of the rabies glycoprotein plasmid in protecting from a lethal virus challenge. Subsequent studies of GM-CSF plasmid co-inoculated with DNA vaccines against HIV-1 (Kim et al. 1997a), influenza (Iwasaki et al. 1997a), encephalomyocarditis virus (Sin et al. 1997) and HCV (Geissler et al. 1997) have confirmed the boosting effect that this cytokine has on both humoral and cellular responses to plasmid-encoded antigens. This effect may be dependent, however, on the route of immunization (Conry et al. 1996).

IL-12 is a prototypic Th_1 cytokine that is known to be a potent inducer of cellular immunity leading to production of IFN-γ and enhancement of NK and cytotoxic T cell activity (Gately et al. 1992, Trinchieri 1995). Kim and colleagues examined the effects of IL-12 gene coadministration on the immune response to plasmids encoding HIV-1 env, gag, pol, and two accessory proteins, nef and vif (Kim et al. 1997a). As expected, IL-12 induced a Th_1-type response with decreased antibody production and increased T cell proliferation as well as markedly enhanced CTL responses to all antigens. In fact, IL-12 codelivery could induce direct CTL activity in the absence of any preliminary in vitro stimulation. Iwasaki and colleagues demonstrated that co-immunization with an IL-12-encoding plasmid can convert a weak plasmid DNA immunogen into one that induces a strong CTL response (Iwasaki et al. 1997a). Other groups (Okada et al. 1997, Tsuji et al. 1997a) have confirmed this activity of IL-12 as a powerful inducer of cell-mediated immunity to DNA vaccines given intramuscularly or intranasally, although when given intranasally the suppression of humoral immunity was not seen (Okada et al. 1997). The effects of cytokine gene adjuvants on the modulation of protective immune responses to lethal HSV-2 challenges were also studied in a murine model (Sin et al. 1998). A DNA expression construct encoding the HSV-2 gD protein was co-delivered with plasmids encoding Th_1-type (IL-2, 12, 15, 18) and Th_2-type (IL-4, IL-10) cytokines and the vaccine modulatory effects were analyzed with regard to the resulting immune phenotype and the mortality and morbidity of the immunized animals following a lethal HSV challenge. It was observed that Th_1 cytokine gene (especially IL-12) co-administration not only enhanced the survival rate, but also reduced the frequency and severity of herpetic lesions following an intravaginal HSV challenge. On the other hand, co-injection with Th_2 cytokine genes increased the rate of mortality and morbidity in challenged mice.

Other cytokines have also been investigated as potential adjuvants for DNA vaccination. The proinflammatory cytokines IL-1, TNF-α, and TNF-β are important mediators of the host response to tissue injury or infection. When these cytokine genes were co-injected into mice with HIV-1 env or gag/pol plasmids, all three significantly boosted specific antibody responses compared to immunization with the HIV-1 plasmids alone. In addition, both TNF-α and TNF-β enhanced T cell proliferation. Another proinflammatory cytokine, TCA3, a chemotactic factor for monocytes, macrophages and neutrophils, has also been reported to increase Th and CTL activity when co-administered with a DNA vaccine, though it did not enhance antibody activity (Tsuji et al. 1997b). In another study, enhancement of antigen-specific Th cell proliferation was seen with TNF-α co-injections (Kim et al. 1998c). In addition, a significant enhancement of the CTL response was observed with the co-administration of TNF-α and IL-15 genes with HIV-1 DNA immunogens. These increases in CTL response were both MHC class I-restricted and CD8+ T cell-dependent.

Similar to cytokine gene co-delivery, the co-immunization with chemokine genes along with DNA immunogen constructs can modulate the direction and magnitude of induced immune responses (Kim et al. 1998a). Co-immunization with IL-8 and MIP-1 alpha genes increased the antibody response in a similar manner to IL-4 and GM-CSF co-immunization. In addition, co-injection with IL-8 and RANTES resulted in a dramatic enhancement of Th proliferation response. Among all combinations, RANTES and MCP-1 co-injections resulted in a high level of CTL enhancement, almost as significant as IL-12, a known CTL inducer for DNA vaccines.

Costimulatory Molecules

Another strategy for strengthening the effectiveness of genetic immunization is through the codelivery of genes for costimulatory molecules such as CD80 (B7.1), CD86 (B7.2), CD40, and CD40 ligand (CD40L) with the goal of improving the antigen-presenting capabilities of transfected cells.

CD80 and CD86 are expressed on APCs and deliver potent costimulatory signals, a necessary second signal, through CD28/CTLA-4 on T cells, resulting in activation of both $CD4^+$ and $CD8^+$ T cells (Linsley et al. 1990, June et al. 1994, Lanier et al. 1995). Studies in mice have shown that intramuscular injection of a CD86 gene expression cassette along with cassettes for the influenza nucleoprotein (Iwasaki et al. 1997a) or HIV-1 proteins (Kim et al. 1998b) results in a significant enhancement of CTL responses to the encoded antigen. This effect was seen when the CD86 gene was delivered in the same plasmid as the antigen gene or in a separate plasmid (unpublished data). The effect of CD80 is less clear-cut. Although codelivery of CD80 plasmids with viral protein plasmids have not demonstrated significant enhancement of immune responses (Iwasaki et al. 1997b, Kim et al. 1997b) two groups have reported that codelivery of CD80 with a tumor-associated antigen led to increased protection from subsequent tumor challenge (Conry et al. 1996, Corr et al. 1997). The reason for this difference in activity is not clear, but it has been suggested that CD80 and CD 86 may differentially induce T cells down the Th_1 or Th_2 pathway (Kuchroo et al. 1995).

It has been investigated whether the bone marrow-derived professional APCs or muscle cells were responsible for the enhancement of CTL responses following CD86 co-administration. Accordingly, CTL induction was analyzed in bone marrow chimeras. In vaccinated chimeras, we observed that only $CD86^+$ MHC class I^+ animals developed detectable CTLs and enhanced IFN-γ production in an antigen-specific manner as well as a dramatic tissue invasion of T cells. These results support that CD86 plays a central role in CTL induction in vivo enabling non-bone marrow derived cells to prime CTLs (Agadjanyan et al. 1999).

CD40 is a member of the TNF receptor superfamily and is expressed on B cells, monocytes, and dendritic cells (Alderson et al. 1993, Caux et al. 1994). CD40 ligand (CD40L or CD154) is not expressed on resting T cells, but is induced by CD3-TCR crosslinking during T cell activation. Activated T cells then stimulate CD40-bearing APCs to express molecules which facilitate antigen presentation to T cells, thereby enhancing antibody responses and proinflammatory cytokine production (Lane et al. 1992, Noelle et al. 1992, Ranheim and Kipps 1993, Kiener et al. 1995, Shu et al. 1995, Kato et al. 1996). Co-administration of CD40L with the DNA immunogen pLacZ has been shown to enhance antigen-specific humoral and cellular immune responses, particularly CTL responses (Mendoza et al. 1997).

The potential roles of adhesion molecules in the expansion of T cell-mediated immune responses in the periphery were also examined (Kim et al. 1999). It was observed that antigen-specific T cell responses can be enhanced by the co-expression of DNA immunogens and adhesion molecules ICAM-1 and LFA-3. Co-expression of ICAM-1 and LFA-3 molecules along with DNA immunogens resulted in a significant enhancement of Th cell proliferative responses. In addition, co-immunization with ICAM-1 (and more moderately with LFA-3) resulted in a dramatic enhancement of CD8-restricted CTL responses. These observations were further supported by the finding that co-injection with ICAM-1 dramatically enhanced the level of IFN-γ and β–chemokines MIP-1α, MIP-1β, and RANTES produced by stimulated T cells. Through comparative studies it was shown that ICAM-1/LFA-1 T cell costimulatory pathways are independent of CD86/CD28 pathways, and they may synergistically expand T cell responses in vivo.

Therapeutic Possibilities

Vaccination targets, almost by definition, tend to be infectious diseases. Indeed, some of the earliest experiments with DNA vaccines were targeted at influenza (Fynan et al. 1993, Ulmer et al. 1993) and HIV-1 (Fynan et al. 1993, Wang et al. 1993). Since then, genetic immunization has been investigated in numerous infectious disease models including hepatitis B (Davis et al. 1995), HIV-2 (Agadjanyan et al. 1997, Yasutomi et al. 1997), HSV-1 (Manickan et al. 1995), HSV-2 (Bourne et al. 1996), rabies (Xiang et al. 1994), hepatitis C (Geissler et al. 1997), tuberculosis (Lowrie et al. 1994), malaria (Mor et al. 1995), mycoplasma (Barry et al. 1995), leishmania major (Xu and Liew 1995), cytomegalovirus (Gonzales-Armas et al. 1996), toxoplasma gondii (Angus et al. 1996), rotavirus (Hermann et al. 1996), and most recently, ebola (Xu et al. 1998).

It may be possible to exploit the ability to induce an immune response in skin demonstrated by DNA vaccination to manipulate the immune system in other therapeutic ways. In addition to infectious disease applications, genetic immunization may have a potential use as a means of cancer immunotherapy. Many cancers have tumor specific markers; it may be possible to stimulate an immune response through DNA vaccination against such markers. In fact, injection of plasmid DNA encoding tumor-associated antigens has been shown to cause a tumor-antigen-specific immune response, and could protect mice from a lethal tumor challenge (Conry et al. 1995, Wang et al. 1995, Kim et al. 1998 d).

Tissue repair is another area in which DNA delivery may have therapeutic application (Eming et al. 1997). DNA delivery to wounded skin has been shown to occur with much higher efficiency than intact skin raising the possibility of DNA delivery to augment tissue repair in acute and chronic skin wounds or burns. Finally, as discussed elsewhere in this volume, gene delivery to skin is an active area of investigation by researchers involved in gene therapy directed at both cutaneous and systemic diseases.

References

Agadjanyan MG, Trivedi NN, Kudchodkar S, Bennett M, Levine W, Lin A, Boyer J, Levy D, Ugen KE, Kim JJ, Weiner DB (1997) An HIV type 2 DNA vaccine induces cross-reactive immune responses against HIV type 2 and SIV. AIDS Res Hum Retroviruses 13:1561–1571

Alderson MR, Armitage RJ, Tough TW, Strockbine L, Fanslow WC, Spriggs MK (1993) CD40 expression by human monocytes: regulation by cytokines and activation of monocytes by the ligand for CD40. J Exp Med 178:669–674

Andree C, Swain WF, Page CP, Macklin MD, Slama J, Hatzis D, Eriksson E (1994) In vivo transfer and expression of a human epidermal growth factor gene accelerates wound repair. Proc Natl Acad Sci USA 91:12 188–12 192

Angus CW, Klivington D, Wyman J, Kovacs JA (1996) Nucleic acid vaccination against Toxoplasma gondii in mice. J Eukaryotic Micro 43:117S

Bagarazzi ML, Boyer JD, Javadian MA Chattergoon M, Dang K, Kim G, Shah J, Wang B, Weiner DB (1997) Safety and immunogenicity of intramuscular and intravaginal delivery of HIV-1 DNA constructs to infant chimpanzees. J Med Primatol 26:27–33

Barry MA, Lai WC, Johnston SA (1995) Protection against mycoplasma infection using expression library immunization. Nature 377:632–635

Bourne N, Stanberry LR, Bernstein DI, Lew D (1996) DNA immunization against experimental genital herpes simplex virus infection. J Infect Dis 173:800–807

Casares S, Inaba K, Brumeanu TD, Steinman RM, Bona CA (1997) Antigen presentation by dendritic cells after immunization with DNA encoding a major histocompatibility complex class II-restricted viral epitope. J Exp Med 186:1481–1486

Caux C, Massacrier C, Vanbervliet B, Dubois B, Van Kooten C, Durand I, Banchereau J (1994) Activation of human dendritic cells through CD40 cross-linking. J Exp Med 180:1263–1272

Chattergoon M, Boyer J, Weiner DB (1997) Genetic immunization: a new era in vaccines and immune therapeutics. FASEB J 11:753–763

Chattergoon MA, Robinson TM, Boyer JD, Weiner DB (1998) Specific immune induction following DNA-based immunization through in vivo transfection and activation of macrophages. J Immunol 160:5707–5718

Cheng L, Ziegelhoffer PR, Yang NS (1993) In vivo promoter activity and transgene expression in mammalian somatic tissues evaluated by using particle bombardment. Proc Natl Acad Sci USA 90:4455–4459

Chow Y, Huang W, Chi W, Chu YD, Tao MH (1997) Improvement of hepatitis B virus DNA vaccines by plasmids coexpressing hepatitis B surface antigen and interleukin-2. J Virol 71:169–178

Ciernik IL, Krayenbuhl BH, Carbone DP (1996) Puncture-mediated gene transfer to skin. Hum Gene Ther 7:893–899

Conry R, LoBuglio A, Loechel F, Moore SE, Sumerel LA, Barlow DL, Pike J, Curiel DT (1995) A carcinoembryonic antigen polynucleotide vaccine for human clinical use. Cancer Gene Ther 2:33–38

Conry RM, Widera G, LoBuglio AF, Fuller JT, Moore SE, Barlow DL, Turner J, Yang NS, Curiel DT (1996) Selected strategies to augment polynucleotide immunization. Gene Ther 3:67–74

Corr M, Lee DJ, Carson DA, Tighe H (1996) Gene vaccination with naked plasmid DNA: mechanism of CTL priming. J Exp Med 184:1555–1560

Corr M, Tighe H, Lee D, Dudler J, Trieu M, Brinson DC, Carson DA (1997) Costimulation provided by DNA immunization enhances antitumor immunity. J Immunol 159:4999–5004

Davis HL, Michel ML, Mancini M, Schleef M, Whalen RG (1995) Direct gene transfer in skeletal muscle: plasmid DNA based immunization against the hepatitis B virus surface antigen. Vaccine 12:1503–1509

Doe B, Selby M, Barnett S, Baenziger J, Walker CM (1996) Induction of cytotoxic T lymphocytes by intramuscular immunization with plasmid DNA is facilitated by bone marrow-derived cells. Proc Nat Acad Sci USA 93:8578–8583

Domashenko A, Cotsarelis G (1999) Transfection of human hair follicles using topical liposomes is optimal at the onset of anagen. J Invest Dermatol 112:552

Eming SA, Morgan JR, Berger A (1997) Gene therapy for tissue repair: approaches and prospects. Brit J Plas Surg 50:491–500

Eriksson E, Yao F, Svensjo T, Winkler T, Slama J, Macklin MD, Andree C, McGregor M, Hinshaw V, Swain WF (1998) In vivo gene transfer to skin and wound by microseeding. J Surg Res 78:85–91

Fan H, Lin Q, Morrissey GR, Khavari PA (1999) Immunization via hair follicles by topical application of naked DNA to normal skin. Nat Biotechnol 17:870–872

Felgner PL, Ringold GM (1989) Cationic liposome-mediated transfection. Nature 337:387–388

Feltquate DM, Heaney S, Webster RG, Robinson HL (1997) Different T helper cell types and antibody isotypes generated by saline and gene gun DNA immunization. J Immunol 158:2278–2284

Fuller DH, Haynes JR (1994) A qualitative progression in HIV type 1 glycoprotein 120-specific cytotoxic cellualar and humoral immune responses in mice receiving a DNA-based glycoprotein 120 vaccine. AIDS Res Hum Retroviruses 10:1433–1441

Fynan EF, Webster RG, Fuller DH, Haynes JR, Santoro JC, Robinson HL (1993) DNA vaccines: protective immunizations by parenteral, mucosal and gene-gun inoculations. Proc Nat Acad Sci USA 90:11478–11482

Gately MK, Wolitzky AG, Quinn PM, Chizzonite R (1992) Regulation of human cytolytic lymphocyte responses by interleukin-12. Cell Immunol 143:127–142

Geissler M, Gesien A, Tokushige K, Wands JR (1997) Enhancement of cellular and humoral immune responses to hepatitis C virus core protein using DNA-based vaccines augmented with cytokine-expressing plasmids. J Immunol 158:1231–1237

Gerloni M, Baliou WR, Billetta R, Zanetti M (1997) Immunity to *Plasmodium falciparum* malaria sporozoites by somatic transgene immunization. Nat Biotechnol 15:876–881

Gonzalez Armas JC, Morello CS, Cranmer LD, Spector DH (1996) DNA immunization confers protection against murine cytomegalovirus infection. J Virol 70:7921–7928

Haensler J, Verdelet C, Sanchez V, Girerd-Chambaz Y, Bonnin A, Trannoy E, Krishnan S, Meulien P (1999) Intradermal DNA immunization by using jet-injectors in mice and monkeys. Vaccine 17:628–638

Hartmann G, Weiner GJ, Krieg AM (1999) CpG DNA: a potent signal for growth, activation, and maturation of human dendritic cells. Proc Natl Acad Sci USA 96:9305–9310

Hengge UR, Chan EF, Foster RA, Walker PS, Vogel JC (1995) Cytokine expression in epidermis with biological effffects following injection of naked DNA. Nat Genet 10:161–166

Hengge UR, Walker PS, Vogel JC (1996) Expression of naked DNA in human, pig, and mouse skin. J Clin Invest 97:2911–2916

Herrmann JE, Chen SC, Fynan EF, Santoro JC, Greenberg HB, Wang S, Robinson HL (1996) Protection against rotavirus infections by DNA vaccination. J Infect Dis 174:S93–S97

Heufler C, Koch F, Schuler G (1988) Granulocyte/macrophage colony-stimulating factor and interleukin 1 mediate the maturation of murine epidermal Langerhans cells into potent immunostimulatory dendritic cells. J Exp Med 167:700–705

Horner AA, Ronaghy A, Cheng PM, Nguyen MD, Cho HJ, Broide D, Raz E (1998) Immunostimulatory DNA is a potent mucosal adjuvant. Cell Immunol 190:77–82

Irvine KR, Rao JB, Rosenberg SA, Restifo NP (1996) Cytokine enhancement of DNA immunization leads to effective treatment of established pulmonary metastases. J Immunol 156:238–245

Iwasaki A, Stiernholm BJ, Chan AK, Berinstein NL, Barber BH (1997a) Enhanced CTL responses mediated by plasmid DNA immunogens encoding costimulatory molecules and cytokines. J Immunol 158:4591–4601

Iwasaki A, Torres CAT, Ohashi PS, Robinson HL, Barber BH (1997b) The dominant role of bone marrow-derived cells in CTL induction following plasmid DNA immunization at different sites. J Immunol 159:11–14

Janeway CA, Travers P (1994) Immunobiology: the immune system in health and disease. Current Biology Ltd, London 7:31–32

June CH, Bluestone JA, Nadler LM, Thompson CB (1994) The B7 and CD28 receptor families. Immunol Today 15:321–331

Kato T, Hakamada R, Yamane H, Nariuchi H (1996) Induction of IL-12 p40 messenger RNA expression and IL-12 production of macrophages via CD40-CD40 ligand interaction. J Immunol 156:3932–3938

Kiener PA, Moran-Davis P, Rankin BM, Wahl AF, Aruffo A, Hollenbaugh D (1995) Stimulation of CD40 with purified soluble gp39 induces proinflammatory responses in human monocytes. J Immunol 155:4917–4925

Kim JJ, Ayyavoo V, Bagarazzi ML, Chattergoon MA, Dang K, Wang B, Boyer JD, Weiner DB (1997a) In vivo engineering of a cellular immune response by coadministration of IL-12 expression vector with a DNA immunogen. J Immunol 158:816–826

Kim JJ, Bagarazzi ML, Trivedi N, Hu Y, Kazahaya K, Wilson DM, Ciccarelli R, Chattergoon MA, Dang K, Mahalingam S, Chalian AA, Agadjanyan MG, Boyer JD, Wang B, Weiner DB (1997b) Engineering of in vivo immune responses to DNA immunization via codelivery of costimulatory molecule genes. Nat Biotechnol 15:641–646

Kim JJ, Nottingham LK, Sin JI, Tsai A, Morrison L, Oh J, Dang K, Hu Y, Kazahaya K, Bennett M, Dentchev T, Wilson DM, Chalian AA, Boyer JD, Agadjanyan MG, Weiner DB (1998a) CD8+ T cells influence antigen-specific immune responses through the expression of chemokines. J Clin Invest 102:1112–1124

Kim JJ, Nottingham LK, Wilson DM, Bagarazzi ML, Tsai A, Morrison LD, Javadian A, Chalian AA, Agadjanyan MG, Weiner DB (1998b) Engineering DNA vaccines via co-delivery of co-stimulatory molecule genes. Vaccine 16:1828–1836

Kim JJ, Trivedi NN, Nottingham LK, Morrison L, Tsai A, Hu Y, Mahalingam S, Dang K, Ahn L, Doyle NK, Wilson DM, Chattergoon MA, Chalian AA, Boyer JD, Agadjanyan MG, Weiner DB (1998c) Modulation of amplitude and direction of in vivo immune responses by co-administration of cytokine gene expression cassettes with DNA immunogens. Eur J Immunol 28:1089–1103

Kim JJ, Trivedi NN, Wilson DM, Mahalingam S, Morrison L, Tsai A, Chattergoon MA, Dang K, Patel M, Ahn L, Boyer JD, Chalian AA, Schoemaker H, Kieber-Emmons T, Agadjanyan MA, Weiner DB (1998d) Molecular and immunological analysis of genetic prostate specific antigen (PSA) vaccine. Oncogene 17:3125–3135

Kim JJ, Tsai A, Nottingham LK, Morrison L, Cunning DM, Oh J, Lee DJ, Dang K, Dentchev T, Chalian AA, Agadjanyan MG, Weiner DB (1999) Intracellular adhesion molecule-1 (ICAM-1) modulates β-chemokines and provides costimulatory signals required for T cell activation and expansion in vivo. J Clin Invest 103:869–877

Klinman DM, Yamshchikov G, Ishigatsubo Y (1997) Contribution of CpG motifs to the immunogenicity of DNA vaccines. J Immuol 158:3635–3639

Krieg AM (1996) An innate immune defense mechanism based on the recognition of CpG motifs in microbial DNA. J Lab Clin Med 128:128–133

Krieg AM (1999) CpG DNA: a novel immunomodulator. Trends Microbiol 7:64–65

Kuchroo VK, Das MP, Brown JA, Ranger AM, Zamvil SS, Sobel RA, Weiner HL, Nabavi N, Glimcher LH (1995) B7-1 and B7-2 costimulatory molecules activate differentially the Th₁/Th₂ developmental pathways: application to autoimmune disease therapy. Cell 80:707–718

Kupper TS (1990) The activated keratinocyte: a model for inducible cytokine production by non-bone marrow-derived cells in cutaneous inflammatory and immune responses. J Invest Dermatol 94:146 S-150 S

Lane P, Traunecker A, Hubele S, Inui S, Lanzavecchia A, Gray D (1992) Activated human T cells express a ligand for the human B cell-associated antigen CD40 which participates in T cell-dependent activation of B lymphocytes. Eur J Immunol 22:2573–2578

Lanier LL, O'Fallon S, Somoza C, Phillips JH, Linsley PS, Okumura K, Ito D, Azuma M (1995) CD80 (B7) and CD86 (B70) provide similar costimulatory signals for T cell proliferation, cytokine production, and generation of CTL. J Immunol 154:97–105

LeClerc C, Deriaud E, Rojas M, Whalen RG (1997) The preferential induction of a Th$_1$ immune response by DNA-based immunization is mediated by the immunostimulatory effect of plasmid DNA. Cell Immunol 179:97–106

Letvin NL, Montefiori DC, Yasutomi Y, Perry HC, Davies ME, Lekutis C, Alroy M, Freed DC, Lord CI, Handt LK, Liu MA, Shiver JW (1997) Potent, protective anti-HIV immune responses generated by bimodal HIV envelope DNA plus protein vaccination. Proc Natl Acad Sci USA 94:9378–9383

Linsley PS, Clark EA, Ledbetter JA (1990) The cell antigen, CD28, mediates adhesion with B cells by interacting with activation antigen, B7/BB-1. Proc Natl Acad Sci USA 87:5031–5035

Lowrie DB, Tascon RE, Colston MJ, Silva CL (1994) Toward a DNA vaccine against tuberculosis. Vaccine 12:1537–1540

Li L, Hoffman RM (1995) The feasibility of targeted selective gene therapy of the hair follicle. Nat Med 1:705–706

Maecker HT, Umetsu DT, DeKruyff RH, Levy S (1998) Cytotoxic T cell responses to DNA vaccination: dependence on antigen presentation via class II MHC. J Immunol 161:6532–6536

Manickan E, Rouse RJD, Yu Z, Wire WS, Rouse BT (1995) Genetic immunization against herpes simplex virus: protection is mediated by CD4+ T lymphocytes. J Immunol 155:259–265

Mendoza RB, Cantwell MJ, Kipps TJ (1997) Immunostimulatory effects of a plasmid expressing CD40 ligand (CD154) on gene immunization. J Immunol 159:5777–5781

Mor G, Klinman DM, Shapiro S, Hagiwara E, Sedegah M, Norman JA, Hoffman SL, Steinberg AD (1995) Complexity of the cytokine and antibody response elicited by immunizing mice with *Plasmodium yoelii* circumsporozoite protein plasmid DNA. J Immunol 155:2039–2046

Morrissey PJ, Bressler L, Park LS, Alpert A, Gillis S (1987) Granulocyte-macrophage colony-stimulating factor augments the primary antibody response by enhancing the function of antigen-presenting cells. J Immunol 139:1113–1119

Noelle RJ, Roy M, Shepherd DM, Stamenkovic I, Ledbetter JA, Aruffo A (1992) A 39-kDa protein on activated helper T cells binds CD40 and transduces the signal for cognate activation of B cells. Proc Natl Acad Sci USA 89:6550–6554

Okada E, Sasaki S, Ishii N, Aoki I, Yasuda T, Nishioka K, Fukushima J, Miyazaki J, Wahren B, Okuda K (1997) Intranasal immunization of DNA vaccine with IL-12- and granulocyte-macrophage colony-stimulating factor (GM-CSF)-expressing plasmids in liposomes induces strong mucosal and cell-mediated immune responses against HIV-1 antigens. J Immunol 159:3638–3647

Pardoll DM, Beckerleg AM (1995) Exposing the immunology of naked DNA vaccines. Immunity 3:165–169

Pertmer TM, Eisenbraun MD, McCabe D, Prayaga SK, Fuller DH, Haynes JR (1995) Gene gun-based nucleic acid immunization: elicitation of humoral and cytotoxic T lymphocyte responses follwing epidermal delivery of nanogram quantities of DNA. Vaccine 13:1427–1430

Pertmer TM, Roberts TR, Haynes JR (1996) Influenza virus nucleoprotein-specific immunoglobulin G subclass and cytokine responses elicited by DNA vaccination are dependent on the route of vector DNA delivery. J Virol 70:6119–6125

Pisetsky DS (1999) The influence of base sequence on the immunostimulatory properties of DNA. Immunol Res 19:35–46

Prayaga SK, Ford MJ, Haynes JR (1997) Manipulation of HIV-1 gp120-specific immune responses elicited via gene gun-based DNA immunization. Vaccine 15:1349–1352

Ranheim EA, Kipps TJ (1993) Activated T cells induce expression of B7/BB1 on normal or leukemic B cells through a CD40-dependent signal. J Exp Med 177:925–935

Raz E, Watanabe A, Baird SM, Eisenberg RA, Parr TB, Lotz M, Kipps TJ, Carson DA (1993) Systemic immunological effects of cytokine genes injected into skeletal muscle. Proc Nat Acad Sci USA 90:4523–4527

Raz E, Carson DA, Parker SE, Parr TB, Abai AM, Aichinger G, Baird AM, Rhodes GH (1994) Intradermal gene immunization: the possible role of DNA uptake in the induction of cellular immunity to viruses. Proc Nat Acad Sci USA 91:9519–9523

Raz E, Tighe H, Sato Y, Corr M, Dudler JA, Roman M, Swain SL, Spiegelberg HL, Carson DA (1996) Preferential induction of a Th1 immune response and inhibition of specific IgE antibody formation by plasmid DNA immunization. Proc Natl Acad Sci USA 93:5141–5145

Roman M, Martin-Orozco E, Goodman JS, Nguyen MD, Sato Y, Ronaghy A, Kornbluth RS, Richman DD, Carson DA, Raz E (1997) Immunostimulatory DNA sequences function as T helper-1 promoting adjuvants. Nat Med 3:849–854

Sato Y, Roman M, Tighe H, Lee D, Corr M, Nguyen MD, Silverman GJ, Lotz M, Carson DA, Raz E (1996) Immunostimulatory DNA sequences necessary for effective intradermal gene immunization. Science 273:352–354

Shu U, Kiniwa M, Wu CY, Maliszewski C, Vezzio N, Hakimi J, Gately M, Delespesse G (1995) Activated T cells induce interleukin-12 production by monocytes via CD40-CD40 ligand interaction. Eur J Immunol 25:1125–1128

Sin JI, Sung JH, Suh YS, Lee AH, Chung JH, Sung YC (1997) Protective immunity against heterologous challenge with encephalomyocarditis virus1 by VP1 DNA vaccination: effect of co-injection with a GM-CSF gene. Vaccine 15:1827–1833

Sin JI, Kim JJ, Boyer JD, Ciccarelli RB, Higgins TJ, Weiner DB (1998) In vivo modulation of immune response and protective immunity against herpes simplex virus-2 infection using cDNAs expressing Th1 and Th2 type cytokines in gD DNA vaccination. J Virol 73:501–509

Smith KA (1988) Interleukin-2: inception, impact, and implications. Science 240:1169–1176

Swain SL, Bradley LM, Croft M, Tonkonogy S, Atkins G, Weinberg AD, Duncan DD, Hedrick SM, Dutton RW, Huston G (1991) Helper T-cell subsets: phenotype, function and the role of lymphokines in regulating their development. Immunol Rev 123:115–144

Torres CAT, Iwasaki A, Barber BH, Robinson HL (1997) Differential dependence on target site tissue for gene gun and intramuscular DNA immunizations. J Immunol 158:4529–4532

Trinchieri G (1995) Interleukin-12: a proinflammatory cytokine with immunoregulatory function that bridges innate resistance and antigen-specific adaptive immunity. Annu Rev Immunol 13:251–276

Tsuji T, Hamajima K, Fukushima J, Xin KQ, Ishii N, Aoki I, Ishigatsubo Y, Tani K, Kawamoto S, Nitta Y, Miyazaki J, Koff WC, Okubo T, Okuda K (1997a) Enhancement of cell-mediated immunity against HIV-1 induced by coinoculation of plasmid-encoded HIV-1 antigens with plasmid expressing IL-12. J Immunol 158:4008–4013

Tsuji T, Fukushima J, Hamajima K, Ishii N, Aoki I, Bukawa H, Ishigatsubo Y, Tani K, Okubo T, Dorf ME, Okuda K (1997b) HIV-1 specific cell-mediated immunity is enhanced by co-inoculation of TCA3 expression plasmid with DNA vaccine. Immunology 90:1–6

Ulmer JB, Donnelley JJ, Parker SE, Rhodes GH, Felgner PL, Dwarki VJ, Gromkowski SH, Deck RR, Dewitt CM, Friedman A, Hawe LA, Leander KR, Martinez D, Perry HC, Shiver JW, Montgomery DL, Liu MA (1993) Heterologous protection against influenza by injection of DNA encoding a viral protein. Science 259:1745–1749

Wang B, Ugen K, Srikantan V, Agadjanyan MG, Dang K, Refaeli Y, Sato AI, Boyer J, Williams WV, Weiner DB (1993) Gene inoculation generates immune responses against HIV-1. Proc Nat Acad Sci USA 90:4156–4160

Wang B, Dang K, Agadjanyan MG, Srikantan V, Li F, Ugen KE, Boyer J, Merva M, Williams WV, Weiner DB (1997) Mucosal immunization with a DNA vaccine induces immune responses against HIV-1 at a mucosal site. Vaccine 15:821–825

Williams RS, Johnston SA, Riedy M, DeVit MJ, McElligott SG, Sanford JC (1991) Introduction of foreign genes into tissues of living mice by DNA-coated microprojectiles. Proc Natl Acad Sci USA 88:2726–2730

Wolff JA (1997) Naked DNA transport and expression in mammalian cells. Neuromusc Dis 7:314–318

Xiang A, Ertl HCJ (1995) Manipulation of the immune response to a plasmid-encoded viral antigen by coinoculation with plasmids expressing cytokines. Immunity 2:129–136

Xiang ZQ, Spitalnik SL, Tran M, Wunner WH, Cheng J, Ertl HC (1994) Vaccination with plasmid vector carrying the rabies virus glycoprotein gene induces protective immunity against rabies virus. Virology 199:132–140

Xiang ZQ, Spitalnik SL, Cheng J, Erikson J, Wojczyk B, Ertl HC (1995) Immune responses to nucleic acid vaccines to rabies virus. Virology 209:569–579

Xu D, Liew FY (1995) Protection against leishmaniasis by injection of DNA encoding a major surface glycoprotein gp63, of L. major. Immunology 84:173–176

Xu L, Sanchez A, Yang Z, Zaki SR, Nabel EG, Nichol ST, Nabel GJ (1998) Immunization for Ebola virus infection. Nat Med 4:37–42

Yasutomi Y, Robinson HL, Lu S, Mustafa F, Lekutis C, Arthos J, Mullins JI, Voss G, Manson K, Wyand M, Letvin NL (1997) Simian immunodeficiency virus-specific cytotoxic T-lymphocyte induction through DNA vaccination of rhesus monkeys. J Virol 70:678–681

Yu WH, Kashani-Sabet M, Liggitt D, Moore D, Heath TD, Debs RJ (1999) Topical gene delivery to murine skin. J Invest Dermatol 112:370–375

Zhang L, Li L, Hoffmann GA, Hoffman RM (1996) Depth-targeted efficient gene delivery and expression in the skin by pulsed electric fields: an approach to gene therapy of skin aging and other diseases. Biochem Biophys Res Commun 220:633–636

Subject Index

Printing (Computer to Film): Saladruck, Berlin
Binding: Stürtz AG, Würzburg